Sexual Health for Men

Sexual Health for Men

The Complete Guide

RICHARD F. SPARK, MD, F.A.C.E.

Associate Clinical Professor of Medicine,
Harvard Medical School

Director, Steroid Research Lab
Beth Israel Deaconess Medical Center, Boston, MA

PERSEUS PUBLISHING
Cambridge, Massachusetts

Portions of this book appeared in *Male Sexual Health,* a Consumer Reports Book published in 1991 by Consumers Union.

Illustrations on the following pages were created by Harriet R. Greenfield: p. 37 (figure 6.1), p. 39 (figure 6.2), p. 73 (figure 10.1), p. 91 (figure 10.7), p. 93 (figure 10.8), p. 142 (figure 12.1), p. 242 (figure 18.2), p. 254 (figure 19.1), p. 255 (figure 19.2), p. 266 (figure 20.1), p. 316 (figure 23.1), p. 317 (figure 23.2), p. 352 (figure 25.1), p. 359 (figure 25.2)

A CIP catalog record for this book is available from the Library of Congress.
ISBN 0-7382-0206-1

Perseus Publishing is a member of the Perseus Books Group

Find us on the World Wide Web at http://www.perseuspublishing.com

Perseus Publishing books are available at special discounts for bulk purchases in the U.S. by corporations, institutions, and other organizations. For more information, please contact the Special Markets Department at HarperCollins Publishers, 10 East 53rd Street, New York, NY 10022, or call 1-212-207-7528.

Text design by Jeff Williams
Set in 11-point Minion by the Perseus Books Group

First printing, March 2000

1 2 3 4 5 6 7 8 9 10—03 02 01 00

Contents

Sexual Health for Men

1

Prologue

When future historians seek to understand why once-taboo topics such as a man's sexual function, sexual peccadilloes, and impotence made the transition from backyard gossip to front-page news, they will inevitably and inextricably be drawn back to the extraordinary political and scientific events of 1998.

Male sexuality, never mentioned in polite circles throughout most of the twentieth century, quite suddenly became *the* number-one topic of conversation as we inched toward the millennium. In January 1998, the world learned of President Clinton's relationship with "that woman"—Monica Lewinsky—and almost everyone from media pundits to citizens on the street weighed in with their insights on men and their sexual behavior.

Two months later, the Food and Drug Administration (FDA) approved sildenafil (Viagra), a pill to treat impotence. Overnight the word "Viagra" was embraced and instantly incorporated into the lexicon of daily living.

"Pure theatrical Viagra," one critic enthused in his review of *The Blue Room* when the erotic play was first staged in London.

"Who put Viagra in the thermometers?" another wag wanted to know as he described the relentless upward thrust of daily temperatures during that summer's torrid Texas heat wave.

CBS television's Leslie Stahl, speaking at a luncheon, quipped that someone must have spiked the floral displays with Viagra to account for the rigid upright blooms in all the guest-table centerpieces.

Maureen Dowd, the witty columnist for the *New York Times*, decried the gender inequity of the FDA's eagerness to approve Viagra for men, shortly after the same agency had axed Phen-Fen, the diet-pill combination so popular among women.

Late-night comedians like Jay Leno had a field day. Capitalizing on our national anxiety about sex, he and his writers fashioned a series of one-liners and, by incorporating the word "Viagra" into every punch line, kept his audience roaring with delight.

The seamy and sordid details of the Clinton-Lewinsky relationship were played out on national television. Congressmen insisted it was not the sex but the *lying about the sex* that was of most concern to them. They then impeached the president, not for his sexual behavior, which everyone agreed was reprehensible, but for his dishonesty.

Yet few in Congress, even those braying the loudest for impeachment, qualified as "first-stone casters."

Disclosure of other men's sexual peccadilloes, previously off-limits, was now fair game and worthy of front-page coverage. This was true not just for tabloids but for mainstream newspapers and media outlets as well. We learned that Representative Henry Hyde, chairman of the House Judiciary Committee, so eager to impeach the president, had himself been embroiled in a five-year clandestine sexual escapade with a woman, a relationship he dismissed as a "youthful indiscretion" (he was forty-one when the affair began.)

Then Representative Robert Livingstone, heir apparent to House Speaker Newt Gingrich, and another one of those calling for the president's impeachment, was "outed" as a four-time adulterer by, of all people, Larry Flynt, the publisher of *Hustler* magazine.

Interwoven with all of the revelations of sexual shenanigans in Washington was worrisome news about Viagra. It now seemed that some men had died shortly after they had used Viagra, and enthusiasm for the "sex pill," as Viagra came to be known, temporarily started to wane.

But men continued to have sexual problems. For them and their sexual partners, this was a year of significant change. Now that a simple remedy—*a pill to cure impotence*—was available, many who had suffered with and endured sexual impairment in silence for years were suddenly emboldened to discuss their problems openly at least with their physicians. For some, Viagra was the answer. For others, different specialized treatments were in order. But now that Viagra *legitimized male sexuality* as a valid health-care issue, more and more men were willing to examine and discuss their own sexual capabilities and limitations.

Sex was only one of the issues men were eager to talk about. Uniquely male concerns about personal health, long held in check, suddenly resurfaced both in real life and in fiction.

In his novel *American Pastoral*, Philip Roth uses his alter ego, Zuckerman, to vividly chronicle events at his fortieth high-school reunion where he and his male classmates obsess about their prostate glands. As a coalition of concerned middle-aged men, all bond to reassure each other that salvation for each of them lies in having *the test*—referring to the prostate specific antigen (PSA) blood test used to detect prostate cancer in its earliest stages.

The fictional Zuckerman has already had both *the test* and life-saving prostate cancer treatment but bemoans the price he had to pay. Following prostate cancer treatment, Zuckerman has survived as a partial man, totally deprived of his sexual vitality. In contrast, real-life prostate cancer victims like former senator Bob Dole seem to be more fortunate. In a stunning departure from a man's traditional reticence to engage in a frank discussion of his own sexuality, former senator Dole went public on the *Larry King Live* show. There he explained how prostate cancer treatment first robbed him of his ability to have sex and then how, when he used Viagra, his sexual function was miraculously restored.

But prostate cancer has not been the only cancer of concern to men. Cancer of the testicle has become more common. Men with malignant tumors of the testicle tend to be much younger than those with prostate cancer. Newer treatments do improve survival, but as is the case with prostate cancer, care has to be taken to ensure that the man who survives testicular cancer does so with his sexuality and fertility intact.

The link between smoking and lung cancer prompted many men now concerned about their own mortality to suddenly start shelling out millions of dollars for new treatments designed to help them kick the nicotine habit. California's clever "Still think smoking is sexy?" ad campaign struck a responsive note and prompted more men to be wary of smoking. The television spots showed handsome tuxedoed men, all with limp cigarettes dangling from their lips, to emphasize the connection between cigarette smoking and impotence. The linkage between smoking and impotence has had more impact than the decades-long surgeon general's warning labels on cigarette packs. When male smokers faced the prospect of a loss of erectile function with continued cigarette use, they started a stampede for Zyban and other smoking-cessation programs. A follow-up *60 Minutes* broadcast provided a national forum for the "smoking causes impotence" message.

At about the same time, other previously squelched male concerns and men's health issues were gaining new currency. Personal grooming, long a mainstay of women's magazines, all of a sudden emerged as a worthy topic for men as well. Do-it-yourself hair-coloring products flew off the shelves of local pharmacies into the hands of men with prematurely, and not so prematurely, graying hair. Two medications, one a rub-on lotion (Rogaine) and the other a prescription pill (Propecia) were now available to help men stem the tide of male-pattern baldness. Finding products exclusively intended to cater to men became a priority for the pharmaceutical industry. (See Table 1.1.)

Uniquely male hormones (androgens) were also in the news. Testosterone, the granddaddy of all male hormones, was a *Newsweek* cover story. Other androgens such as DHEA (dehydroepiandrosterone) vaulted into prominence because of claims that this enigmatic adrenal gland hormone had extraordinary previously unrecognized curative, healing, and anti-aging powers. Then eyebrows were raised when it was revealed that Mark McGwire, the burly St. Louis Cardinals slugger, relied on yet another ob-

TABLE 1.1   Catering to Men's Needs

Product	Purpose	Actual Sales year to date 1998	Total Sales projected for 1998
Propecia	Hair growth	$45 million	33% below expected
Rogaine	Hair growth	$71 million	8% above 1997
Nicoderm	Stop smoking	$216 million	13% below 1997
Nicotrol	Stop smoking	$33 million	48% below 1997
Ncorette	Stop smoking	$318 million	19% above 1997
Zyban	Stop smoking	$84 million	50% above expected
Viagra	Impotence Rx.	$524 million (6 mo.)	>$1 billion first year

SOURCE: Adapted from the *New York Times*, 11/11/98 C 1 , "The Elixirs of Life Style"

scure male hormone, androstenedione, as part of his daily training regimen. Once again, male hormones became a hot topic of conversation.

Male sexuality remained in the headlines right up to the very last day of the year.

Health maintenance organizations (HMOs) fumed over the *cost* of Viagra from the beginning. The Kaiser Foundation Health Plan, which had campaigned vigorously to avoid paying for any Viagra prescriptions, was finally thwarted by California's health-care regulators. On December 31, 1998, the State of California ruled that Kaiser could not isolate male sexuality as unworthy of medical attention. Nor could Kaiser unilaterally exclude Viagra or any other treatment to improve men's sexual function from their benefits package. The ruling will likely have widespread implications, for Kaiser was not the only health-care insurer to impugn sexually impaired men and deny them access to proper treatment.

Today as we begin the millennium, the most personal and intimate of a man's health issues—his sexuality, virility, fertility, and health-care choices—are being discussed with renewed intensity and refreshing candor. Men have an eagerness for answers and direction. Options for improvement in all spheres of men's health are expanding. Opportunities abound. We still have much to learn, but we have come so far, in such a short period of time.

Let us begin.

2

What Do Men Want?

How do you really know what is good for you? Even if it comes with a money-back guarantee, does every product claiming to make a man bigger, stronger, or sexier really work? Do those in the advertising business think of all men as chumps who are willing to shell out cash to fulfill their sexual fantasies? In this chapter you will learn how much reliance to place on claims, which are basically marketing devices, hearsay evidence, anecdotes, testimonials, the power of the placebo, and the value of placebo-controlled clinical trials.

What do men want?

To be better, have more, and not be frightened.

It is as simple as that.

But be *better* how, have *more* what, and what on earth could possibly *frighten* a man?

Let's start with *better*.

No matter what our age or circumstances, we men are forever striving to be better—*stronger, faster, smarter, richer, sexier*. Maybe it is the competitive spirit instilled in all of us from the time we were little boys. As youngsters we pester our parents to buy the "Breakfast of Champions," hoping that if we wolf down enough cereal flakes each morning we will turn into remarkable athletes. Some do, but most don't.

Yet we never seem to outgrow our little boy's naïveté and remain steadfast in the belief that there will always be *something on the shelf* that will help improve our virile profile. The only difference is that as grown-ups we do our own shopping, if not for cereal then for any other product to help us be better men.

Consider for example, our desire for *more*.

When we learn that there is an item called the "Stud Pill for Men," which is said to be "safe . . . proven . . . FDA legal . . . increases serum testosterone levels . . . reverses male aging" and also "burns fat . . . builds muscle . . . boosts strength, energy and sex drive" our natural reaction is "Wow!"

The "Stud Pill for Men" is the brainchild of Wayne Josephson, who, according to a story in the *Wall Street Journal* (January 27, 1999), left his job in Minneapolis and, adrift in the doldrums of inactivity, wandered into a health food store, purchased some androstenedione capsules, and immediately cheered up. Then sensing an entrepreneurial opportunity, he created a web site to repackage, relabel, and then market androstenedione as the "Stud Pill for Men."

Business was brisk, and in the first month, 1,000 bottles of the "Stud Pill for Men" were sold via electronic commerce. Emboldened by his sudden success and gifted with a knack for nifty names, Josephson expanded his line, offering the "Passion Pill for Women," and "Herbal Trim," a dietary supplement for those eager to lose weight. With all three items in his inventory, Josephson is expected to have first year web-based sales of $500,000. (According to the *Wall Street Journal*, Josephson's clientele are mostly "weary middle-aged stock brokers.")

There is only one problem.

No one has ever proven that the Stud Pill is either "safe, proven, FDA legal, can reverse male aging or will burn fat, boost strength, energy or sex drive." The medication was *never FDA-approved*, because the FDA never heard of the Stud Pill until after it went on-line.

Then how can Josephson claim that the Stud Pill does all these remarkable things? Because:

1. There is no one to stop him.
2. Many men are eager, some desperately eager, to believe him.
3. Androstenedione is relatively innocuous and unlikely to do any real harm.
4. Men who are anxious to believe in the value of this or any other men's product are unusually susceptible to the power of the placebo and become "placebo responders."

What's a placebo responder?

A placebo responder is someone who feels poorly, takes a pill, and immediately gets better even though the pill—a placebo—contained no medicine. We men are notorious placebo responders.

For example, during the very first stages of testing sildenafil (Viagra) as a remedy for erectile dysfunction, some men were given Viagra and others were given placebo pills that looked just like Viagra but had no active medication. Neither group of men knew whether they were taking Viagra or placebo. Twenty-four percent (24%) of placebo-treated impotent men reported stronger, firmer erections and improved sexual intercourse. They did not know that the tablets they were taking were dummy pills.

Almost three times as many (70%) of those using the real Viagra pills had improved erectile and sexual function. These studies comparing placebo pills to Viagra not only validated Viagra's effectiveness but also told us something very interesting about men. Almost one in four men using *any new pill, vitamin, herb, or diet* will swear that they do indeed have more gusto even if that treatment is a medicinally inert sugar pill or placebo.

Hold on a second! Josephson was taking androstenedione pills, the real "Andro," and not a placebo. He told us this made him feel better. And what about Mark McGwire, who led us all to believe that it was his use of androstenedione that allowed him to hit those seventy home runs? Is that just a coincidence?

It could be.

In matters of health, all of us, men and women alike, depend on information from many sources, but for the most part we rely on:

1. Claims, anecdotes, and hearsay evidence
2. Testimonials

Doctors may not want to admit it, but they also rely on claims, anecdotes, and hearsay evidence, yet are more influenced by dramatic new findings from:

1. Medical case reports or
2. Placebo-controlled trials

ANECDOTES OR HEARSAY EVIDENCE

These are part of the currency of daily living. We all turn to our friends, neighbors, or colleagues to give us advice and share with us their feelings about the best place to shop or dine, and when it comes to health-related issues, we ask what doctor or hospital is the best. Chances are we take our friends' advice and, if pleased, continue to patronize that doctor or hospital. Anecdotes are little more than one neighbor helping another. The marketing of the Stud Pill relies on what is the equivalent of an "on-line" claim or anecdote. Josephson swears he "feels ten years younger" since he started taking androstenedione. If we believe him, we will send him money and buy his product.

TESTIMONIALS

In contrast to hearsay evidence, testimonials are a little more of a hard sell. The pitch to men relies on our preoccupation with our maleness and being better, stronger, or more athletic. We men are, for the most part, insecure and envy others who are more muscular, physically fit, or skilled at sports. This makes us vulnerable to testimonials from star athletes, who *for a fee* will tell you that they look and perform as well as they do because they use a particular nutritional supplement, cereal, or athletic shoe. The implication is that you can be just as attractive, appealing, or athletic if you also use the nutritional supplement, eat the cereal, or buy the athletic shoes. Testimonials are an excellent way to increase sales of a product but are not necessarily an effective way of improving your jump shot or physique. McGwire's endorsement of "Andro" has the same effect as a testimonial.

Until recently, other celebrity testimonials have not been pressed into service to endorse men's health products, but all of that changed when former senator Bob Dole was hired by Pfizer, the manufacturer of Viagra, to encourage men with erectile dysfunction to "speak with their doctor."

MEDICAL CASE REPORTS

When doctors develop a truly novel therapy they will describe their experience treating one single patient in a medical journal. On occasion their innovative approach is so dramatic that it changes the nature of medical treatment forever. Two examples come to mind immediately.

The case of Leonard Thompson, the first diabetic to receive insulin, and "Baby Louise," the first child born after in vitro fertilization (IVF), are notable examples of how a *single case report* altered the course of medical history. Doctors still share information by publishing case reports describing their experiences, but as the demands for proof of efficacy intensify, physicians have increasingly relied on more rigorous criteria to be convinced that treatment is effective and, in particular, that one treatment is safer and better than another. To do this they have increasingly relied on the placebo-controlled trial.

THE PLACEBO-CONTROLLED TRIAL

In the past when the range of effective treatments was limited but the extent of disease and suffering infinite, physicians were willing to try any treatment that they knew about from their own *personal anecdotes,* a colleague's *hearsay evidence,* or *testimonials* from their professors.

For example, the common head cold, with its fever, runny nose, sneezing, and frequently accompanying cough is the result of an infection caused by a *virus.* Penicillin, a potent antibiotic, lethal for many bacteria, has no effect on viruses. Yet for years patients with head colds were treated with penicillin, and when they recovered, improvement was attributed to the penicillin. The only way to really know whether the improvement in symptoms was due to the penicillin or to the body's own defenses fighting off the cold was to do a placebo-controlled trial, comparing penicillin to a placebo.

Doctors find a group of cold sufferers who have comparably severe head colds and treat half with placebos and half with penicillin, then track their progress.

- If penicillin-treated patients stop sniffling, sneezing, and coughing in two days and the placebo-treated patients remain sick for another week, then it would be fair to conclude that penicillin worked because it shortened the duration of illness from seven to two days.

- But if both the placebo and penicillin-treated patients symptoms cleared up within five days, this would indicate that penicillin therapy was *no better than a placebo,* proving to doctors that penicillin was not effective for the common cold. It is this type of placebo-controlled study that persuaded physicians to shy away from prescribing penicillin for the common cold.

- Today, placebo-controlled trials are the "gold standard." Before it will approve any new medication, the FDA demands that the sponsoring pharmaceutical company conduct a series of placebo-controlled trials to prove that their new medication (1) does what it is intended to do, for example, lower blood pressure or relieve depression, and (2) is more effective than a placebo in achieving these goals.

- Further, placebo-controlled trials also provide an opportunity to assess side effects. If headaches are reported by 5 percent of those taking the new medication and 5 percent on placebos, then it is fair to say that you are no more likely to have a headache on medication than on placebo, but if the headache percentages are 12 percent with medication and 4 percent with placebo, then headache must be considered a medication side effect.

Thus, as a result of FDA-mandated placebo-controlled trials, we know that a medication does what it is intended to do and has a well-defined side-effect profile.

- Not all currently available pills have to go through the same rigorous procedure. Many new tablets containing herbs, vitamins, male hormones, and dietary supplements are exempted from the FDA's oversight and can be sold without having to prove they work at all or are better or safer than placebos because they are only rarely compared to placebos. For these readily available over-the-counter products, the claim "clinically proven" does not have the same ring of authority (see Chapter 21).

PLACEBO-CONTROLLED TRIALS FOR MEN

Placebo-controlled studies have been particularly helpful in determining whether therapies are effective or ineffective in men with a wide range of problems. They have demonstrated, for example, that yohimbine tablets are more effective than previously believed for men with psychogenic impotence (Chapter 17), that a medication called alprostadil inserted directly into the penis made it easier for impotent men to have erections (Chapter 19), and that two medications, terazosin (Hytrin) and doxazosin (Cardura), both originally developed to treat high blood pressure, also alleviate bladder spasm and improve urine flow in men with big prostate glands. Neither Hytrin nor Cardura decreases prostate size, but finasteride (Proscar) does. (See Chapter 23.)

Curiously, placebo-controlled trials also proved that finasteride, given in a smaller dose and sold as Propecia, helps slow down a man's tendency to lose scalp hair and is useful as a treatment for male-pattern baldness. (See Chapter 15.)

Finally, as we continue to explore the many uses of male hormones, we have been able to establish that enormous doses of testosterone do indeed increase a man's muscle bulk and weight-lifting capacity. Men taking large doses of testosterone gain weight and become stronger even without exercise, but when testosterone is combined with an intensive training program, they become even stronger (Chapter 13).

Throughout this book, results of the most reliable placebo-controlled clinical trials will be described to help you decide what are the most effective traditional or alternative medicine treatments needed to maintain and sustain your health, sexuality, and fertility.

WHAT FRIGHTENS MEN?

Men and women share the same concerns regarding major illness, death, and disability, but for each gender some illnesses, especially those that pose a threat to their own sexuality, hold a special terror. Women fear breast cancer not just because of the potentially deadly implications of the diagnosis but also because breast cancer treatment, no matter how carefully done, distorts a woman's sense of femininity. By analogy, some uniquely male problems heighten a man's level of anxiety either because the diagnosis is so ominous or the required treatments so harsh that they threaten to deprive a man of his virility.

Common conditions such as benign prostate hyperplasia (Chapter 23) and prostate cancer (Chapter 24) can be managed with some facility today. But for each uniquely male condition, lifesaving therapy can wreak havoc with a man's sense of masculinity, sexuality, and fertility. Fortunately, the range of remedies is now sufficiently mature so that for the individual man with prostate or testicular cancer, a personalized palette of options can be devised to not only quell his short-term anxieties but also help him plan for the future. And the future is becoming more and more important. Today as we enter the millennium, all of us men face the prospect of a longer and more productive life. Each one of us should be able to continue to look forward to, and enjoy, an enhanced quality of life as we mature (Chapter 28).

3

Thirty Million Men

Why are men so difficult when they have to confront personal issues? We do not hesitate to take charge of established businesses and start up new ones or help our children and neighbors cope with their own crises, but when we have a private problem, an intimate sexual one, we suddenly feel all alone and adrift without any sense of where to turn. This self-imposed isolation is no longer warranted. If you have a sexual problem, you should know that you are not alone. You are one of 30 million American men who can be helped to regain their sexual function and vitality.

Boys will be boys. So goes the wisdom of mothers.

Men will be men. Ask any man's wife or lover.

There are times, however, when an individual man cannot be quite the man he would like to be—or once was.

If it is just his status at work, income, or physique that is below expectations, opportunities for improvement are immediately apparent and readily available. He can always seek out a more satisfying job to resolve work-related problems. Financial consultants, eager to advise on income enhancement, will somehow materialize to help him "grow his money," and if he craves a better body, equally ardent exercise buffs will surface to tout the benefits of working out at the local Y or gym to firm up, tone up, and build bigger muscles.

But what if his problem is not fiscal or physical but sexual? What if he is not the man he once was because he is no longer able to have sexual intercourse with his wife or sexual partner? What does he do then?

After all, every man has been taught from the time he was quite young that sex is not just a source of pleasure but was so important that it was ordained in the Bible. The scriptural directive is clear and unambiguous: "A man . . . shall cleave unto his wife and they shall be one flesh" (Genesis 1:23). For a man to cleave, his penis must swell and achieve an erection sufficient to allow for vaginal penetration. Then his penis remains firm during a period of thrusting until he ejaculates.

We assume this is a universal fact of life applicable to all species, but in reality *on-demand* sex is a luxury enjoyed only by the human species.

Men and women are unique in the animal kingdom. Most mammals are obliged to restrict their sexual activity to well-defined cycles when climate and availability of food and water are favorable for breeding. This is not true for humans, for as explained in *The Marriage of Figaro,* "that which distinguishes man from the beast is drinking without being thirsty and making love at all seasons."[1]

Some men cannot make love in any season because they are impotent. They can neither achieve nor sustain an erection satisfactory for intercourse. The loss of erectile function can have a profound effect on a man—and not only in the way he thinks about sex. The word "impotent" also means lacking power or vigor, ineffective. Impotence can so undermine a man's self-esteem and confidence that it affects all his other relations—with his partner, family members, and friends. Mistimed ejaculation or infertility can have similar consequences.

Faced with any other health issue such as pain, fever, or bleeding, a man would ordinarily turn to his doctor to find out why he aches, has a high temperature, or is shedding blood. After all, these are real symptoms and must be caused by "real physical problems."

But sexual problems have always been somehow different, not something easy to talk about because they are frankly "too personal or private." Now this reticence transcends a man's natural anxiety about his anatomy, for there are other exquisitely personal and private health problems unique to a man's genital function that do not impose comparable constraints on consultation.

A man who finds that he is urinating too often during the day (sometimes an indication of bladder infection or diabetes mellitus), has trouble expelling urine from his bladder (a clue to the presence of prostate trouble), notices a lump in his testicle (possibly caused by a testicular tumor or an inflammation of the epididymis), or experiences burning pain during urination as well as pus oozing from the tip of the penis (a common symptom of a sexually transmitted disease) will not hesitate to go directly to his doctor with expectations that treatment will be available to provide relief from these annoying and occasionally frightening genital symptoms (Table 3.1).

In contrast, when a man's problem is not related to the role of his penis as a passageway for expulsion of urine from his bladder but as a sexual instrument, his thinking and actions change dramatically. If his penis balks at becoming or staying erect when he attempts to have sex, he does not, as a rule, automatically call his doctor for advice. This is not surprising, because for years men, women, and even many doctors have been led to believe that male sexual problems were not likely to be caused by "real" physical prob-

---

[1]Pierre de Beaumarchais, *Le Mariage de Figaro* (1784), act 2, scene 21.

TABLE 3.1   Man's distressing private symptoms and their possible causes

Symptom	Possible Cause
Urinating copiously and often	Diabetes mellitus
Urinating often but in small amounts	Enlarged prostate
Painful urination	Sexually transmitted disease or prostatitis
Lump in the testicle	Testicular tumor or epididymitis
Urinating frequently at night	Enlarged prostate, diabetes mellitus, sexually transmitted disease

lems but rather were the consequence of ill-defined "mental" factors or worse yet were an indication of his individual weakness as a male, a misguided perception that persists even today.

When former senator Bob Dole went public to describe his own sexual problems, he was properly applauded for having the courage to step forward and discuss a delicate personal issue in public. But former senator Dole could be at ease talking about this, for his erectile dysfunction was caused by surgical treatment of his prostate cancer *and was not his fault.*

The concern that impotence is an indication of a man's inadequacy as a male persists as the major misconception and an obstacle to proper care. Even more damaging is the erroneous belief that once lost, a man's sexuality or "male sexual life force" could never be reclaimed.

Awash in a sea of misinformation, humiliated and paralyzed by a sense of grieving about no longer "being a man," the impotent man tries to ignore his problem, becomes reclusive, and more often than not does not seek help. So he and other men like him suffer in silence, too embarrassed to seek help. Swaddled in this unwarranted self-imposed isolation, this man would be surprised to learn that he is not alone.

Today, there are at least *30 million other American men with similar sexual problems.*

Thirty million is quite an extraordinary number of sexually impaired men. Why haven't we heard more about this problem? Frankly, because nobody, not even the individual man struggling to make sense of his sudden loss or his gradual ebbing of sexual powers, could bring himself to talk about his problem, even with a family physician.

Paradoxically, in an age smug with a sense of heightened sexual enlightenment, the only ones left "in the closet" are men—impotent men. Closeting their shame may have been their only recourse in years past when doctors had only a primitive understanding of the physical foundations of normal male sexual function and limited treatment options to reinvigorate men's sexual capabilities.

That is no longer true.

Scientists have cast aside their own prejudices and unraveled the intricate details of male sexuality. They did this first by defining the components of normal male sexuality to establish the template for sexual competence. Now, when a man's sexual function falters, doctors can look for weak links in the system. It is in principle no different than first knowing what it takes to make an automobile engine run smoothly and then figuring out what to do when the engine starts to stall or sputter.

You would think that doctors, of all people, would learn this in medical school, but in reality, talk about sex has for the most part been ignored or trivialized in most medical schools until quite recently.

WHAT WE HAVE LEARNED RECENTLY
ABOUT MALE SEXUALITY

Within the past two decades, stunning developments have provided doctors with refreshing new insights about the causes of, and treatments for, a range of male sexual problems including impotence, now more genteelly defined as "erectile dysfunction" (ED), premature or delayed ejaculation, and male infertility. An increasing number of doctors specializing in reproductive medicine now acknowledge that a "male factor" is partially or entirely responsible for about 50 percent of infertile marriages. Even men beyond what would normally be considered peak reproductive years have come under new scrutiny.

We now have a better understanding of *what stimulates* and *what stifles* both a man's sexual desires and his ability to participate in and not only enjoy but revel in his natural sexuality. Until doctors understood the details of a man's unique sexual chemistry, they could offer only limited treatment. Remember, as recently as 1980, doctors believed that 90 percent of all sexual problems were "primarily psychic in origin."

We live, we learn.

Emotional problems can prevent normal sexual function in both men and women, and "psychogenic impotence" does remain as one of the many deterrents to normal male sexual function. However, today *physical* conditions dominate as the most common impediments to male sexual satisfaction.

The pie graphs in Figure 3.1 illustrate how rapidly medical thinking has evolved. Up until 1980, medical textbooks taught, and most doctors believed, that a man's loss of sexual function was invariably the result of a problem in his mind. The term "psychogenic," already in vogue as a legacy of Sigmund Freud's pioneering work on the psyche, was never challenged. In the absence of any contrary evidence, it was believed that all, or at least most (90 percent), impotence was of "psychogenic" origin. If this premise were indeed true, then doctors skilled in delving into the labyrinthine maze

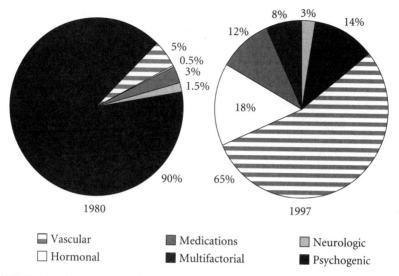

FIGURE 3.1 Change in understanding of causes of impotence (erectile dysfunction) between 1980, when a psychologic basis dominated, and 1997, when physical forces were recognized as more important.

of a man's psyche (that is, psychiatrists and psychologists) would be best equipped to restore the sexual function of impotent men.

They were not.

Indeed, by their own admission, psychologists and psychiatrists had a dismal record in the treatment of impotent men.

Why?

Normal male sexual function required something more than just a healthy psyche. Sure, it is important to have the proper mindset, but the ability to translate that attitude into effective sexual behavior requires some quite specific alterations in a man's anatomy, like the transformation of his penis from a limp to an erect state. The erection a man needs to be sexually successful seems to occur spontaneously but involves a coordinated effort starting with impulses originating in the brain, moving through other nerve tracts, and eventually culminating in an unfettered flow of blood into the penis to create an erection. This flurry of activity that is required for a man to have an erection is ultimately dependent on his unique male sexual chemistry, which links his hormones and vital body chemicals called neurotransmitters.

WHAT ELSE IS IMPORTANT?

Some medications commonly used to treat high blood pressure, depression, ulcers, and high cholesterol levels interfere with normal male sexual function. In addition, nonprescription chemicals like alcohol and nicotine can also wreak havoc with a man's sexual response cycle. (See Chapter 16 for details.)

For the 30 million men in the United States suffering from impotence, either chronic or intermittent, now is the time to come forward. In most cases, once the problem or problems causing impaired sexual function have been identified, physicians can develop effective treatments. Sildenafil (Viagra) is one such treatment useful for many, but not all, impotent men. There are other options, for what was once an arid therapeutic landscape is now awash with remedies.

Today's man with sexual problems is not alone. Men, after all, have been grappling with concerns about their own sexuality since biblical times. Consider how far we have come.

4

The Sexual Man from the Bible to Viagra

Impotence is not a new problem; only our willingness to discuss it more openly is new. As far as we know, the sexuality of man was first described in detail in a biblical tale involving a king, a married woman, her husband, and a virgin. This chapter traces the history of the evolution of our understanding of a man's sexuality from biblical times to the present.

DAVID AND BATHSHEBA, URIAH, AND ABISHAG

David, slayer of Goliath, singer of psalms, and king of Judea, was a passionate man reputed to have ten concubines and several wives. Yet one day he grew restive and "arose from off his bed, and walked upon the roof of the king's house: and from the roof he saw a woman washing herself; and the woman was very beautiful to look upon" (II Samuel 11:2). David was so stirred by the vision of Bathsheba that he summoned her to his chambers and "lay with her" and impregnated her. In the heat of their passion, Bathsheba may have neglected to mention that she was a married woman.

Uriah, Bathsheba's husband and one of David's most loyal captains, was at the time waging war in a distant land. In an effort to disguise the paternity of Bathsheba's child, David arranged for Uriah to be summoned home on furlough. The king assumed that Uriah, weary of battle and in need of a rest, would rejoice at being reunited with Bathsheba and sleep with her. Then when her child was born, she could attribute the pregnancy to that union. But Uriah demurred. He would not even enter Bathsheba's house, let alone sleep with her, for like many men of his time, he believed that by having sexual intercourse and ejaculating he would be sapped of his strength and ill-prepared to return to battle.

When his ruse failed, David saw to it that Uriah was placed in a combat position that would inevitably result in his death. Only then could David take the "recently widowed" Bathsheba as his wife and claim to be the rightful father of their son Solomon.

In the biblical account, David's action angered the Lord and he was punished. "Wherefore hast thou despised the commandment of the Lord, to do evil in his sight? Thou hast killed Uriah the Hittite with thy sword, and has taken his wife to be thy wife" (II Samuel 12:9). David's *sword* was taken from him in more ways than one. He became despondent, ineffective, and impotent. David's impotence was a cause of concern to those closest to him. In an effort to resurrect the king's flagging sexual function, David's advisers sent for a young virgin, Abishag, to rekindle his desires. "And the damsel was very fair, and cherished the king, and ministered to him: but the king knew her not" (I Kings 1:4). David had lost the power to have erections, and by inference, it was presumed that he lacked the power to rule.

Why did David become impotent? The conventional biblical interpretation is that it was punishment for his philanderings with Bathsheba. Others argue that David, riddled with guilt over the entire affair and humiliated by his transgressions, became depressed, leading one to suspect that psychologic factors contributed to his sexual dysfunction. (See Chapter 17.) It is also of some interest that David's impotence first occurred when he was seventy. Was his impotence merely a natural consequence of his aging? (See Chapter 26.)

The story of David's impotence illustrates a prevalent attitude at that time: Man is naturally blessed with the gifts of potency and fertility and forfeits them only by his own indiscretions or the malicious acts of others.

WITCHES AND CURSES

The belief that impotence was caused by malicious acts became prominent during the Middle Ages, when the church developed a proprietary interest in sexual dysfunction, primarily because impotence served as an impediment to procreation. The most thorough early descriptions of sexual problems and possible remedies appeared in the fifteenth century in *A Short Treatise About the People Who, Impeded by Spells, Are Unable to Have Intercourse with Their Wives*. The text describes details of reversing impotence-causing curses invoked by witches, including placement of "testicles of a cock under the bed." A sequence of remedies that might alleviate the spells includes ridding the house of diabolical substances, adequate confession, sprinkling the wall of the house with dog's blood, and carrying bile of fish. Finally, the text suggests that the couple abstain from intercourse for three days. Controlled abstinence is a recommendation still made today to alleviate a condition known as performance anxiety. (See Chapter 17.)

Perhaps the most notorious medieval writing delving extensively into the problems of sexual function is the 1489 *Malleus Maleficarum, or The Witches Hammer*. The text is unequivocal: Impotence results from spells cast by witches under the direction of the devil. Here, too, a series of remedies is described, and if all fails, one may "approach the witch." Witch hunts followed.

By the sixteenth century, some people were beginning to consider that factors other than diabolical spells might be responsible for male sexual dysfunction. Dr. Johann Weyer, in 1563, speculated that impotence could result from natural causes or from the inappropriate use of medicines. This was the first indication that medication might impede sexual function. (See Chapter 16.)

THE ROOSTER EXPERIMENT

It was not until the nineteenth century that meaningful scientific inquiries into certain aspects of male sexual function were reported. In 1849, a Belgian cleric, August Berthold, made critical observations by studying the behavior of common barnyard fowl. He noted that roosters chased hens but capons did not. (A capon is a rooster whose testicles have been removed to encourage development of tender flesh and a plump bird.) Berthold found that if he reimplanted testicles in the capon, the bird promptly resumed its innate roosterly behavior and started chasing chickens again. This elegant and unusual avian experiment offered the first convincing evidence of a physiologic role for the testicle in normal male sexual function.

Forty years later, the French neurologist Claude Brown-Sequard attempted to provide a clinical counterpart to Berthold's studies. He reported that he and other older men were revitalized by injections of watery extracts of animal testes. Since testosterone, the active hormonal component of the testis, is not water soluble, it remains unclear exactly what testicular products Dr. Brown-Sequard injected to achieve this salutary response. Perhaps the study served only to illustrate the confounding role of the placebo in the treatment of older men with diminished virility. Nevertheless, his experiments were the last scientific inquiries into the subject of male sexual function and dysfunction for decades. Other scientists working in this era found themselves oppressed by the stultifying influences of the Victorian age, a period when investigation of matters relating to sex was neither encouraged nor condoned.

FREUD AND OEDIPUS

In the early twentieth century, the overpowering influence of Sigmund Freud resurrected interest in sexual problems. Freud's achievements, although extraordinary, were so intimidating that they stifled research in other disciplines for a considerable period. Freud believed that men became impotent because they linked their sexual partners with their mothers, yet Freud himself had difficulty reconciling this concept with his own observations. He was convinced that *all men* experienced oedipal conflict but recognized that impotence was not universal.

Nonetheless, the belief that impotence was primarily a problem of *psychogenic* ("it's all in your head") origin dominated medical teaching until the early 1980s. Before that time, it had been recognized that vascular, neurologic, and occasionally hormonal disorders might be associated with impaired sexual functioning. But prevailing dogma dictated that these physical disorders were rarely found in impotent men.

Today, a more realistic appraisal stipulates that although psychologic factors unquestionably contribute to impotence in some instances, *physical* causes of impotence must also be considered. Psychologic issues are critical, but they no longer supersede a comprehensive diagnostic evaluation to explore the possible role of such factors as problems with blood flow, nerve damage, hormone deficiencies, and, quite commonly, side effects of prescription and nonprescription medications, and commonly used products like cigarettes and alcohol.

THE WHALE AND THE WALRUS

In the late 1930s and early 1940s, several physicians were preoccupied with the mechanics of the erectile process and tried to solve the problem of impotence by inserting a stiffening agent inside the flaccid penis of impotent men. Other mammals had solved this problem during evolution by developing a permanent bonelike structure within their erectile tissue. Referred to as an *os-penis*, this can acquire formidable dimensions. For example, the os-penis of the whale is six feet long, and a similar structure in the walrus is two feet in length.

Surgeons searching for a way to help men who had suffered penile mutilation decided to create a human os-penis. They were of the opinion that if they could devise an operation that would provide the penis with permanent, rodlike firmness, then penetration of the vagina would always be possible. In 1936, two surgeons, one in Russia and the other in Germany, exploited this concept by using the cartilage from a man's rib to provide the penile rigidity required for vaginal penetration. Unfortunately, there were multiple technical problems with the cartilaginous implants, and the technique was soon abandoned. Still, this inventive surgical technique anticipated and heralded the future development of the currently popular silicone penile prostheses. (See Chapter 18.)

It was the plight of individual men who had experienced penile trauma that prompted surgical efforts to implant rib cartilage. These physicians were unaware of the numbers of nontraumatized healthy men who were unable to acquire erections satisfactory for sexual intercourse. That information emerged after the studies conducted by Alfred Kinsey.

KINSEY

In 1948, Dr. Alfred Kinsey scandalized the public by publishing *Sexual Behavior in the Human Male*. In this landmark work, Kinsey catalogued different patterns of male sexual function and reported that 2 percent of American men under the age of forty suffered from impotence. His data implied that 10 million men were experiencing sexual problems. (These estimates were probably on the low side.) Despite his findings, research into male sexual dysfunction proceeded only slowly for the next two decades.

THE TURNING POINT

The early 1970s were watershed years. Researchers schooled in disparate disciplines proved to be unusually productive and broadened our basic knowledge of normal male sexual function. Each step forward led to the development of innovative therapies for men suffering from impotence, ejaculatory disorders, or infertility.

Masters and Johnson

William Masters and Virginia Johnson studied the physiology of sex by direct observation and, in 1970, published their results, defining what they termed the "normal male sexual response cycle." Their innovative treatment for sexual dysfunction involved both partners in several weeks of specific exercises to restore sexual communication, intimacy, and satisfaction. (See Chapter 17.)

The Vascular Steal Syndrome

Medical research had been making strides in related areas. A French surgeon, Dr. René Leriche, discovered that when severe atherosclerosis (hardening of the arteries) partially blocked some branches of the abdominal aorta, the normal flow of blood into the penis did not occur. In 1973, Czechoslovakian surgeon Dr. V. Michal described a somewhat different vascular problem, which he termed the "pelvic steal syndrome." In this disorder, a man can acquire and sustain an erection as long as he doesn't move his legs. Moving the legs drains—"steals"—blood away from the pelvis, so the erection collapses. This type of impotence can now be corrected with surgery that unblocks the affected artery. Then blood can flow freely to the genitalia and remain there throughout intercourse. Other forms of impotence due to blood-vessel blockage are now attributed to impaired blood flow through still smaller blood vessels. This, too, can be corrected by surgery. (See Chapter 10.)

Erections and the Electroencephalogram

Neurologists, aware of the role of the central, peripheral, and autonomic nervous systems in erectile process, provided new insights into the neurophysiology of erections. It had long been known that most men wake in the morning with an erection. Although the erection occurs coincident with a full bladder and disappears after urination, filling the bladder with urine does not cause the erection. Rather, this early-morning erection is associated with specific electrical changes occurring in the brain during sleep.

Most men, independent of sexual desire, experience spontaneous erections while sleeping. These nocturnal erections coincide with the onset of a particular type of sleep called rapid eye movement (REM) sleep. Using an electroencephalogram (EEG), which measures electrical activity in the brain, and direct observation, physicians can monitor the brain-wave patterns identifying the onset of REM sleep and the appearance of erections. The procedure, referred to as nocturnal penile tumescence (NPT) monitoring, is one diagnostic test often employed in the early evaluation of men complaining of impotence. Until recently, NPT testing was restricted to the domain of hospital sleep labs, an expensive site for testing and an unnatural environment for any man to have a good night's sleep. Advances in technology have now made it possible to evaluate the precise number, vigor, and duration of a man's nighttime erections at lower cost as he sleeps in the comfort of his own bed. Other neural reflexes critical to erection can also be assessed by direct testing to determine whether there is an underlying neurologic cause for impaired erectile function. (See Chapter 10.)

Urologists "Cut to the Chase"

Another critical development in the early 1970s involved two groups of urologic surgeons who independently proposed that the most direct way to help men suffering from impotence was to unburden them of the anxiety associated with first acquiring and then sustaining an erection satisfactory for intercourse. The urologists reasoned that if they provided the man's flaccid penis with a mechanical device that gives it permanent rodlike firmness, vaginal penetration could be achieved on demand, independent of sexual desire or arousal. In essence, this device would allow men to be perpetually prepared for sexual intercourse. This was basically similar to the thinking that led to the first attempts to use cartilage as a penile stiffening agent. But this time there was a difference, for *silicone* had been refined and was readily available. Using silicone, the first penile prostheses were designed, developed, and then implanted. (See Chapter 18.)

DR. BRINDLEY GOES TO LAS VEGAS

Urologists continued to make major advances in understanding the nature of men's erections. The American Urologic Association (AUA) holds a meeting each year to discuss the most recent advances in the field. In 1985, the AUA's annual meeting was in Las Vegas, and at that meeting one of their scientists, Dr. G. S. Brindley described an unusual discovery. He knew that the natural tendency of the penis is to remain limp and flaccid because nerve signals called *alpha impulses* prevent the penis from enlarging. A man's penis only becomes erect by shutting off or blocking these alpha impulses. This is what occurs spontaneously during normal sexual arousal and when men experience spontaneous erections during sleep. Dr. Brindley found a way to block these erection-inhibiting alpha impulses and claimed he could create an erection in the absence of sexual arousal. He could do this by injecting a common alpha-blocking drug called phentolamine directly into a man's penis. Dr. Brindley went on to say that he *had just injected phentolamine into his own penis* and was willing to demonstrate how well it worked. Then he dropped his pants, displayed his firm rigid penis and invited all in attendance to check how natural his medication-induced erection looked and felt. Women in the audience may have fainted, and AUA members in attendance were said to have gasped at Dr. Brindley's audacity. But shortly after this bold presentation, all were finding ways to reproduce his feat. Within less than a year, the concept of intrapenile injection became a well-established and recognized treatment for men with erectile dysfunction. (See Chapter 19.)

MORE RECENT ADVANCES IN ENDOCRINOLOGY

Two pivotal developments in the field of endocrinology once again emphasized the role of hormones in normal male sexual function. Researchers identified and analyzed a new hormone, gonadotropin-releasing hormone (GnRH). GnRH is made in a portion of the brain called the hypothalamus, from which the hormonal regulation of male sexual function is orchestrated. Later, it was determined that the pattern of GnRH release is critical; "pulsatile GnRH secretion" is a prerequisite for normal testosterone and sperm production and, as a consequence, is vital for male sexual and reproductive success.

By the early 1980s, my colleagues and I had accumulated enough experience to publish "Impotence Is Not Always Psychogenic." In a group of 105 men with complaints of impotence, we found thirty-five who had specific hormonal abnormalities. Recognition of the abnormality and institution of appropriate treatment resulted in prompt restoration of potency. By the end of the decade, the role of the pituitary gland and of a portion of the brain called the temporal lobe as well as the role of testosterone as regulators of male sexual function was appreciated. (See Chapter 12.)

SEX, MEN'S BODY CHEMISTRY, AND VIAGRA

We know now that there is more to a man's sexual life than his testosterone. What could be more important than this manliest of all male hormones?

Nitric oxide. What is nitric oxide?

Nitric oxide (NO) is the chemical instigator of a man's erection. NO is not a hormone but a *neurotransmitter*. Unlike hormones, which are produced in endocrine glands and released into a man's bloodstream to exert their influence all over his body, neurotransmitters have more modest ambitions. Neurotransmitters influence the behavior of neighboring cells. The neurotransmitter NO allows blood to flow into the penile erectile bodies and is crucial for a man to develop early penile swelling, a condition called *tumescence*.

Full *rigid erections* require a second, locally produced chemical called cyclic GMP (cGMP). A man's penis remains erect and rigid as long as the local cGMP levels remain elevated. When cGMP levels diminish, so does a man's erection. Sildenafil (Viagra) increases cGMP, and this is why it works to improve the stamina of a man's erections.

Thus, the combination of locally produced *NO is needed to initiate* a man's erection, and *cGMP is required to sustain* it. When cGMP levels fall, a man's erection fades. As long as penile-tissue cGMP levels remain high, erectile vigor persists. Sildenafil (Viagra) is effective because it helps maintain high cGMP levels.

It is as simple as this.

1. Deplete cGMP and a man loses his erection
2. Buttress cGMP levels and man can maintain his erection.
3. Sildenafil (Viagra) stabilizes cGMP levels and increases erectile vigor.

Is Viagra foolproof and guaranteed to improve every impotent man's erections and sexual performance all the time? Unfortunately not.

There is a yin and yang to a man's erections. Just as some neurotransmitters turn the erectile process on, others turn it off. For example, adrenaline-like chemicals (always lurking in the body and spewed out during stress) can siphon blood out of a man's penis with lightning speed, causing his erection to collapse.

Thus, the NO cGMP signal "turns on" a man's erection, whereas adrenaline "tuns it off." NO and cGMP, as well as the potential side effects, proper

---

use, cost, and controversy surrounding Viagra, are discussed in more detail in Chapter 11.

Sildenafil (Viagra) has been very effective in allowing many impotent men to experience erections and enjoy sexual function once again. However, for the 30–35 percent of impotent men who do not have improved erections with Viagra, other treatment strategies are likely to be more effective.

HELP IS ALWAYS AVAILABLE

Physicians in many specialties are now equipped to take initial exploratory steps in diagnosing male sexual problems. Detailed evaluation and effective treatment can be developed when the patient's own personal physician works in close collaboration with doctors trained in urology, sexual therapy, or endocrinology. Today we have more treatment options than ever before.

5

You Are Not Alone

Whether he calls it impotence or ED—erectile dysfunction—the man experiencing a sexual problem often believes his predicament is unique to him. As we start to talk honestly about sex, it is becoming increasingly apparent that more and more men and women are having sexual difficulties. This chapter provides answers to the most frequently asked questions about male sexual dysfunction, or ED, including these: How common is it? Is aging a factor? Do common medical problems like hypertension, diabetes, and depression cause impotence, or is it the medications used to treat these conditions that disrupt a man's sexual function? Can you do anything to prevent impotence?

When a man is unable to achieve an erection satisfactory for intercourse, he is considered impotent. Today the term "erectile dysfunction," or "ED" has supplanted "impotence," probably because ED is a less emotionally charged term. This is not surprising because the dictionary defines the word "impotent" as (1) lacking physical strength or vigor: weak, (2) powerless; ineffectual, (3) incapable of sexual intercourse. This definition is more than just demeaning, for it strikes at the very fabric of a man's maleness.

Generally speaking, the phrase "erectile dysfunction," or "ED," has been promulgated by those who are frankly promoting different impotence treatments and are themselves more comfortable saying that they have a new product to correct ED than a novel impotence treatment. However, the individual man with sexual problems rarely comes to the doctor saying, "My primary problem is that I have ED" or "Doc, now that you've helped lower my blood pressure, I wonder if I could discuss my erectile dysfunction with you." Men, if they discuss their sexual difficulties at all, either resort to euphemisms such as "I can't get it up anymore" or fall back on the embarrassing admission "I guess I've become impotent."

However you choose to label it, the truth is that many men, if not all men, have at one time or another experienced isolated episodes of ED, or impotence. Often this is transient, a result of fatigue, excessive drinking, or preoccupation with business or family problems. Under these circumstances, it would be inappropriate to saddle the man with a diagnosis of complete impotence; instead he is said to have experienced situational erectile dysfunction. Criteria established by Masters and Johnson indicate that a diagnosis of impotence is appropriate only when a man experiences failure more than 25 percent of the time during attempted intercourse.

HOW COMMON IS IMPOTENCE?

It was not until the middle of the twentieth century that reliable information on the prevalence of impotence was available. As previously noted, Dr. Alfred Kinsey, in his *Sexual Behavior in the Human Male,* estimated that impotence occurred in less than 2 percent of men under the age of forty. The incidence increased gradually with age, so that, according to Kinsey, 6.7 percent of men were impotent by age fifty-five and almost 25 percent at seventy. Recent data suggest that Kinsey's report significantly underestimated the total. Current surveys indicate that impotence plagues 30 million American men.

Part of the problem in collecting accurate data relates to men's lack of candor when discussing sexual problems. Most men are more than willing to answer questions about their income, general health, smoking, and drinking habits. They are often disarmingly frank about their extramarital relationships, sexual preferences, and sex life. Still, the same men are recalcitrant when confronted with a questionnaire asking for truthful and accurate answers regarding sexual impairment. As noted, in a prior chapter, these times of extraordinary sexual enlightenment, impotence may be the only subject remaining in the closet.

Because it is important to have some estimate of the prevalence of impotence, investigators have devised a series of questionnaires with sufficient ingenuity to provide information that may have been overlooked in the past.

For example, two investigators, Drs. Anthony Reading and William Weist, recruited subjects in London, England, by proposing to examine attitudes relating to the development of a male contraceptive. During the course of the extensive interview, information was elicited relative to the volunteers' current sexual function and dysfunction. The investigators found that among a group of presumably healthy, sexually active, heterosexual Englishmen (age twenty to thirty-five) involved in a stable relationship, 8.25 percent admitted having difficulty achieving and maintaining an erection satisfactory for sexual intercourse, and 18.5 percent said that they did not achieve an erection satisfactory for masturbation.

Dr. Ellen Frank and her associates at the University of Southern California decided that the optimal way to verify descriptions of male sexual function was to direct the same questions to *both* husband and wife. Dr. Frank, like others, recognized that reliable descriptions of sexual function are most likely to be obtained by using a subtle approach. Her extensive fifteen-page questionnaire, therefore, contained only one and one-half pages relating to sex. In her survey of one hundred married couples in their mid-thirties, Dr. Frank identified surprisingly high levels of sexual dysfunction reported by the men and confirmed by their wives. Sixteen percent of the men reported difficulty acquiring or sustaining an erection. In addition, 36 percent felt they ejaculated too quickly, and 4 percent were unable to ejaculate at all. This number is roughly *twenty times Kinsey's estimate* for a similar age group.

Dr. Michael Slag of the Minneapolis Veterans Administration expanded on Frank's observations, providing data from a different perspective. He interviewed men attending a Veterans Administration outpatient clinic for problems unrelated to sexual function and found that of 1,180 men, 401 (34 percent) complained of impotence. But this patient population differed in several respects from the couples studied by Dr. Frank.

The men in Dr. Slag's study were older; the average age was fifty. In addition, all had some medical problem that prompted them to visit the clinic. In many cases the illness itself was the primary cause of sexual dysfunction. It is also worth noting that men attending any clinic can be expected to receive medication, and many medications can affect sexual function. In fact, Dr. Slag was able to incriminate medications as a direct cause of the impotence in 22 percent of the impotent men in his study.

Dr. Leslie Schover, a psychologist at the State University of New York at Stony Brook, surveyed 300 men with a mean age of 55 and reported that 21 percent of them complained of impotence.

DOES AGING CONTRIBUTE TO IMPOTENCE?

Kinsey's observation that older men experience problems with sex more often than younger men is accurate. But the reasons remain the subject of considerable controversy. Gerontologists have been studying a group of healthy older men age sixty to seventy-nine as part of the Baltimore Longitudinal Study (BLS) on aging. Men in the study were queried about their sexual activity during the course of a year. They were then divided into those who had "least," "medium," and "most" sexual events (intercourse and/or masturbation). Roughly equal numbers of men fell into each category. This suggested that some independent factor—not age alone—determines the level of sexual vigor for men over sixty. In this population of healthy men, only 25 to 35 percent reported difficulty achieving a functional erection.

Other investigators have challenged the BLS observations, maintaining that they are not reproducible. Dr. Alexander Vermeulen of Belgium arrived at a diametrically opposite conclusion. His data indicate that among sixty-to eighty-year-old men, only 25 to 35 percent do *not* have problems; rather, fully 65 to 75 percent do have problems. Some argue that it is not the aging process per se but other concomitant factors that are responsible for the diminished sexual ability of older men. The BLS study may be faulted because only men who were unusually healthy and free of common medical problems such as high blood pressure and diabetes mellitus qualified for inclusion. Since both high blood pressure and diabetes are common in older men, many investigators believe it is inappropriate to generalize observations from the BLS experience to other geriatric populations.

AN UPDATE ON
MALE SEXUAL DYSFUNCTION

Important new information regarding the numbers of men who experience sexual problems emerged in 1994 with the publication of the Massachusetts Male Aging Study (MMAS). The respondents, 1290 men forty to seventy years old, answered a brief sexual questionnaire and indicated whether they had: no "sexual problems" (never impotent) or "minimal impotence" (rare erectile failures but still able to have sexual intercourse most of the time); "moderate impotence" (difficulty acquiring or maintaining an erection but still able to have sexual intercourse periodically); or "complete" impotence (never able to acquire or maintain an erection and unable to have sexual intercourse).

The MMAS results were surprising, for it turned out that impotence surfaces as a problem for more men *much earlier in life than expected.* Forty percent of men admitted to minimal, moderate, or complete impotence at age forty. The numbers of men plagued by some degree of erectile dysfunction increase by about 10 percent with each succeeding decade, so that at age fifty, no less than 50 percent of men admitted to some erectile failures, 60 percent acknowledged some sexual problem at age sixty, and 70 percent were sexually impaired at age 70.

Complete impotence—present in only 5.1 percent of forty-year-olds, increased threefold to 15 percent for seventy-year-old men. The numbers of men describing moderate impotence increased from 17 percent to 34 percent between age 40 and 70, and episodes of minimal impotence remained remarkably constant at 17 percent for all age groups studied. Although 60 percent of forty-year-old men could say they were "not impotent," only 33 percent of the seventy-year-olds could provide a similar answer.

Increasing age is not the only problem. Several factors—some within, and others beyond the individual man's control—increase the impotence risk. In this survey, the probability of developing complete impotence was 56 percent for current smokers compared to 8.5 percent for nonsmokers. Diabetes mellitus, high blood pressure, use of antihypertensive medications, and cardiac drugs independently and collectively augmented the chances of developing impotence. Only a few men go through life without ever having experienced one or more episodes of impotence.

EFFECTS OF HYPERTENSION, DIABETES, AND MEDICATIONS

High blood pressure (hypertension) by itself has a negative effect on male sexual activity. Untreated hypertensive men are three times more likely to experience potency problems than men of similar age with normal blood pressure. Unfortunately, antihypertensive medication can cause further deterioration in erectile or ejaculatory function.

To overcome problems caused by medications, the patient can describe the unpleasant and unwanted effects to his physician in detail (being forthright about potency problems) and the physician can adjust drug dosage or prescribe alternative medication to control high blood pressure without negative sexual (and other) side effects. The same approach holds true for many other medications routinely used to treat a spectrum of common problems such as peptic ulcer, gastrointestinal disturbances, depression, and a wide range of psychiatric conditions. Many of these can interfere with normal erections. (See Chapter 16 for a comprehensive list of prescription medications and chemicals that adversely affect male sexual function.)

Diabetes mellitus can have a devastating effect on a man's sexual function. As many as 35 percent of diabetic men twenty to sixty years old experience impotence, whereas only 9 to 10 percent of nondiabetic age-matched controls (that is, men in the same age bracket who do not have diabetes) are similarly affected.

Diabetes is associated with an increased predisposition to two types of vascular disease. One affects the large blood vessels that supply blood to the pelvis. The other involves the smaller blood vessels in the penis that must dilate to become engorged with blood so that an erection can occur. If an impotent, diabetic man has evidence of either macro- or microvascular disease in body organs distant from the genital area (heart, eyes, kidney, and so on), he most likely has vasculogenic impotence. Effective treatment depends on pinpointing the specific defect responsible for the erectile failure; treatment for vasculogenic impotence differs from that for neurogenic impotence.

PREVENTION OF IMPOTENCE

There is no way to stave off aging, but some modifications in behavior can help minimize risks of sexual dysfunction. Smoking, heavy drinking, obesity, high levels of serum cholesterol, and elevated blood-sugar levels, as well as the use of narcotic or other mood-altering drugs, can all contribute to impotence. Early investments in weight reduction, temperance in alcohol consumption, and avoidance of nicotine and drugs during youth may provide significant sexual dividends later on.

6

The Six Phases of Normal Male Sexual Function

It is tempting to think of sexual intercourse as a seamless process flowing effortlessly from arousal to erection to ejaculation. This level of understanding suffices only for those men fortunate enough never to have experienced sexual problems. In this chapter, you will find a discussion of the individual components that make it possible for a man to want to have sex and then see how he can render that desire into a complete and pleasurable experience for him and his partner.

One way of understanding the cycle of a man's sexual responsivity is to look at the individual steps that make it possible for him to have sex. The six critical stages are: *libido, erection, plateau, ejaculation and orgasm, detumescence, and refractory period.* Proper sequencing and integration of these phases is critical.

- *Libido* describes the intensity of sexual desire or drive.
- *Erection* refers to the transition of the penis from a limp to an erect state. Increased blood flow into specialized chambers in the penis is necessary for this transition to occur. Nerve signals that originate in the spinal cord are responsible for activating increased blood flow.
- The *plateau* phase occurs at the peak of sexual excitement and is associated with increases in pulse, blood pressure, and respiration rate.
- *Ejaculation,* the pulsatile release of semen, is entirely under neurologic control. *Orgasm* is the pleasurable feeling and sense of relaxation following ejaculation.
- *Detumescence* is the loss of erection after ejaculation.
- During the *refractory period,* men are unable to acquire another erection.

LIBIDO

Psychologic factors and the hormone testosterone, which is produced by the testicles, regulate male libido. Studies in animals have demonstrated that removal of the testicles, a procedure called castration, results in a precipitous decline in testosterone levels in the bloodstream. Shortly thereafter, the castrated animal loses sexual interest.

Castration has the same effect on adult men, and loss of sexual desire is commonplace among men with advanced prostate or testicular cancer who have had to sacrifice their testicles to save or prolong their lives.

Some impotent men still have some, but not enough, testosterone. Their testicles no longer work as efficiently as they once did. As a consequence, they produce inadequate amounts of testosterone and have lower than normal serum testosterone levels. These men notice a gradual but progressive diminution in sexual desire. Potency may be preserved during brief interludes of subnormal serum testosterone levels, but when testosterone production remains chronically low, impotence is inevitable. Treatment with testosterone usually restores sexual desire and potency.

Emotional setbacks as a result of clinical depression, loss of a loved one, or a business reversal can also result in a decline in libido. For these men, whose testosterone levels are normal, testosterone treatment is neither warranted nor effective. Rather, recognition and treatment of the depression, the grief, or the self-doubts are more appropriate. Counseling or psychotherapy is often helpful in restoring sexual desire.

ERECTION

Men acquire erections by fantasy or when confronted with erotic stimuli (psychogenic erections), after direct stimulation of their genitals (reflex erections), and spontaneously during sleep (nocturnal erections).

Psychogenic erections occur in response to any one of a variety of sensory stimuli, usually visual or auditory. Visual and auditory cues are so reliably consistent in provoking psychogenic erections that behavioral therapists often use them to learn more about what stimulates or inhibits erections in normal and sexually dysfunctional men.

All such studies share a traditional experimental "stimulus-response" design. The stimulus is either an audio- or videotape describing or showing heterosexual sex acts. The response is an erection, which is recorded by attaching a sensor, somewhat like a blood pressure cuff, to the volunteer's penis. The device measures changes in penis size and can be used to determine what conditions enhance or inhibit erection. A normally potent man exposed to an erotic audio- or videotape will develop an erection. When, for example, the content of the audiotape is held constant but the subject is distracted and asked to complete an innocuous questionnaire, he loses his

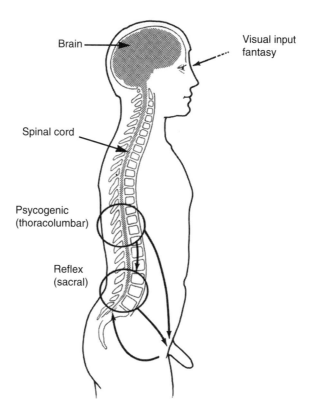

FIGURE 6.1   Nerve impulses originating at two different levels of a man's spinal cord allow him to have psychogenic and reflex erections.

erection. Similarly, if the videotape is replaced by a neutral travelogue, the subject loses his erection.

This stimulus-response model has provided some predictable as well as some unexpected insights into the interaction between psychologic influences and physical responses. The observation that for heterosexual men, an audiotape narrated by a female is more effective in provoking an erection than a similar script narrated by a male is not surprising. Less intuitive is the observation that although mildly threatening cues result in diminution of the erection, more aggressive cues paradoxically enhance arousal.

NEURAL CONNECTIONS

Two centers in the spinal cord serve as important junctions for *psychogenic* and *reflex* erections. (See Figure 6.1.) The first site, located in the upper back, is the thoracolumbar erection center. It appears to be a critical way station for psychogenic erections. The second site, in the lower back, or sacrum, is the sacral erection center. Nerve routes from this area receive and send impulses to the genitalia to facilitate reflex erections.

The Six Phases of Normal Male Sexual Function

Reflex erections are initiated by local nerve impulses originating in the genital area. Manual or oral stimulation of the penis or scrotum will evoke a reaction in bundles of nerve fibers in the penis called pacinian corpuscles, activating the first segment of a reflex circuit. (The tip, or glans, of the penis contains the greatest concentration of these pressure-sensitive corpuscles.) Neural impulses arising in local or genital nerves travel with lightning speed to the lower spine. Once received at this site, the circuit is completed by transmission of nerve messages back to the cavernosal nerve in the penile erectile bodies to set in motion the series of events that increase blood flow into the penis to create an erection.

Still another set of neurologic signals originating in the lower spine travel to the prostate and seminal vesicles. These structures are the source of the seminal fluid that is released during ejaculation. Impulses from the lower sacral areas also activate muscles in the pelvis to help maintain the strength of both psychogenic and reflex erections. The same muscles will be called on later to contract rhythmically during ejaculation.

VASCULAR REACTIONS

The foregoing describes the neurologic connections necessary for normal erectile function. The actual process depends on events that stimulate blood vessels in the penis to dilate or widen to accommodate the massive influx of blood required for an erection.

The penis contains three cylindrical bundles of blood vessels (two corpora cavernosae and one corpus spongiosum) uniquely designed to trap blood. (See Figure 6.2.) The spongy tissues fill and become engorged with blood to create the erection.

Normally, when blood flows into a portion of the body, it enters and exits promptly, providing nourishment and removing wastes. This inflow and outflow is efficient for all organs of the body but is not conducive to the development and maintenance of an erection. Blood must flow into and be held captive within the penile corporal bodies to allow for initial swelling. Then another process must inhibit outflow so that a rigid erection develops and is maintained. Small blood vessels in the penis swell and exert pressure on the veins that normally allow blood to drain out of the penis. The blood in the penis is thus "trapped," and the erection can be maintained until orgasm or stimulation ceases.

PLATEAU

Following erection, most men reach a plateau. During the plateau phase, which may last from thirty seconds to two minutes, a rapid series of events occurs.

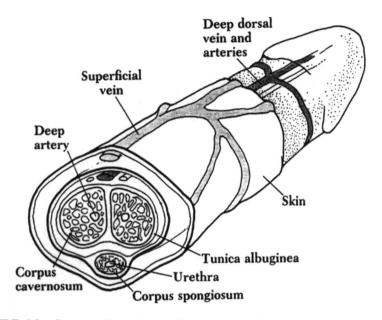

FIGURE 6.2   Cross-section of penis illustrating penile erectile bodies: the corpora cavernosae and corpus spongiosum.

Men experience a flushing of the face and an increase in heart rate up to 150 to 175 beats per minute. At the same time, distinct rises in both systolic (pressure when heart contracts) and diastolic (pressure in between heart contractions) blood pressure are evident. Testicular size increases by 50 percent. Then, fluid from the accessory sexual organs, the prostate and seminal vesicles, begins to discharge. This preclimactic stage is under neural control and prepares the man for ejaculation. Signals from the nervous system facilitate the movement of sperm-rich fluid from the seminal vesicles and prostate into the urethra in anticipation of ejaculation. The urethra is a hollow tube in the center of the penis that allows urine to be eliminated from the bladder.

EJACULATION AND ORGASM

Ejaculation and orgasm occur as pelvic muscles contract to propel seminal fluid through and out the urethra. At the culmination of sexual excitement, carefully timed neurologic impulses act to close the internal bladder valve (sphincter). This allows all the ejaculated seminal fluid to be pushed *forward* through the urethra (*antegrade ejaculation*).

If the bladder sphincter does not close, ejaculated semen is forced *backward* into the bladder. This abnormal ejaculation, called *retrograde ejaculation*, occurs in some paraplegics, in men treated with some antihypertensive medications (such as guanethidine), and often after prostate or bladder surgery or radiation treatment to the pelvis. Men who lose the capacity to have antegrade ejaculation can retain erectile function and experience orgasm, but they often become alarmed when they do not sense fluid passing through the urethra. Some become depressed over their inability to complete this phase of the male sexual response cycle. Impotence may follow.

Orgasm is distinct from ejaculation. Orgasm is the pleasurable phenomenon experienced at a conscious level that is associated with the rhythmic contraction of certain pelvic muscles (the bulbocavernosus and ischiocavernosus muscles); a sense of relaxation follows.

DETUMESCENCE AND REFRACTORY PERIOD

Following ejaculation, blood drains out of the penis, which then reverts to its normal resting state. The penis remains limp and flaccid for a period of time during which neither erection nor ejaculation is possible. The penis is considered to be unresponsive (refractory) to stimulation during this interval. The duration of the refractory period seems to vary with age; younger men may experience reflexogenic erections thirty to forty-five minutes after ejaculation, whereas older men may require two to three hours or more before doing so.

7

Defining the Problem: What Disrupts a Man's Normal Sexual Response Cycle?

A man who develops a sexual problem tends to concentrate his energy on his recalcitrant penis, which does not become erect when it should. But riveting attention on the penis is not the best way to resolve the problem.

The inability to achieve an erection is most commonly traced to a specific problem in three of the six phases (libido, erection, ejaculation) of the normal male sexual response cycle (see Chapter 6). Psychiatrists, psychologists, and sex therapists use a language that differs slightly from the terminology used elsewhere in this book. In their vernacular, *sexual desire* takes the place of libido; *arousal* is used instead of erection; and *orgasm* is substituted for ejaculation.

There are several avenues through which these individual areas of sexual vulnerability can be explored. Only by teasing apart the individual components of the male sexual response cycle can the cause of ongoing sexual failure be revealed. Then a focused treatment plan can be formulated.

DESIRE-PHASE (LIBIDO) PROBLEMS

Two desire-phase problems, *low sexual desire* and *aversion to sex*, are now recognized. When psychologists and sex therapists talk about low sexual desire, they do so in a global fashion. If a man complains of reduced desire, it is important to know whether it is partner specific. Has the man lost interest in having sex only with his partner? Does he have any interest in, or fantasize about, having sex with other partners? Is he having erotic dreams? Does he have any sexual fantasies? Do spontaneous erections occur under any circumstances?

If the answer is yes to any of the above, the diagnosis is not low sexual desire. That diagnosis is reserved for men who answer "no" to all these questions. Men with genuine low sexual desire often state that they cannot remember the last time they experienced any sensation of lust, horniness, or true sexual desire.

LOW SEXUAL DESIRE

Four readily recognizable events—death of a spouse, physical illness, recent surgery, and divorce—result in a predictable loss of sexual desire. Blunting of desire is also a common but transient phenomenon after any physically or emotionally stressful episode. The sexual problems of men who have suffered an acute medical illness or recent surgery are, for the most part, of limited duration. Desire and potency will return slowly but steadily. For widowers and divorced men, the sequence of events is more protracted but usually resolves with time alone or with limited reassurance and counseling.

In other instances, the precipitating factors responsible for the loss of sexual desire are less apparent. Additional effort is required to unravel the chain of events that singly or collectively served to quench the libido.

A lack or progressive diminution in sexual desire may also be the harbinger of depression. Depressions are complex medical problems and require more detailed evaluation and treatment. Potency returns to depressed men only when their depression is alleviated. Often, antidepressant medications are necessary to help cope with symptoms of depression. (See Chapter 16.)

AVERSION TO SEX

Aversion to sex is an uncommon and poorly understood subcategory of impaired sexual desire. This diagnosis implies not just a lack of interest in sex but an overall repugnance concerning all sexual activities. The man suffering from sexual aversion finds sex a disgusting, anxiety-provoking experience and the cause of severe guilt and shame. Aversion to sex is often reported by men with primary impotence (men who have never been potent). It is rarely seen in the man with secondary impotence (a man who was potent in the past but is now having difficulty achieving erections), though it may occur if he discovers a shift in gender preference. Recently recognized homosexual feelings may evoke a so-called selective impotence. In this case, a previously heterosexual man may develop an aversion to sex with females only.

AROUSAL-PHASE DISORDERS

Psychologists classify problems achieving and sustaining erections as arousal-phase disorders. Men with inadequate arousal insist that they have normal desire, a persistent passionate sexual feeling. They complain primarily of the inability either to achieve or to maintain an erection satisfactory for sexual intercourse. They are frequently troubled by the fact that they don't enjoy sex as much as they used to.

It is important to determine whether the impotent man still has erections and, if so, under what circumstances. Normally, erections occur spontaneously during sleep. The impotent man may be aware of his spontaneous nighttime erections only when he wakes up in the morning and finds that his penis is fully erect. This implies that the neurologic signals and blood flow to the penis are still operating normally. A phase of normal sleep known as rapid eye movement, or REM, sleep seems to be critical for the initiation of early-morning erections. Men who sleep fitfully do not have REM sleep and will not have erections when they wake in the morning; this is no cause for alarm.

If a well-rested man does not have erections when he arises, it is important to determine whether he can get an erection under any other circumstances. Can he bring his penis to an erection when masturbating? Does his penis become erect when he views sexually explicit material or an erotic film? Is there someone other than his wife or primary partner who can stimulate him to an erection? If the answer is yes to any of those questions, blood flow (vascular) and neurologic signals to the genitals are likely intact.

The ability to have a brief but not lasting erection is characteristic of men who have penile venous incompetence. With this condition, the blood vessels fail to close off the veins that carry blood from penile chambers so that the blood drains from the penis shortly after the initial erection is achieved. The problem can be corrected by surgery. However, surgery is not necessary for all men who have difficulty maintaining an erection.

Sometimes erections occur and then disappear as the man loses concentration on the sexual act. This so-called lack of sensate focus is common in middle-aged men. It can be corrected relatively easily with a series of sensate focus exercises described in Chapter 17.

Many older men have difficulty acquiring an erection and become disheartened when it seems to fade prior to penetration. Surgery is not necessary for these men, either. Continued local genital stimulation generally restores erectile vigor.

An unusual medical condition referred to as Peyronie's disease may eventually cause the erect penis to bend into a "J" shape that renders it virtually useless for intercourse. The growth of fibrous bands in the outer sheaf (tunica albuginea) of the penis is responsible for the deviation in shape. This can be repaired by surgery to release restricting bands or, as a last resort, by insertion of a penile prosthesis.

Men who are unable to have an erection with a partner often have spontaneous erections during sleep or in the early morning. This is vital information because it indicates that both neurologic nerve impulses and blood flow to the penis are adequate. The selective erectile failure may be a manifestation of performance anxiety, a common condition usually amenable to treatment through counseling or sensate focus exercises. (See Chapter 17.)

ORGASM-PHASE PROBLEMS

Orgasm-phase axis problems include premature, inhibited, or retrograde ejaculation.

Premature Ejaculation

It is often difficult to determine exactly when ejaculation is premature, for in nature the ability to ejaculate rapidly is valued, and in the animal world, rapid ejaculation after vaginal penetration is a desirable trait. Such activity ensures an efficient evolution of the species and also allows the coupling creatures to spend little time in the defenseless posture of sexual intercourse. As soon as their reproductive act is completed, they can go on with the more critical business of day-to-day living, like foraging for food and defending against predators.

Such is not the case with man, since the advent of the supermarket has greatly simplified food gathering, and if one discounts the distracting influence of a small child at the bedroom door requesting a glass of water, no meaningful predators threaten extended human sexual activity.

Certainly, ejaculation can be considered premature if it occurs prior to vaginal penetration. Thereafter, the precise amount of thrusting time necessary to achieve ejaculation varies. From a *reproductive* perspective, no problem exists as long as ejaculation occurs intravaginally. In terms of the sensual experience, couples find that a more prolonged period of intravaginal pelvic thrusting prior to ejaculation maximizes sexual excitement and increases opportunities for female orgasm. Exercises can condition men to put off ejaculation for a longer period. Such "squeeze" and "start-stop" techniques are discussed in detail in Chapter 17 under "Exercises to Delay Ejaculation."

Inhibited Ejaculation

Some men who are able to have erections cannot ejaculate. The condition responsible for this may be readily apparent. Paraplegic men cannot ejaculate because the nerves in the spinal cord responsible for ejaculation have been destroyed. A common side effect of many antidepressant medications is an inability to ejaculate. The ejaculatory nerves remain intact but are inactivated.

Spinal-cord injuries and antidepressants are not the only causes of an inability to ejaculate. Psychologic factors can play a prominent role. Delayed or inhibited ejaculation is often attributed to a man's subconscious desire to withhold something valuable from his sexual partner. The reasons for this vary, but they usually involve a man's repressed anger toward his sexual partner. Withholding semen by inhibiting ejaculation is one means of establishing absolute and ultimate control during the sexual act.

More often, men who do not ejaculate have a more specific agenda, specifically a dread of initiating a pregnancy. Even when contraceptive methods are more than adequate (she is taking birth control pills and he is using a condom), *fear of fathering a child* has led some men, consciously or unconsciously, to find it difficult to ejaculate intravaginally.

Problems arise when a man perceives, rightly or wrongly, that he alone has been forced to shoulder what should have been a mutual burden. A partner's lack of support or interest in the midst of a career crisis, a failure to share the anguish of a serious illness in a family member, or the inability to recognize a man's need to be engaged in some meaningful work even when retired are among the areas of conflict identified in men who are unable to ejaculate.

Therapy directed at understanding and rooting out the underlying disaffection toward the sexual partner is usually effective in allowing the normal ejaculatory process to resume.

Retrograde Ejaculation

A woman may believe that her partner has not ejaculated if she does not sense a pulse of semen in her vagina at the conclusion of intercourse. What she perceives as a lack of ejaculation may in fact be only a loss of the ability to ejaculate forward. Some men experience orgasm and ejaculate, but the semen they ejaculate squirts *backward* into their bladder (retrograde ejaculation) instead of *forward* through their penis (antegrade ejaculation). This is a common occurrence in men who have had prostate or bladder surgery or radiation treatments to the pelvis.

Retrograde ejaculation is also a problem for hypertensive men who are treated with the antihypertensive medication guanethidine (Ismelin). In contrast, some medications useful in the treatment of depression and low sexual desire may restore sexual desire and the ability to achieve erections. But they do so at the expense of the ability to ejaculate. (See Chapter 16.)

8

Finding the Cause

When a man's sexual function declines, all he knows is that he can't perform and wants the problem fixed right away. Treatment follows diagnosis. The medical history and a series of directed questions, followed by a physical exam and some lab tests, are all that is required. Your physician will ask a series of questions to understand when and why you first started to have sexual problems. He will also want to know your general medical history, current medications, and something about your habits. Then he will do a physical exam, obtain a blood sample for some laboratory tests, review the results, and then determine what treatment is best for you. The types of questions your doctor will ask and the physical exam he will perform are outlined in this chapter.

THE MEDICAL HISTORY

When did your sexual problems begin?

For most men, sexual problems evolve as an insidious stuttering process characterized by intermittent loss and restoration of sexual function over several years. As the condition responsible for the original sexual failure becomes more firmly entrenched, a man struggles to maintain some sexual interest and potency. Eventually, he experiences a complete loss of sexual capabilities.

Sometimes, however, an impotent man may describe a different scenario and give a history of sudden loss of sexual potency that then becomes persistent and unremitting, as in the following case: "I can tell you the exact date and time that the problem happened. It was 11:00 P.M. on my wife's birthday. Four months earlier, on my birthday, sexual function was fine. When her birthday rolled around, I was unable to perform and have been unable to get an erection from that date on."

Psychologic problems are the most likely cause of impotence for this man and other men with similar histories. With the exception of acute penile or spinal-cord trauma, no physical or physiologic process causes a sudden and permanent disappearance of male sexual function.

When was the last time your sexual function was normal?

Men with sexual problems are frequently so despondent about their loss of potency that they cannot recall a moment when their sexual function was normal. The definition of "normal" may also be elusive. A man of sixty may feel that sexual function was truly satisfactory only when he was in his twenties and capable of prodigious feats of sexual prowess. If he expects treatment to allow him to recapture the sexual glory of his youth, he will be disappointed. A more reasonable baseline estimate for normal sexual function can be obtained by reviewing his level of sexual activity five to seven years ago. It is possible that during those years, he considered sexual function satisfactory if he could make love about once a week or even once every two weeks. If he has no sexual capability now, a more appropriate therapeutic goal may be to aim for a return to weekly or biweekly sexual intercourse.

Do you still have erections?

If a man has fully rigid erections during sleep, when he wakes up in the morning, or under any circumstances, the doctor will assume that the neurologic impulses for triggering an erection and the vascular channels leading to the penile erectile cylinders are intact. If, on the other hand, erections are totally absent, then nerve damage or vascular insufficiency must be suspected. Erections that occur briefly and then fade suggest other diagnoses, including penile venous incompetence (see Chapter 10), lack of sensate focus (see Chapter 17), or presbyrectia (the normal pattern of change with aging) (see Chapter 26). Treatments are available for all of these conditions.

Have your feelings toward your partner changed?

Conflict sets the stage for a common, usually reversible, type of male sexual dysfunction. Squabbles, disagreements, and arguments are an inevitable component of any close relationship. Discussion, mediation, some old-fashioned bellowing, or even weeping may be called into play to arrive at a satisfactory resolution. Not all discord is resolved to each partner's satisfaction.

When waters churned up during an argument are eventually stilled, the calm may be confined to the surface. Bruised feelings, submerged in the interest of restoring harmony, do not disappear; they linger to fester in the fertile fields of the subconscious. It is here, in the subconscious, that gnawing anger, insecurities, and resentments form a powerful coalition to cripple male sexual function.

Sometimes the areas of conflict seem almost childish and superficial, as in the case of Sam, a fifty-two-year-old man who had been impotent for about three years. The circumstances surrounding the development of his impotence were not apparent to him at first, but after reflecting about it, he recalled that just before the age of fifty he had had a passionate desire to own a sports car at a cost somewhere in excess of $40,000. He had discussed this with his wife, who pointed out that they could not afford that sort of indulgence. Not swayed by her logic, he countered that he had worked hard all his life, sacrificed for others, and now, as he was approaching fifty, was entitled to this one little luxury. Apparently her rejoinder was something like this: "A little luxury? A car like that is nothing but a penis extender for small boys." From that moment on, he was unable to have an erection.

Is there someone else?

Not all relationships are forever. When a married man finds himself attracted to another woman and engages in an extramarital affair, he may remain fully potent with his wife and mistress, or he may reserve his potency for his mistress and display a selective impotence with his wife. Only when he has sexual problems with both his wife and mistress will he feel compelled to seek medical assistance. Guilt is usually responsible for his impotence. The dynamics are not complex.

A man may be attracted to the other woman because she is younger, slimmer, prettier, sexier, or just different from his wife. He is consumed with but also ashamed of his passion for her. Potency can be restored only by resolving his guilt. Counseling or therapy can be helpful for this and other forms of impotence caused by emotional or psychologic conflict. Treatment, however, is effective only if the man is willing to accept the notion that the therapeutic process is, first, not a threat to his masculinity and, second, will take some time, usually several months, before positive results can be achieved.

Have you been under unusual stress?

A variety of life stresses associated with work, job insecurity, financial pressure, personal strife, or an illness in a family member can consume so much of a man's attention that he becomes preoccupied with his worries and loses all interest in intimate sexual activity. Onerous daily burdens drain sexual energy and must be disposed of so that he can recapture and refocus his sexual life. This plan is more readily outlined than implemented.

Do you have any problems with ejaculation?

Discharge of semen out of the penis sooner than expected or desired is referred to as premature ejaculation. Ordinarily, ejaculation occurs only after a prolonged period of intravaginal penile thrusting. Ideally, the duration of thrusting will be sufficient to allow the man and his partner to achieve orgasm at about the same time. Ejaculation that occurs immediately after penetration minimizes both male and female sexual pleasure.

Exercises are available to allow the man to contain his ejaculate for a longer period of time. The so-called squeeze and start-stop techniques are discussed in Chapter 17.

An inability to ejaculate is another source of concern. Some medications routinely used in the treatment of the common cold, nasal congestion, and depression inhibit the reflexes that allow ejaculation to occur. Cold medications can be abandoned, but antidepressant drugs are not so readily discarded. Adjustment in the type of antidepressant drug prescribed may help restore normal ejaculation.

Is ejaculation painful?

Some men experience pain when they ejaculate. The anticipation of intense pain with ejaculation is understandably a powerful disincentive to sex. Ejaculatory pain originates in the rectum and passes like a bolt of electricity through the penis at the moment of orgasm. An inflammation or infection in the prostate is often responsible. Treatment with antibiotics or warm baths usually diminishes the inflammation and infection and allow ejaculation to occur without pain.

Is their blood in your semen?

The sudden appearance of bloody seminal fluid is an alarming symptom requiring prompt medical attention and urologic evaluation. Frightened by this symptom, men hope that the problem will go away by itself if they abandon sexual intercourse. This is foolhardy behavior. A visit to the doctor will help uncover the reason for the bloody semen. Often, bladder or prostate infection and occasionally prostate cancer are responsible for the appearance of blood in the semen. Prompt treatment can be instituted and then sexual function will return.

Does your partner enjoy sexual intercourse?

Sexual intercourse should be a shared pleasure. If the partner views sex only as an obligation and merely accommodates the man, then his pleasure will be diminished. For older women who have gone through menopause, sexual intercourse can be unpleasant. This is because the postmenopausal lack of estrogen hormones affects female sexual tissues, resulting in a narrowing or shrinking (atrophy) of the vaginal lining. Further, without estrogen, inadequate mucus is produced by the glands in the crypts of the vagina, and the vagina fails to lubricate normally, making intercourse painful. Treatments include local lubricating ointments or estrogen hormones. The advisability of either of these treatments should be discussed by the woman with her physician or gynecologist.

What form of contraception are you using?

For the younger woman, fear of pregnancy can be a major impediment to her continued enjoyment of sexual intercourse. Some women are likely to shy away from sexual activity unless they can be reassured that they will not become pregnant. A review of the couple's current contraceptive practices is in order. If fear of impregnation looms as a factor diminishing the enjoyment of sex, alternative contraceptive options should be considered.

Have you had any injury to or inflammation of your testicles?

It is in the testicles that the hormone testosterone is manufactured and then released into the bloodstream. Adequate circulating testosterone levels are needed to maintain sex drive or libido. If the testicles are injured or attacked by a virus, their capacity to generate sufficient testosterone may be diminished. Then serum testosterone levels and sex drive decline. Inflammation of the testis ("orchitis" is the medical term) is usually exquisitely painful and not readily dismissed. However, there are some more furtive forms of testicular inflammation that cause only a flulike illness with characteristic muscle aches and pains. In such cases, the pain is often mistakenly identified as a groin muscle pain and considered merely an integral part of the flu.

When a virus invades the testicle, it causes first a swelling and then a shrinkage in testicular volume. A man may be aware that his testicle is smaller than it used to be. Recollection of "normal" testicular size can be a perilous and slippery slope. The passage of years has a magnifying effect on our memory. In retrospect, the genital size of our youth seems to be more substantial than it actually was.

Are you having trouble sleeping?

Depressed, impotent men have difficulty sleeping (insomnia). They fall asleep readily but cannot stay asleep. They usually say they go to bed at about 11:00 P.M., then wake up in the middle of the night and are unable to fall back to sleep.

While it is true that older men frequently awaken in the middle of the night, they do so to urinate. Usually when they return to bed, they fall asleep promptly. Depressed men do not. Recognition and treatment of the depression is a priority if sexual function is to return.

Routine questions regarding general health are now in order; issues of critical importance relate to a history of high blood pressure (hypertension), diabetes, heart disease, pelvic surgery or X-ray therapy, prescription medications, or other chemical use.

High Blood Pressure

Hypertension can impair male sexual function. Impotence is about three times more common in untreated hypertensive men than in men of similar age who have normal blood pressure. We are not sure why. Persistent high blood pressure possibly invites hardening and narrowing of the small blood vessels in the penis. When this occurs, blood cannot flow with the same freedom into the erectile bodies, making it difficult for men with hypertension to achieve or sustain erections.

Almost all men with high blood pressure are treated with antihypertensive medications, some of which have sexual side effects (see Chapter 16).

Diabetes Mellitus

Impotence is a common problem for diabetic men. Sexual problems do not surface when diabetes first appears, but after some years, the diabetic process can damage blood vessels and nerves needed for erections. The large or medium-size arteries become clogged, and blood cannot reach the penis with sufficient force to create an erection. Diabetes can scar smaller arteries, restricting the "breathing room" of the penile erectile cylinders so they cannot expand sufficiently for a fully rigid erection.

Diabetes also disables the nerves that normally signal penile blood vessels to start trapping blood to hold an erection. Symptoms and signs of this diabetic nerve damage (neuropathy) include numbness or tingling of the legs and feet and difficulty in fully emptying the bladder.

Heart Disease

During sex, heart rate and blood pressure increase. The heart requires additional oxygen. If the arteries leading to the heart are narrowed because of atherosclerosis (hardening of the arteries), they cannot provide a sufficient supply of oxygenated blood to accommodate those increased demands of the heart. When this occurs, a frightening chest pain called angina pectoris can develop. The pain acts as a powerful countervailing force to continued sexual activity. If a man has experienced such pain during sexual intercourse, his physician will want to schedule diagnostic studies to determine whether the pain is due to coronary artery disease or other problems.

The increase in heart rate and blood pressure during sex is so predictable that sexual activity can be thought of as a "stress test" that stretches the limits of cardiac reserve. But bear in mind that men who have had heart attacks and even those who have had cardiac surgery can, after a period of recuperation, return to a normal sex life. However, an appropriate amount of time must elapse to allow the damaged heart muscle to recover and surgical wounds to heal.

An extensive patient-doctor discussion of the wisdom of continued sexual activity is prudent. Then a collaborative decision to develop a plan for an appropriate and safe pace of physical activity leading to the resumption of sexual intercourse is sensible.

Surgery or X-ray Treatment

Surgery, particularly in the lower abdomen, may restrict blood flow or neurologic signals needed for normal erections and ejaculation. Of specific interest is a history of vascular or arterial surgery that focuses on restoring blood flow to leg muscles without attending to a man's sexual needs. The aorta pumps blood to the lower extremities and pelvis. Blood cannot flow freely through blood vessels narrowed by atherosclerosis. This limits the supply of blood to the penis and legs (see Chapter 10). Surgery intended to restore blood flow to the legs may result in inadvertent injury to the smaller blood vessels or nerves required for full erectile vigor.

Prostate surgery sometimes injures the systems required for normal forward ejaculation.

Malignancies that have spread to the lower abdomen are often treated with surgery or radiation therapy (X-ray treatment). Neurologic control of the systems responsible for normal erections is disabled by these treatments. This causes impotence or an inability to ejaculate.

Prescription Medications

Several drugs, specifically antihypertensives and antidepressants, as well as those commonly used to treat ulcers, can impair sexual responsiveness. Frequently, an adjustment in medication type or dosage is all that is needed to restore sexual potency. (See Chapter 16.)

Other Chemical Use

The chemicals in prescription medications are not the only substances responsible for disrupting male sexual function. Thus, the routine medical history contains questions concerning alcohol consumption, cigarette smoking, and use of marijuana, cocaine, and heroin. All these substances, when used in excess, can sabotage the operation of internal systems responsible for sex drive, erections, and ejaculation. (See Chapter 16.)

THE PHYSICAL EXAM

After taking the medical history, the doctor will perform a physical exam and will look for previously undiagnosed high blood pressure, diabetes, heart disease, and prostate problems. In addition, there are several unique features of the exam when sexual difficulties are involved.

Visual Field Exam

This test helps determine whether any loss of vision has occurred in the corner of the eyes. Pituitary tumors press on the portion of the eye nerves responsible for lateral or peripheral vision. They may also interfere with testosterone production, resulting in impotence.

Thyroid

The thyroid gland sits in the neck in front of the windpipe (trachea). The thyroid regulates virtually all the metabolic processes of the body and, when not functioning properly, can have a profound effect on desire and potency. The doctor can feel whether the thyroid is large or lumpy; patients whose impotence is caused by an over- or underactive thyroid (hyper- or hypothyroidism) have distortions in thyroid anatomy that can readily be detected.

Pulses

As noted, adequate blood flow to the penis is essential for normal erections to occur. The easiest way to evaluate blood flow is to feel a patient's pulse, particularly in the arteries in the groin and lower legs. Men with atherosclerosis or other problems that restrict blood flow have dampened pulses. If weak or absent pulses are found, blood flow to the genitals may also be inadequate.

Neurologic Exam

Signs of nerve damage (neuropathy) can be detected by simple maneuvers. Decreased sensation to the touch of a feather or a pinprick or sluggish or absent knee and ankle reflexes suggest a defect in the nerves that normally carry sensation and activate reflexes.

Penis and Testicles

The penis is checked for any firm, fibrous bands or distortions in shape that would indicate underlying Peyronie's disease (see Chapter 19.) Testicular size is estimated. A substantial variation exists. Nevertheless, testicles less than 3.5 centimeters (one and one-half inches) are considered small. Truly atrophied testicles appear as pea-size nubbins in the scrotum.

It is also important to determine whether both testicles have descended fully into the scrotum. Normally, the testicles descend immediately before birth. Some testicles do not complete the migration; they become nonfunctional and can produce neither adequate amounts of testosterone nor sperm.

The length of the penis is rarely a factor in sexual dysfunction. For the very few men whose erect penis is too small for penetration, reconstructive surgery is possible.

9

Getting Started: Understanding a Man's Sexual Frustrations and Failures and Their Treatment

How does a man begin dealing with something as embarrassing as impotence? He will make an appointment to see his doctor in the hope that he will leave with a prescription for Viagra. That alone may solve his problem. If it does not, then more has to be done. His physician, who is interested in uncovering the cause of his current problem, may ask some specific questions. Talking about what has happened—technically known as the medical history—is the starting point. What invariably unfolds is a remarkable story. Men and women usually reveal their personal histories in the privacy of a doctor's office setting. My office, I suspect, is no different than those of my colleagues.

Picture one weathered brown desk, three comfortable chairs: two for my patients, another for me, all upholstered in a tweedy gray, the obligatory diploma array on the wall, medical reference books, some at my fingertips, others in bookcases, photos of my family—the space is about as cozy as you can make a space for men and women to feel at ease discussing sensitive subjects.

Still, there are times when anger and frustration, long held in check, erupt in even the most tranquil office setting. But seemingly insurmountable problems can be resolved as long as men and their partners are willing to work together with each other and their physician. It really is quite gratifying to find a way to help.

DETECTIVE WORK

Introductions then.

"Please tell me how I can help you."

"We're having a little sexual problem," confessed Bernard, a diminutive man attired in men's wear meticulously designed not to offend or cause a passerby to even take notice. With his pale tan button-down shirt, Pablum-colored slacks, gray tie, and crushed penny loafers, Bernard could easily have been mistaken for someone in clandestine intrigue rather than what he was, a forty-year-old accountant, more at ease analyzing someone else's spread sheet than describing what he has come to recognize as his own "sexual shortfall."

"A little problem! Tell him Bernard, tell him everything. If you don't, I will," fumed Ellen, an ample, impatient woman whose scrupulous attention to her own appearance, a gold scarf accenting a smart black business suit, stylish pumps, meticulously applied rose-petal lipstick, and just-from-the-hairdresser "big hair" coiffure, stood out in stark contrast to Bernard's conspicuously beige—looking to blend into the woodwork—persona. Ellen's appearance and demeanor demanded attention. She would no longer remain silent, for she was determined to plow straight ahead scattering the seeds of her sexual discontent in my office.

Bernard was considerably more circumspect. He fidgeted in the gray armchair, crossing and uncrossing his legs, then blurted out, "I find it difficult to talk about our problem."

"Our problem! It's not *our* problem, it's *your* problem" came from the other chair. "This is not the first time we've been through this. Remember when we went all the way out to that fancy sex clinic in the Midwest where they did all those tests? They proved there was nothing wrong with me, nothing. I'm fine, my sex drive is normal, not excessive, and I am not oversexed! Bernard, *not oversexed*!" Her voice was getting shrill now.

"I have a perfectly normal libido for a thirty-four-year-old woman. The problem is yours, *all yours*, or at least the way you relate to me."

"Or you to me," whimpered the by now thoroughly deflated and sheepish Bernard.

"Let's start with something we can all agree on. How long have you two known each other?"

"Five years," said Ellen; a silent nod from Bernard.

"How did you two meet?"

"We were fixed up. It was right after Bernard got out of the hospital."

"I was having some trouble with my eyesight, but that's all better now."

"What we, I mean what I really want to talk about is why I can't make love to Ellen even though I love her very much."

"If he really loves me that much, why can't we have sex? I mean, is that too much to ask?"

I have learned to anticipate the rancorous verbal interplay whenever I see couples. Invariably, the sexually functional partner finds my office a convenient and acceptable arena for cataloging the extent and depth of his or her sexual frustration. But this is a good sign.

Actually what was required for this one couple's relationship to be refloated on a sea of sexual equanimity and compatibility was not all that difficult. It was just necessary to pay attention to the proper clues.

Clue 1

Bernard and Ellen have had long-standing sexual problems, yet they are still eager to work together to find a solution. Not all couples are this patient. All too often, sexual inadequacy in a man or a lack of sexual responsiveness in a woman is enough to scuttle the entire relationship. Yet Bernard and Ellen have persevered and remain eager to solve their problem.

The two of them were in my office years before Viagra was available. Even if we had had this remarkable medication back then, Viagra would not have been helpful to Bernard. To know why we have to move on to the second clue.

Clue 2

What caused Bernard's vision to falter and could that old problem be responsible for any of his current sexual difficulties? Yes, it could.

Bernard's eyesight was compromised because something—an enlarged pituitary gland—had butted up against the nerve carrying visual signals from the back of his eye to his brain. This blocked his ability to see out of the corners of his eyes. Full vision returned after radiation treatment broke the grip of the pituitary tumor on his eye nerves. But the X-ray treatment that allowed him to see normally also damaged Bernard's pituitary gland. That tiny structure is charged with regulating a man's hormone output throughout his body. Testosterone is one of those hormones that depends on a healthy pituitary gland. With a damaged pituitary gland, Bernard could no longer generate the normal amounts of testosterone required for sexual competence.

Once testosterone and other hormone levels were replenished, Bernard's sexual function returned to normal. Other doctors caring for Bernard and Ellen never looked at his blood testosterone levels, for in those years, psychologic problems and relationship conflicts were the only recognized causes of impotence. Today we know better.

SEX AFTER DEATH:
THE MOST-COMMON WIDOWER'S PIQUE

George came alone on a stormy winter day. Frost from the winter chill had steamed and fogged his glasses, temporarily blinding him so that he took some time getting oriented in the office waiting room. Snow medallions and epaulet icicles dotted his black storm coat, then coalesced into rivulets that puddled beneath his chair. Tall, gray-haired, and weary, he was unable to contain himself, so his words came in a gush of passion and grief. He began in the middle.

"It was worse every day," George sobbed as he recounted the horror of watching someone he loved waste away and deteriorate. Doris, it seems, had developed one of those terrible unrelenting neurologic diseases that caused a slow steady physical and mental deterioration. George was as devoted to Doris as she was to him. For a while he structured his life so that he could spend time caring for her. Leaving work early, he would rush home to feed and bathe her and also clean her when she could no longer control her bladder or bowels. During the day when he had to be at work, he paid a neighbor, Estelle, or Estelle's recently divorced and temporarily unemployed daughter Diane a few dollars to look in on his wife, braid her hair, and provide a simple lunch. As Doris became more and more incapacitated, George, Estelle, and Diane, alone or in combination, became unable to cope, and arrangements were made to transfer responsibility for Doris's care to a nursing home. There she lingered for another year or so, with George visiting daily or nearly every day. Then, some would say mercifully, she just did not wake up one morning.

The wake was worse than George could have imagined, even though he had been making preparations for this moment ever since Doris entered the nursing home. He had provided Callahan's Mortuary with Doris's favorite blue dress, but even with a tuck here and there and carefully applied makeup and rouge, Doris still looked gaunt and grim in her coffin.

They all came to pay respects, Doris's younger sister, Louise, a birdlike woman given to perpetual preening, eyelash fluttering, and a syncopated hand thrashing as if preparing to lift off to some celestial realm to be reunited with her husband, Patrick, whose conviction for real-estate fraud had just been overturned, albeit posthumously.

"Poor George," Louise gushed, as she offered her perfumed cheek for the brother-in-law's obligatory peck while assiduously exempting any other part of her body from physical contact. Widowed, alone for years since her Patrick's untimely demise, she was there not so much to console as to share with George the misery of her widowhood.

"No matter how miserable and alone you feel now, you should be prepared to cope with even more loneliness with each passing year. We who have had our loved ones taken from us are the only ones who understand." She reassured him that she would always "be there for him" to talk by phone or join him whenever he felt ready have dinner or go to the movies together. Then she patted him on the arm, whispered, "Courage," and fluttered off to chat with someone else. He was not reassured.

Others came, old friends—men to clasp his arms, give him a hug, and offer veiled references about getting together sometime, and women like Louise, offering their rouged cheeks for kissing with promises to deliver casseroles sometime in the future. Business associates, even his boss, showed up and suggested he take a few days off, with pay of course. He thanked them and told them how much he appreciated their coming; then as soon as they could gracefully exit, they did. It was already a dismal experience. His sister-in-law, old friends, and business buddies, even his neighbor Estelle, were all wearing the same shade of ash gray, dark gray, or black, as they said, "Out of respect for the dear departed, you understand."

Diane was not. She now had a full-time job, came directly from work, and did not have time to drab down. In her new position as a restaurant hostess, greeting and then escorting diners to their seats at Stefan DeTruit's newly renovated Jardin des Viands et Legumes, "Proper dress and grooming," Stefan himself told her, "was essential."

"We have only one chance to make a first impression, n'est-ce pas, Miss Diane?" he oozed. Diane was nearing forty and needed the job. So she took his advice, invested in a small wardrobe, and that day seated the lunchtime and "early-bird special" evening crowd and then came directly to the wake. Her dark black hair, remarkably still in place, framed her cheerful face, which was accented only by a blaze of lipstick. Her brightly colored blue-and-white print dress flowed over her supple young body. The mere sight of her moving swiftly toward him immediately raised George's spirits. When she came to embrace him, she did so with her entire slender body arching her pelvis against his groin, which raised something else as well.

"My God, what is the matter with me," George thought. "Here I am with my wife not yet in the grave, holding another woman in my arms and responding with an enormous erection?"

Embarrassed that Diane would be offended by his swollen penis, he tried to arch his groin aft to back his body away.

Sensing his arousal, Diane pulled him closer and whispered in his ear, "Call me at work, we need to talk about this some more." His erection stiffened.

During his wife's illness, Raymond had been willing, even eager, to extinguish his own sexual desires. He would become celibate if that's what it took to make Doris well, and he had not even allowed himself to think about sex for the past four years. Now here he was clearly and unexpectedly aroused in the arms of another woman with his wife's corpse laid out just over his shoulder. Consumed with guilt, he glanced back at the coffin, uttered yet one more "Omigod," and his erection vanished.

His recitation of events at the wake was vivid and impassioned. It was as if Doris's illness had left him a physically, emotionally, and sensually bankrupt hull of a man. He expected to suffer forever for his late wife. Now as a result of Diane's brazen behavior, his resolve to grieve was stunningly sidetracked by his feelings of sexual arousal. He sought counsel from his pastor, who was understanding but could not help him cope with his resurrected passion. He was frightened and for a while avoided all contact with Diane. She phoned him at home and then at work and left messages, but he never returned her calls. Erotic dreams made his sleep fitful. He was frantic, desperately missing Doris and eager to mourn her for a decent amount of time, and had no intention of sullying her memory by being "unfaithful."

Widowers like George have difficult times putting their lives back together. They invariably mourn their wives, usually plunge into work to keep their minds focused on something other than their own sadness, and more often than not are desperately lonely. There comes a time when they crave company and start to see other women. Occasionally companionship is enough, but sooner or later, sex becomes important in the relationship. Men like George who start to have erotic dreams and wake up with rigid erections are ready for such a relationship but may have difficulty functioning sexually for two reasons.

First, they feel guilty, sensing they are being adulterous. Second, sexual insecurities loom large, and they worry that their own sexual performance will not meet their new lover's expectations. Only a conviction that grieving has gone on long enough will assuage guilt. Sexual self-confidence is quite another matter. Fear of sexual failure, a condition known as performance anxiety (Chapter 17), is common. For some, a dose or two of Viagra is all that is needed to allow them to regain their sexual confidence and resolve the most-common widower's pique. George was just such a man.

WINSTON'S WOEFUL INADEQUACY

Winston, né William, was neither a happy child nor a cheerful tycoon. This, his biographers reckoned, was what allowed him to be so dominant a figure in the business world. His trademark Churchill-like scowl, perfected in his preteen years, descended frequently and predictably on what was by nature a cherubic countenance. Like a wild buffalo's flared nostrils, the "cherub-to-Churchill" transformation alerted both casual and not-so-casual onlookers to impending danger.

The Canadian photographer Yosuf Karsh had to pluck a cigar clenched in Winston Churchill's lips to capture the original, now-classic image of the glowering British prime minister for *Life* magazine. All that was needed initially to catalyze William's transmogrification into Winston was a mother's compulsive tidying up and reordering of a young boy's carefully arranged convoy of toy trucks.

Winston embraced, or rather glommed on to, his new British persona so ferociously and with such tenacity that he realigned his speech, demeanor, and family history by sheer force of will. He carried this pretension to extremes, even seeking to reconstruct his own genealogy. He often referred to his parents, who had come from Kiev to Trenton and operated a fruit and vegetable stand, as "humble but honest greengrocers from a land far away."

Slight of build—he preferred the term "dapper" over "small"—Winston was always dressed in impeccably tailored usually double-breasted suits of the finest English cloth and weave. He had for many years been something of a legend, having acquired considerable notoriety not only for his remarkable talent for orchestrating a string of worldwide mergers and acquisitions but also for his enduring passion for British vernacular and style. This permeated his entire persona and business demeanor. At his local office he hired men and women from all over the world who were fluent or conversant in several languages and dialects to handle international business negotiations with the utmost efficiency. He was particularly dependent on his private secretary, a man called Nigel, to deal with matters of the utmost delicacy.

Indeed, it was Nigel who called to persuade my secretary that Mr. Winston "was frightfully busy" and had many "awfully" important meetings to attend. If he was to be scheduled for an afternoon appointment, he expected to be seen precisely at 14:00 hours so that his driver could pick him up and bring him back to the office for a "dreadfully" vital conference call at 14:30 hours.

"We'll do our best" was my secretary's reassurance.

"That may not be good enough" was Nigel's imperious rejoinder.

"Must be out by 2:30" was penciled in over Winston's name in the appointment book.

He arrived a little after the appointed hour. Dapper was indeed the proper adjective for this man who was a commanding presence as soon as he entered a room. Just over five feet four inches tall, with neatly groomed dark brown hair just starting to thin, he was dressed in his trademark double-breasted black-and-gray glen plaid suit, highlighted by a precisely knotted gold silk tie, overlaying a custom-tailored pearl-gray-and-white striped shirt. Ever so slight lifts in his highly polished shoes completed his ensemble. My secretary recognized him from his frequent TV appearances and gushed, "You must be Mr. Winston." His response: "Of course I am, dear woman."

Winston was ushered into my office, where he spent some time, in what for him was small talk, cataloging past, present, and future business triumphs. Having established his string of successes, he had made it quite clear that he was a man who was now in a position to get anything he fancied, except what he wanted most—a child and heir.

"You see, old chum," he told me after a few minutes, "it appears that I will be forever without issue, a fearfully embarrassing situation for Felicity and me." He rolled the tumblers on his combination-lock briefcase, deftly extracted and then thrust in my direction a sheaf of papers. Printed reports from laboratories in Boston, London, and Lucerne described sperm counts of a Mr. W. All indicated that his ejaculate contained more than enough sperm, but unfortunately, most of the sperm present, although normal in appearance, lacked the vital vigorous forward-swimming patterns of sperm from fertile men.

"Look at the report from Guys," he instructed, alluding to Guys Hospital, a prominent medical center in Great Britain. "Do you see that? 'Woefully inadequate sperm motility.' Nobody has ever used the term 'woefully inadequate' about me, never!" he snorted.

He was fifty-two, had been married for six years, and was still reeling from the term "woefully inadequate" when I asked him about his wife.

"Well, that's what started the whole ball rolling, don't you see."

"Dear Felicity was nearing thirty-four and starting to fret about her biologic clock, and that's when we decided to give it a go, but month after month she kept having her period, so the first thing I thought was that there was something wrong with her, but she checked out just fine. It was Felicity's gynecologist who suggested that I might be the problem. That's when the sperm counts started."

Although he had married later than most of his contemporaries, he insisted that he had led a quite vigorous and active sex life "with nary a complaint, I tell you, nary a complaint" from the many different women who had shared his bed, grateful to have been his sexual partner.

"Woefully inadequate, indeed!" he snorted.

We spent some time making the distinction between sexual and reproductive competence, noting that while orgasmic gratification was maintained, the majority of married men rarely heard complaints until fertility became an issue.

"Do you know if any of your partners ever became pregnant?" I asked.

"They always took precautions," was his response. "Except . . . " he paused. "Say . . . how long do you think I've been like this, you know—woefully inadequate," he wanted to know.

"It looks like this problem with your sperm count has been present for some time," I conjectured. "It certainly did not occur over night."

"Bitch!"

"I beg your pardon," I blurted, thinking that he was referring to his wife, when in reality he was festering over payments currently being made to a young Chilean woman who had been insisting that "Mr. Winston" was the father of her one-year-old child.

"Let me examine you now, because my secretary told me you had to be out of here by 2:30 for an important conference call."

"Oh, that can wait," he snapped back. "Do you really think I could have had this problem for more than a year?" he wanted to know, as he bridled at the deceit of the woman he now described as "that Valparaiso Vixen." He had, it seems, been forced to pay handsomely to support a woman and the child she had conceived while laying with another man, whose sperm could not have been "woefully inadequate."

He was still musing on this throughout the physical exam and only when I was about to check for the presence of a hernia and asked him to cough did he ask:

"Is there a chance I could have a child with Felicity?"

"It is a long shot, but we can give it a try. But we'll need to see you and Felicity together, since the procedure is rather arduous," I responded.

"Schedule a full hour visit for Mr. Winston and . . . Felicity."

"Phyllis, her given name is Phyllis," he confessed.

How can someone turn a "woeful inadequacy" into a healthy newborn baby?

In principle, all that is needed is to find one healthy ovum and a single sperm.

This extraordinary new development can be accomplished by actually slipping a single sperm directly into one egg (ovum) produced by Phyllis. The technique is known as intracytoplasmic sperm injection, or ICSI. To maximize chances of success, doctors will have Winston masturbate and collect a semen specimen in a vial. Then they will examine his semen and then isolate and select the healthiest sperm. They will then use that single sperm for the ICSI procedure. For more details on ICSI and other novel reproductive techniques, see Chapter 25.

TITS

Malcolm had not been to a doctor for over five years.

"They laughed at me, that's why," was his explanation.

When he made an appointment to see me, he told my secretary he had a "personal problem" and wanted a private consultation, gave his name, a call-back home phone number, and a request that he not be contacted at his workplace. He was, it turned out, a real-estate broker catering to the college crowd and made a decent living finding apartments for the hordes of young men and women who descended on New England each fall to attend one of the many colleges, universities, and professional schools sprinkled about the greater Boston area. He arrived early, thumbed through several different issues of *People* magazine, and waited impatiently.

Although his age was listed as twenty-seven, he still had what some would call "boyish good looks," something of an asset when dealing with college-age students. He was wearing a blue blazer, button-down oxford shirt, and striped tie, an outfit identical to that currently draping the mannequin in the college bookstore window. His dark brown neatly parted hair was maintained in place by one of the hair gels favored by college students at that time.

"I would like to discuss a very personal problem with you," he began.

He looked at the door, got up from his chair to make sure it was shut tight, then continued.

"I have large breasts" was his opener.

Looking across the desk, I could tell he was hefty, more than just chubby, and it was possible that mounds of fat tissue accumulated just beneath the skin overlying his chest gave the appearance of breasts, a common occurrence in obese men.

"And milk is leaking out of my breasts," he insisted.

Knowing that mounded fat tissue cannot produce milk, I became intrigued and asked him, "How long have you had this problem?"

"The breasts I've had since I was a teenager, but the milk didn't start until five years ago," he said, then went on to recount the troublesome events of his teenage years.

His preteen pudginess soon gave way to a period of self-loathing and despair over his body's shape. He ate more, moved less, and by the time he was sixteen was overtly obese. As his body began to balloon, he became increasingly repulsed by his image in the mirror and became withdrawn, retreating into his own fortress of flesh. Malcolm assiduously avoided all high-school team sports by having family doctors write notes describing "weakened knees" and "respiratory insufficiency," conditions the doctors attributed to "chondromalacia" and "asthmatic bronchiolitis" respectively, although the doctors' records never actually documented the presence of any of these conditions. They just did it as a favor to Malcolm and his mother. All had recognized by now that the plump young boy was not destined to be a gifted athlete. But it was not concern about faring poorly in any competitive race or test of strength that frightened the young boy. No, Malcolm could have willingly and cheerfully accepted a last-place finish. He was terrified and dreaded the prospect of having to undress in the locker room and risk the inevitable mockery and ridicule he would suffer when other teenage boys saw his bloated body.

It wasn't just that he was fat; Sheldon, a tenth grader, was already more rotund and chunkier, but Malcolm was unique, for he was growing breasts. There was no question about it.

"Honest to God, Doc, I was growing tits! Big ones, too. Some of the girls who were slower to develop would complain and ask advice from other girls on what to do because they weren't big enough up there," he said, pointing to his own chest area, "and I thought to myself, maybe I could work out a trade.

"Then I thought, maybe it's all a horrible mistake made at birth. Maybe I'm really a girl and that is why I'm growing tits," he went on, and sweat began to collect on his forehead as he relived the panic of that period of his adolescence when he was plagued by concerns of gender ambiguity.

"I didn't say anything to my parents, but each night in bed I kept checking myself, you know down there," he said, pointing toward his crotch, "but everything checked out all right. I had what a man is supposed to have. But I also had these damn tits and they seemed to be getting bigger every day." Malcolm was perspiring more heavily now.

"And I had no one to turn to, so I went to the library, found a book about Greek mythology, and that's when I really freaked out."

"The Greeks knew about these half man–half woman people, I forget what they called them."

"You mean hermaphrodites," I ventured.

"Yeah, that's it," he said. "Then I kept thinking each night, what's going to happen to me? Am I going to end up like one of those freaks in the circus, half man–half woman like the bearded lady? Then I realized I couldn't even be the bearded lady because here I was almost seventeen years old, all I had was a little peach fuzz on my face and some of the other boys were already starting to grow beards and mustaches, and I wasn't even shaving yet. And those damn tits kept growing, getting bigger and bigger every day! Oh shit, I thought. What or who am I?"

"I kept pretty much to myself those years. I just did my work, graduated high school, then went on to junior college, then from there, got this job in real estate, and was managing all right until one day I noticed this stain on the front of my undershirt, not like from sweat you know, but something else."

"Then I looked down at my chest, and my tits were squirting milk, real milk. Whenever I touched the nipple in just the right way, the milk would come gushing out. It got so bad I started to wear these pads between my nipple and shirt so that the milk wouldn't leak through. That's when I first went to the clinic doctor five years ago. I showed him the milk coming out of the nipple, and he laughed."

"Damnedest thing I ever saw," he said, and then had me wait while he went to get some of the other doctors who were seeing patients in other offices.

"He made me show them how I could make milk come out of my nipple, and when I did it, they all laughed," Malcolm said, as a tear formed in the corner of his eye, the bitterness of the humiliating experience still fresh in his mind.

"Did they do any blood tests?" was what I wanted to know.

"No, they just stood there, three of them in a circle around me, laughing their heads off."

"I was so upset I just grabbed my clothes, put them on as fast as possible. I wasn't even buttoned or zipped up all the way but I ran out of the doctor's office, went straight home and started crying."

Two days later when he had calmed down enough to get back to work, he had already resolved never to see another doctor again, ever. If those doctors, professional men, could not restrain themselves when they saw his freakish body, how would a date respond? He fantasized young women in his room breaking into peals of laughter as soon as he disrobed. Just conjuring up this mortifying experience was enough to suffuse his face with crimson shame.

"So I never dated, just stayed to myself, did my job, went home and ate."

"But our new health insurance policy required a physician's statement of good health before they would accept any of us in the office, so I went to see the company doctor." He mentioned the name of a primary-care physician here in Boston.

"And he did blood tests?"

"Yes," he said, then handed me a piece of paper.

"And that's why you're here today?"

"I guess so."

"Did he tell you why the blood test results were so important?"

"He said you would do that."

I promised to do precisely that but only after I had the opportunity to examine Malcolm. Everything he had told me was true. He was certainly more than moderately obese, had surprisingly little facial hair, certainly no beard or even the hint of a mustache.

His breasts were more than substantial. They jutted out from his chest wall like a catafalque on which his hopes for a future as a normal man lay in state. On closer examination, his ponderous breasts had surprisingly large nipples, unusual for a man, and from these nipples exuded an unmistakable milky white fluid, unheard of in a man. The rest of the general exam was remarkable only for cascading layers of fat that tumbled like plump aprons to obscure the natural outlines of his bones, joints, and even his genitals. His nocturnal self-groping performed in panic to clarify his gender as an adolescent proved to be accurate. He did have a normally developed penis but small testicles, so there was no question of his gender. That he was a man was not in doubt.

But what had made his breasts grow and leak milk, and why were his testicles, which were normally shaped and positioned in his scrotum, smaller than one would expect for a man of his age?

I am the sort of endocrinologist who is always eager to understand each man's unique body chemistry, and in trying to understand Malcolm's case, I thought about these problems:

1. What hormones can make a man's breasts enlarge and leak milk, cause his testicles to shrivel, and decimate his libido and self-confidence?
2. I knew that two hormones, prolactin and estrogen, when present in excessive amounts can cause a man's breasts to enlarge and produce milk.
3. Further, too much prolactin cripples a man's testosterone-producing apparatus, and when testosterone output is below normal, a man's libido, self-confidence, and beard growth cannot thrive.

Malcolm had all of these hormonal problems—too much prolactin and estrogen and too little testosterone. Treatment lowered his prolactin level and his breast-milk production ceased. Then, once prolactin values were held in check, serum testosterone levels rebounded and muscular strength and libido returned. Malcolm started exercising and took off fifty-plus pounds. As his body became more trim and fit, his breasts didn't. Although they stopped leaking milk, they remained large, unsightly, and a persistent source of embarrassment to him, though it was nothing that a skilled plastic surgeon could not correct. With all of that behind him and feeling and looking "great," he is for the first time in his life starting to date and enjoy a sexual relationship. For more on hormones and male sexuality, see Chapter 12.

SWEETS

Anthony was a large man. Some meeting him for the first time would come away with the impression that he was not only a large man but, more precisely, a large, fat man. He, on the other hand, was more inclined to put a more favorable spin on his substantial bulk.

"I guess you could say I've always been a kinda beefy and brawny guy" was how Anthony put it when we first met.

"I was always eating or drinking something for as long as I can remember, and I'm sure that explains in part how I got to be so big, but then like outta nowhere all of a sudden I'm thirsty like my mouth is constantly parched, so I start drinking anything I can get my hands on, water, soda, juice, but still my mouth feels like sandpaper. No matter what I drink, I can't seem to get enough to drink so I drink more. Then with all that drinking, I have to get rid of the extra water, so I'm constantly running to the bathroom and I'm peeing all the time. I mean every hour I'm in the toilet taking a leak, and almost as soon as I zipper up, I've got to go again."

"It got so bad I went to see the doctor, who told me I have sugar diabetes and he told me to come here, and that's all I know."

"What do you know about diabetes?" I asked him.

"Well, it's caused by eating too many sweets—hell, any fool knows that—so as soon as he told me what I had I started cutting down. I mean I switched right away. Now I put Equal in my coffee, instead of sugar. I only drink Diet Coke now, and I've cut out the sweets completely."

"Tell me what you had for breakfast today."

"There, right there, is a perfect example of how I've changed. Time was I could polish offer a rasher of bacon, two to three eggs over easy, a coupla English muffins, and two or three cups of coffee with plenty of sugar and cream, and more often than not a jelly donut for dessert. But today all I had was some OJ, black coffee with Equal, and a small stack of pancakes, but I cut out the jelly donut for dessert."

"Did you put anything on the pancakes, like butter or syrup?"

"Of course, ya know what flapjacks taste like without butter and syrup?"

So we spent some time going over the importance of portion control and the proper foods to eat to help control his blood-sugar levels and reviewed the importance of trying to bring his diabetes under control. At first a strict diet was recommended, and when his blood-sugar (glucose) levels and weight both remained too high, we added blood-glucose-lowering pills, lots of different ones, and when these proved ineffective, he started insulin injections.

During his initial visit, we discussed among other things Anthony's sexual function, which he assured me was "never better."

"Doc, I tell ya I'm like a forty-five-year-old rutting bull. I could have sex two or three times a night if the wife would allow it, but for her once or twice a week is enough, but I'm on the road a lot and there are, how shall I put it, other opportunities . . . . Ya know what I mean, Doc, there's no keeping the bull down when he's rutting," he said, flashing a salacious grin, and a conspiratorial "guys" wink.

Within five years, his rutting days over, Anthony's bull was put out to pasture.

"I don't know, Doc, I just can't get it up anymore. Edna, she's good to me, but all the things that worked in the past don't work no more, and Edna's getting on my case. Now she wants it more than I do. Ya gotta help me."

Anthony would prove to be quite a challenge. In addition to causing blood-sugar levels to rise, his diabetes also damaged nerves and blood vessels throughout his body, including those that he needed to have a normal erection.

Among doctors who care for diabetics, there is a general belief that nerve and blood vessel injury is less likely to occur in those men who are diligent about controlling their blood-sugar levels with proper diet and exercise. Unfortu-

nately, Anthony was not inclined to be quite as attentive to the dietary, exercise, and insulin schedule needed to keep his diabetes in satisfactory control. He was already starting to show signs of diabetic damage to his nerves and arteries. This in turn blocked the normal nerve impulses and blood flow required for a man to have an erection. Thus, complications of diabetes were responsible for Anthony's impotence. Impotence is a common problem for men with diabetes.

About 65 percent of diabetic men benefit from Viagra, but Anthony was not to be one of them. Rather, he was one who would have to rely on other options such as intrapenile injections, vacuum devices, or surgical insertion of a penile prosthesis. (See Chapters 18, 19, and 20.)

10

Recent Advances in Male Sexuality

What makes it possible for a man to have sex?

The process of acquiring an erection requires a coordinated effort between a man's nervous system, his arteries and veins, and ultimately his hormones.

This chapter will focus first on how impulses from a man's nerves make it feasible for him to respond sexually. The discussion explores the crucial role of the arteries and veins responsible for regulating blood flow, for it is the power with which blood flows into and the swiftness with which blood exits a man's penis that determines whether he will acquire, maintain, or lose his erection.

Later on in Chapter 12, we will explore the role of hormones and their influence on a man's sexuality.

WHAT IS NORMAL?

How Your Nervous System Determines Sexual Responses

Girding for Sex. A man must have an erection to have sex, but his ability to become sexually aroused begins first with signals that originate in his brain, spinal cord, and peripheral nerves. This provides a man with a range of opportunities to be prepared for sex. Not all erections are the same. Different parts of a man's nervous system are called into play to allow him to have spontaneous erections, erections after genital stimulation, and unstimulated nighttime or early-morning erections.

A man's penis can become swollen and rigid only when he is:

1. Sexually aroused by erotic images or sensations—these are *spontaneous,* or *psychogenic, erections.*

2. Stimulated by having his genitals caressed—these are *reflex erections.*
3. Sleeping peacefully during rapid eye movement (REM) sleep—these are *nocturnal erections.*

Spontaneous, or Psychogenic, Erections.   So-called psychogenic erections originate in response to stimuli that excite the senses. Specific sights, smells, sounds, nongenital touching, and even imagination may initiate a psychogenic erection. A man's brain perceives these sensations and then transmits nerve impulses to a relay station in the spinal cord just below the lower chest (thorax) and just above the upper back (lumbar area). This area is known as the thoracolumbar erection center. Nerve signals from this site tell pelvic nerves to start the flow of blood into the penis.

Impulses from the thoracolumbar erection center work together and coordinate with a second erection center located in the lower back (sacral area) to maximize a man's erection. Thus, the impetus for sex relies on signals from the brain and spinal cord to provide the trigger for sexual arousal.

The Trigger to Sexual Arousal (Figure 10.1).   Blood does not flow willynilly into the erectile chambers of the penis. There must be a go-ahead signal, a trigger, which is controlled by impulses originating in a man's nervous system, particularly his brain and spinal nerves. Sexually arousing images, words, or aromas—an attractive woman, an erotic phrase, and an enticing scent—activate the senses of sight, smell, and hearing. Then these signals originating in the eye, ear, and nose are flashed first to the brain so that man is aware that something sexy is in the area. The brain then packages these erotic signals and sets in motion a transfer system to relay this information to a critical site in the mid-spinal cord situated just at the end of the chest just above the lower back. Impulses from the brain arriving here are immediately relayed, activating yet another critical second neural signal, this time dispatched to the genital area. This opens the door so that continued gushes of blood pound with ever-increasing velocity into the penis. As the internal pressure mounts, the veins that would ordinarily siphon blood out of the penis are choked off. It is this vigorous arterial inflow clogging the corpora cavernosae, coupled with the stalled venous outflow, that allows the penis to become swollen, rigid, and then erect.

The entire sequence of events occurs with lightning speed in young men, but for more mature men, visual images, as well as other erotic cues intended to stimulate sexual arousal, are not quite as excitatory. As a consequence, although the capacity to respond to sensually mediated sexual cues remains, translating this sense of arousal into prompt penile engorgement and erections fires off at a more measured and leisurely pace as men age. This age-related disparity in sexual responsiveness is often a great source of

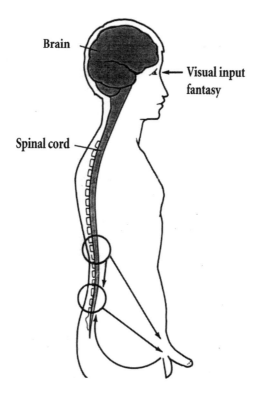

Brain

Visual input fantasy

Spinal cord

FIGURE 10.1   The trigger to sexual arousal. How a man's nervous system responds to erotic cues to stimulate penile erections.

consternation for older men and their partners, who grieve for the loss of sexual spontaneity of their adolescence and young adult years.

The sexual excitement of youth can, and does, occur in response to the slightest provocation. Visual or other sensory stimuli as well as fantasy suffice to activate what has been referred to as a psychogenic, or psychoactive, erection. The brain is particularly well suited to act as the launching pad for this type of erection because it is within the conscious brain that man can sort out which image is sexually arousing (an erotic photo) and which one is not (a head of lettuce). Visualizing or fantasizing about the erotic scene or photo will evoke a psychogenic erection, whereas unless you have an unusual vegetable fetish, looking at lettuce will not.

Men of all ages will respond to erotic stimuli with equivalent interest, but not with comparable degrees of penile swelling and stiffening. Whereas an instant erection is the norm for a man when he is young, the same man may not experience a comparable level of arousal to the same or similar sexual signals as he advances in years. Although stripping a man of his sexual vigor may be unfair and unreasonable, this sexual slippage is, alas, like the age-associated diminution in his sprinting speed, agility, and nimbleness, inevitable. However, men of all ages can continue to enjoy and derive pleasure from sex. The sexuality of aging man is the subject of Chapters 26 and 27.

Reflex Erections. Direct manual or oral genital stimulation can also provoke an erection. This type of erection is referred to as a reflex erection because it can occur in the absence of erotic stimuli. It is, in a sense, the genital equivalent of a knee jerk.

All of us have experienced a knee jerk during a routine physical exam. When the doctor taps your knee with a little rubber reflex hammer, your leg automatically jerks forward. This is a classic example of a *stimulus-response reflex*. The tap of the hammer on the knee is the *stimulus* for the initiation of a nerve impulse that travels with lightning speed to a junction in the spinal cord. Here the reflex arc is completed, and a second signal speeds down another nerve to activate the *response,* a muscle contraction that makes your leg kick forward. The same basic principle can be used to understand how men acquire reflex erections.

Stroking of the scrotum and penis triggers the *stimulus* by activating a local genital nerve called the pudendal nerve. The pudendal nerve then carries the message directly to the spinal-cord sacral erection center, which initiates the *response* by flashing another impulse so that the penis can fill with blood and become erect.

During sex, men probably utilize both the psychogenic and reflex systems and take advantage of both the thoracolumbar and sacral erection centers.

Stimulating and Inhibiting a Man's Sexual Responsivity. Until recently, researchers were stymied in their attempts to understand the phenomenon of psychogenic erections. They have been obliged instead to rely on examining reflex erections. Because they can be readily induced, reflex erections are easier to study.

Normally, reflex erections occur as couples engage in genital foreplay. Researchers have recruited men to participate in a study to determine exactly how reflex erections are achieved and sustained. Volunteer partners for the recruits, however, were not used. Instead, a mechanical vibrator is applied to the genital area to provoke the erection.

Once initiated, a reflex erection can be sustained *as long as the man is not burdened by any competing neurologic demands*. For example, a man who has been stimulated to a full reflex erection will promptly lose his erection when asked to do a nonsexual task such as mental arithmetic. When instructed to discontinue that distracting activity, further genital stimulation can restore his erection.

The real-life counterpart of this occurs every day. A man may become sexually aroused and erect readily, but if in the midst of his lovemaking his mind strays to problems at work, this distraction will have the same effect as mental arithmetic and his erection will vanish. Fortunately, this is not irreversible, for a man can also augment and restore his erection through fantasy. This implies that a reflex-stimulated erection can be enhanced with psychologic input.

These studies demonstrate how readily reflex erections can be induced, lost, and regained. This information has practical take-home value. Impotent men commonly complain about loss of an erection during lovemaking. But if a man is capable of achieving and sustaining an erection in the first place, it is reasonable to presume that both neurologic signals and vascular blood flow into the penis are normal. This implies that his erection can be reactivated with the proper stimulus. Psychogenic and reflex erectile systems allow rigid erections to return as long as there is no distracting or competing neurologic signal.

Nocturnal and Early-Morning Erections: The Body's Sexual Fail-Safe System. A good night's sleep is an involved process. Several predictable stages of sleep are recognized: We become drowsy; fall asleep; fall into a deeper sleep; become more readily arousable and then fall into a still deeper sleep; then wake. Each stage of sleep generates its own distinctive pattern of neurologic signals. We know from studies of sleeping subjects that characteristic shifts in the brain wave or EEG patterns reliably mark each sleep stage. During REM sleep, the eyes dart rapidly back and forth under the eyelids, and the neuroreflexes responsible for spontaneous nocturnal erections are activated.

Interludes of REM sleep occur sporadically throughout the night; normal men have about four episodes nightly. Each interval of REM sleep heralds the development of a new nocturnal erection. (See Figure 10.2.) In fact, the penis may remain erect for a total of two hours each night. A man is usually not aware of most of these REM-sleep intervals during the night unless he wakes during the night and finds that he has an erection. Most commonly, he recognizes only the consequences of last night's REM sleep because he has an erection when he wakes in the morning.

If you are like most men and recognize that your early-morning erection collapses after urination, you will conclude that this erection is due to the accumulation of urine in the bladder. This is not the case, since urine collects in your bladder throughout the day and never triggers an erection, that is, unless you have fallen asleep at your job and have drifted into REM sleep.

A man's capacity to have nighttime erections persists throughout his life. However, in later years not all of his nighttime erections will be dependent on REM sleep. After the age of sixty, men acquire the ability to achieve nocturnal erections during both REM and non-REM sleep. The reason for this

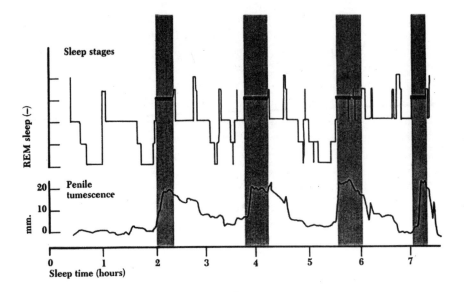

FIGURE 10.2   Nighttime and early-morning erections occur during rapid eye movement (REM) sleep.

age-related shift in nocturnal erections has not been satisfactorily explained. (See Figure 10.3.)

The erections acquired during sleep and after stimulation are generally sufficient to allow for vaginal penetration. However, the sexual act does not end with penetration. Ejaculation must occur.

Ejaculation.   Ejaculation requires a completely different set of neurologic signals. Once again, the spinal cord plays a pivotal role. During the earliest phase, fluid released from the testicle, prostate, and seminal vesicles seeps into ducts that connect to the tube (urethra) in the middle of the penis. Later, as man approaches sexual climax, a second set of nerve impulses initiates vigorous contractions of the muscles of the pelvic floor. It is these muscles and their contractions that propel stored semen out of the genital tract and through the urethra during orgasm.

This elaborate neurologic circuitry is susceptible to different physical and chemical insults that can interfere with the normal transmission of signals and cause neurogenic impotence.

Diagnosing Neurogenic Impotence.   The number of tests currently used to evaluate nerve damage as a cause of erectile dysfunction is increasing. Many of the more sophisticated invasive tests are primarily investigational and are best performed in research centers. For the majority of men, the information provided by these tests is little more than the frosting on the di-

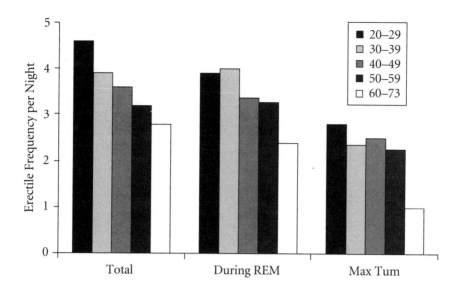

FIGURE 10.3　Nighttime erections occurring in men of different ages. SOURCE: Adapted from I. Karacan, R. L. Williams, J. I. Thornby, and P. J. Salis, "Sleep-Related Penile Tumescence as a Function of Age," *Am. J. Psychiatry* 132 (1975): 932–937.

agnostic cake. Symptoms and signs of neurologic problems can usually be detected in the medical history and physical exam. For example, diabetic men with absent reflexes and diminished sensation in their lower extremities can be presumed to have nerve damage. If they are also impotent, it is reasonable to presume that nerve damage is the cause of their impotence.

However, two types of tests are still in use to develop some more specific information. The most popular test, the nocturnal penile tumescence test, assesses a man's ability to achieve and sustain erections during the night. Other more sophisticated tests evaluate the nerves responsible for reflex erections and ejaculation.

Tests of Nocturnal Penile Tumescence.　The observation that normal men experience spontaneous erections during sleep has been common knowledge since the early 1950s, but this phenomenon was not studied in detail until 1965. In that year, Dr. Ismet Karacan introduced the scientific world to the concept of nocturnal penile tumescence (NPT) monitoring. Dr. Karacan knew that erections occurred during the particularly restful REM sleep. His pioneering studies and those that followed evolved from careful evaluations of normal men in hospital sleep laboratories. The men's brainwave patterns, eye movements, and number, strength, and duration of erections were recorded.

A device something like a blood pressure cuff is placed around the man's penis before he falls asleep. As erections develop, the swelling and enlargement of the penis create pressure, which is recorded to identify those moments when his erections occur. This information is compared to his simultaneous brain-wave pattern to see if erections occur when a man is experiencing REM sleep. Figure 10.3 illustrates the results of NPT testing in healthy men of different ages. Note that for young men, nighttime erections are frequent and vigorous. Nocturnal erections persist in men as they age, although with each advancing decade, there are fewer erectile episodes each night.

The NPT test is often used as the "definitive" diagnostic test to determine whether a sexually dysfunctional man has organic or psychogenic impotence. Men who do not have nighttime erections are classified as having organic impotence, whereas those who have a full complement of nighttime erections are diagnosed as having psychogenic impotence. But results from one night's testing are not always reliable. Often, repeat testing is necessary to establish validity of the diagnosis. This is expensive and not always covered by health insurance. Thus, alternative methods of NPT testing have been developed.

Snap Gauge

The snap gauge is fitted around the shaft of a man's penis at bedtime. The gauge is equipped with three bands of different tensile strength so that an increased degree of penile enlargement is required to break each ring. Minor swelling will break only the first ring; further swelling will break the second ring; but only a fully rigid erection will rupture the third ring.

The snap gauge has the advantage of being relatively inexpensive and does provide limited information about erectile capability. It does not, however, provide any information on the nature and extent of REM sleep or the frequency and duration of nocturnal erections. A single, brief (say, thirty-second) erection would break all three rings but would be inadequate for intercourse.

The Rigi-Scan

The Rigi-Scan is a new device calibrated to provide information on penile rigidity as well as swelling (tumescence). One problem still plaguing standard NPT tests, even those performed in sleep laboratories, is that recordings of tumescence do not provide information about rigidity. The Rigi-Scan seeks to correct that deficiency.

The Rigi-Scan is actually a small computer that can be easily slipped into a pocket in a Velcro cuff that fits easily around a man's thigh. Connected to the computer are flexible wires linked up with two soft cloth-covered loops. One loop is affixed to the tip of the penis and the other to the base. The doctor or technician usually demonstrates the proper placement of the loops. Then the patient is given the attaché case containing the Rigi-Scan unit to take home. When he is ready for bed, he slips the loops over the base and tip of his penis, then goes to sleep. During the night, the Rigi-Scan computer records the number and vigor of his erections. He returns the attaché case containing the Rigi-Scan unit to his doctor in the morning. Then the data can be downloaded onto a standard computer. Results of erectile activity and penile rigidity are generated back on the computer monitor and printed out for analysis.

Rigi-Scan units generate NPT results at a fraction of the cost of a laboratory sleep study done in a hospital. The Rigi-Scan also provides a convenient means of evaluation over several nights.

Information gleaned from this test is immediately available and provides detailed information on the number, vigor, and duration of a man's erections. Further, in the absence of other confounding factors, the results are highly reproducible, so that one man's Rigi-Scan imprint is as constant as his fingerprint. A normal Rigi-Scan recording in Figure 10.4 illustrates multiple erectile episodes of tumescence and rigidity at the base and tip of the penis. Sustained tip and base penile rigidity of greater than 65 percent is considered adequate for vaginal penetration.

The normal Rigi-Scan record in Figure 10.4 stands in contrast to the distinctly abnormal record shown in Figure 10.5, which is characterized by only a few erectile episodes and rigidity of 45 percent, clearly inadequate for vaginal intercourse. A man's Rigi-Scan pattern is fairly constant unless he does something to disrupt his system. Excessive alcohol intake is one such disruptive influence. As little as four ounces of alcohol before retiring can convert the healthy erections into weak erections. Figures 10.6a and b illustrate the nighttime erections of the same man on two successive nights, the first *without* and the second *with* a hefty drink before he went to bed. Note that the normal vigorous erections displayed by this man on one night vanish the next evening after a four-ounce vodka nightcap. (See Chapter 16 for more details on alcohol and sexual function.)

Erections can only occur if both the nerve impulses to the penis and the blood flow within the penile arteries are normal. Thus, it should come as no surprise to note that men with neurologic disorders, for instance, diabetic autonomic neuropathy, multiple sclerosis, or spinal-cord injury, or those with vascular diseases such as high blood pressure or hardening of the arteries, or those who smoke have abnormal Rigi-Scan recordings.

Today, Rigi-Scan recordings are used primarily to segregate those men who have impaired erectile activity from those men who are capable of having normal nighttime erections.

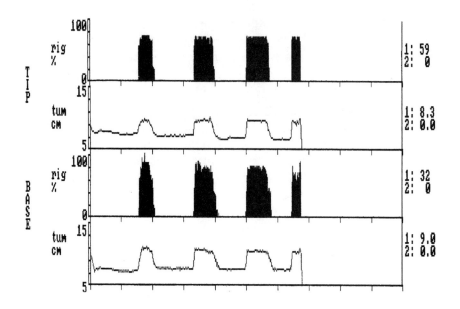

FIGURE 10.4   Rigi-Scan recording illustrating normal pattern of nighttime erections. SOURCE: Courtesy of Dr. Andre Guay Lahey Clinic.

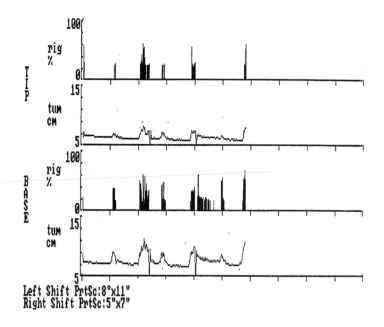

FIGURE 10.5   Abnormal Rigi-Scan recording showing only a few weak nighttime
erections of limited duration. SOURCE: Courtesy of Dr. Andre Guay Lahey Clinic.

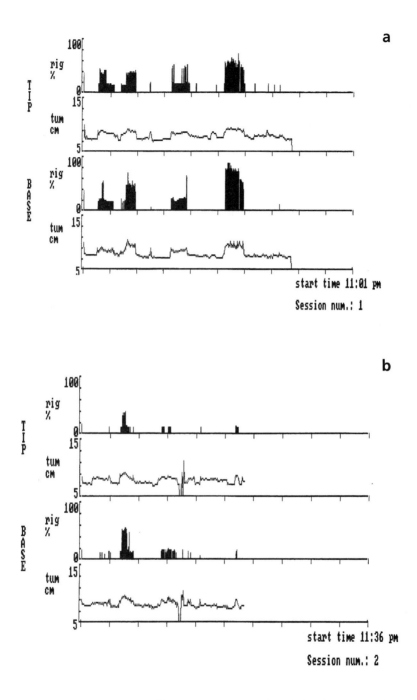

FIGURE 10.6   Rigi-Scan recordings on two successive nights in a normal man with (a) no bedtime cocktail, and (b) the next night after 4 ounces of vodka at bedtime. Note decrease in frequency and vigor of erections after vodka. SOURCE: Courtesy of Dr. Andre Guay Lahey Clinic.

1. A man who has a normal Rigi-Scan recording but is still unable to have sex has emotional problems (psychogenic impotence).
2. If a man's Rigi-Scan reveals an inadequate pattern of nighttime erections, his sexual problems are most likely based on some physical problem (organic impotence). This means he has a physical—a neurologic, vascular, or hormone problem—responsible for his sexual dysfunction.
3. The Rigi-Scan is thus a clearinghouse, allowing physicians to determine whether a given man's impotence is due to psychologic or physical causes. This vital information serves as a critical diagnostic fork in the road, allowing physicians to channel those men with psychogenic impotence to one set of health-care providers and offer different treatment options to men with physical problems.

New Thinking About the NPT.   Although many physicians still rely on NPT results to segregate impotent men into psychogenic and organic categories, others have challenged the basic premise of the NPT test.

What does it mean if a man has involuntary erections at night in a hospital but cannot have an erection when he attempts to have sex? Is there any way to evaluate the ability to achieve an erection in response to sexually provocative stimuli? Several investigators have attempted to refine the NPT test to do precisely that. They have developed techniques to compare results of spontaneous penile tumescence during sleep to the penile tumescence stimulated by erotic arousal.

This new approach requires a two-stage study. Standard NPT testing is done in one night in a sleep lab. On another day, penile tumescence is measured as a man views a series of videotapes. A tape depicting oral and genital heterosexual sex follows a sexually neutral film, usually a travelogue. In addition to the measurement of penile tumescence, subjects are asked to advance a lever to indicate how aroused they were by either film.

All men, potent or impotent, report significant subjective arousal when viewing the erotic videotape. Some men considered to have psychogenic impotence had a normal complement of erections during the night and a normal complement of erections when viewing the erotic videotape. The diagnosis of psychogenic impotence seemed secure. Nevertheless, a substantial number of men who had spontaneous nocturnal erections and described the erotic videotape as arousing did not have an erection when viewing that film.

The addition of the erotic videotape should confirm the NPT results. But this turns out not to be the case. There now appears to be a subset of men originally thought to have psychologic problems who may have spontaneous erections while they sleep but do not have erections in response to standard erotic stimuli. No matter how enticing or alluring their partner, the neurologic systems responsible for initiating psychogenic or reflex erections do not work. Possibly these men have a subtle malfunction in the system responsible for activation of these erections; we do not yet have the answer. But it is likely that a minor disruption in the way the brain receives and processes erotic material is responsible.

The Rigi-Scan test alone or with accompanying erotic videotape must be performed under a doctor's supervision. Today, these are often performed as part of a male sexual-function research study.

However, there are some simple tests a man and a woman can do to find out if the man has any problem with nerve signals to his penis. The first test, called the cremasteric reflex, requires only some gentle stroking and careful observation, whereas the second test, the scrotal reflex, requires a bag of ice. Here's how these other neurologic function tests work.

In the *cremasteric reflex* test, when a man's inner thigh is stroked, that side of his scrotum contracts in a response called a cremasteric reflex. Stroking the thigh sends a signal to the thoracolumbar erection center, which then completes the reflex by transmitting a neural impulse to contract the scrotal muscle. This resembles what happens during a psychogenic erection. The reflex is absent in patients with diabetic neuropathy and multiple sclerosis.

The *scrotal reflex* is less selective. Put any healthy man in a cold room and his entire scrotum will contract, bringing both testicles up toward the groin. Applying ice to the inner thigh can bring about the same reflex. The scrotal reflex is absent in men with certain types of nerve damage like that seen in multiple sclerosis. It is still not clear how vital a normal scrotal reflex is to normal sexual function. Beyond these two tests that a couple can perform in the comfort of their bedroom, other tests, such as the Rigi-Scan, are more elaborate and must be done under a doctor's supervision.

WHAT CAN GO WRONG? NEUROLOGIC PROBLEMS CAUSING IMPOTENCE

Specific Causes of Neurogenic Impotence

The very fact that disparate areas of the central and peripheral nervous system are vital for normal erection indicates that an equal number of sites are vulnerable to injury or malfunction. Impotence is the inevitable consequence of any condition that interrupts the normal flow of neurologic impulses in the brain, thoracolumbar erection center, sacral erection center, and peripheral nerves.

For purposes of discussion, it is convenient to compartmentalize neurologic problems causing impotence into those originating from the brain, the spinal cord, and the peripheral and autonomic nervous systems. (The peripheral nerves govern voluntary actions; the autonomic nerves govern involuntary actions.)

THE BRAIN

Temporal Lobe Epilepsy

Ordinarily, men with neurogenic impotence retain a normal sex drive. However, there is one group of men with a form of neurogenic impotence for whom the primary problem is a lack of sex drive. In their case, the loss of libido is caused by a type of epilepsy that originates in the temporal lobe of the brain. This condition is referred to as either temporal lobe epilepsy (TLE) or complex partial seizures. Unlike patients with conventional epilepsy who suffer periods of unconsciousness and shaking, TLE patients have more subtle symptoms. They may experience periodic rage, occasional unexplained dizziness or fainting, auditory hallucinations, bed-wetting, and lapses of attention (called fugue states).

We are not entirely sure why only the epilepsy that arises in the temporal lobe has such a devastating effect on sexual desire. Recently, researchers determined that a feedback loop exists between the temporal lobe and the hypothalamus, the area of the brain where signals critical for sexual function originate. The control of pituitary and ultimately testicular hormone secretion is dependent on hypothalamic signals. Epileptic discharges originating in the temporal lobe can disrupt normal hormone production.

For men with TLE, treatment of the hormonal abnormalities alone does not restore potency. Hormone treatment must be combined with conventional anti-epilepsy medication. (See Chapter 12.)

The Spinal Cord

Spinal-cord injury at the upper back (thoracolumbar) or lower back (sacral) erection center causes a selective loss of erectile capability. Damage to the thoracolumbar erection center destroys the capacity for psychogenic erections. Men can no longer have erections merely by fantasizing or viewing sexually explicit material. However, they can still have reflex erections with vibrator-induced genital stimulation. This is possible because reflex erections originate in the lower spine and use different nerve tracts from those required for psychogenic erections.

In contrast, men who have had lower-spinal-cord injury—involving the sacral erection center—lose the ability to have reflex erections. If their upper spinal cord remains intact, they can still have psychogenic erections.

Automobile and diving accidents, combat injuries, and gunshot wounds cause trauma severe enough to shatter the spine. These are among the most common disrupters of spinal-cord impulses. The neurologic injuries caused by such violence produce profound defects in other nerve functions. Men with lower-spinal-cord injuries frequently lose the ability to move their legs. They may even lose the ability to empty their bladders. The spinal-cord–injured patient experiences a striking disruption in his daily life. Men with such severe neurologic impairment were until recently considered irrevocably impotent, and their sexual needs were ignored. A new generation has a more positive outlook.

Spinal-cord injuries, although devastating, are not sexually fatal. The man who loses control of muscle function can still retain his interest in sex. He can be stimulated to some degree of erection, depending on the location of the injury. There is, as yet, no way to repair the nerve damage.

Ejaculation is more of a problem, but there are now means of stimulating ejaculation in a fashion similar to that used in animal husbandry. The electroejaculation techniques successful in collecting semen from breeding livestock have been used with some success in men. On rare occasions, patients with spinal-cord injuries have been stimulated to ejaculate so that their semen could be collected and used to inseminate their partners.

In one large study of almost 1,300 men who had suffered spinal-cord injury, 77 percent were able to have erections. Thirty-five percent engaged in sexual intercourse. Spontaneous ejaculation was possible in only 10 percent, however.

Lumbar Discs and Discogenic Impotence

Lumbar disc disease and sciatica are common medical conditions. The bones (or vertebrae) of the spinal column are separated from one another by cushions called intervertebral discs. These discs consist of a soft, gelatinous interior encased by tough, fibrous tissue. As long as the discs remain neatly stacked directly beneath the vertebrae, they cause no problem. But occasionally discs drift from their midline position and press on spinal nerves. If the disc presses on the sciatic nerve, the patient experiences pain down the side of his leg. Other nerves in the spinal cord are responsible for regulating bladder function and erections.

When the location of the disc interferes with a man's ability to have erections, he is said to have discogenic impotence. These men usually have other neurologic symptoms, such as: lower-back pain, difficulty ejaculating, occasional urinary dribbling, and pain radiating to their hips and down their legs.

Computerized axial tomography (CAT scan) reveals the location of a disc and its relation to the spinal cord; surgery frequently alleviates pain and corrects some of the urinary and sexual symptoms. But only about one-third of men with discogenic impotence experience a return of potency after the disc is removed.

Peripheral Nerves and the Autonomic Nervous System

Nerves leave the spinal cord then wend their way through the body to allow us to experience different sensations. When compressed, crushed, damaged by disease, or severed by trauma, nerves do not function properly. All of us have at one time or the other experienced the effects of a compressed or crushed nerve. Cross your left leg over your right and upward pressure from the right knee will compress the nerve traveling down the back of the left leg. After a while, the left leg starts to tingle and become numb. Stand up and walk around and the tingling and numbness disappear.

If pressure on a nerve persists for more than a few moments, the numbness can persist. For example, men who drink heavily and fall to sleep in a stupor will often burrow their head into their armpit, pressing on a vital complex of nerves called the brachial plexus. Deep sleep results in constant pressure from the head on the brachial plexus, and the next morning, arm, hand, and fingers of one side can be numb and weak. This sort of nerve damage referred to in medical parlance as a *Saturday night palsy* may last from several hours to days before normal sensation and function returns.

What do crush injuries to nerves and blood vessels have to do with male sexuality?

Nerves and the blood vessels vital for a man to have an erection are close to the genital surface, and when they are compressed, they can interrupt the normal neural traffic needed for a vigorous erection. See the section on cycling and sex later in this chapter.

Multiple Sclerosis

Multiple sclerosis (MS) is a poorly understood medical condition that can attack nerves throughout the body. The primary problem in MS is a loss of the normal protective sheath (or myelin) around nerves. Without this protective covering, nerves cannot transmit their messages coherently. When the nerves affected are in vulnerable areas of the spinal cord, impotence develops. Current estimates indicate that 50 percent of men with MS are impotent.

Multiple sclerosis is a chronic disease and given to inexplicable periods of sudden improvement (or remission), followed by deterioration (or exacerbation). When MS goes into a temporary remission, sexual function may return. But the course of the disease is capricious, and worsening may come just as suddenly and unpredictably. Therefore, the sexual function of men with MS is always precarious and fluctuates over time. There is as yet no cure for this disease.

Syphilis

The bacteria that cause syphilis are called spirochetes. Because penicillin kills spirochetes, it was believed at one time that it would rid the world of the scourge of syphilis forever. Unfortunately, syphilis remains and has made a resurgence during the AIDS epidemic.

Men infected with syphilis first develop a hard ulcer on the tip or shaft of the penis. If this is ignored and syphilis remains untreated, the spirochete establishes a foothold and spreads to other organs. When syphilis invades the spinal cord, it destroys cells responsible for the neurologic reflexes that control erection and bladder sensation. Late-stage syphilis is treatable with penicillin, but spinal-cord or neural damage is irreversible. Men in this late stage of syphilis cannot have erections or empty their bladders.

Diabetes Mellitus and Diabetic Neuropathy

Diabetes mellitus is a common medical condition affecting 10 million Americans, 4 million of them men. Diabetes sets in motion events that damage the heart, eyes, and kidneys and prevent nerves from transmitting impulses efficiently. The nerve damage is called diabetic neuropathy, and it takes several different forms.

Impotence in diabetic men may be a reflection of a neuropathy affecting several different types of nerves. Some nerves carry messages of sensation, like pain and pleasure. Others transmit impulses that allow the pelvic muscles to contract during ejaculation. One other critical component of the nervous system, the autonomic nervous system, is also vital for sexual function. The autonomic nervous system works silently and effortlessly and helps us get through many daily functions.

For example, in the morning, when we first stand up, our blood pressure drops. This fall is temporary; the autonomic nervous system instigates a battery of neural responses that helps stabilize blood pressure. Diabetic patients with autonomic neuropathy cannot do this. Because diabetes has damaged their autonomic nervous system, they cannot marshal a prompt increase in blood pressure. Diabetics' blood pressure often falls to very low levels, occasionally causing fainting.

The autonomic nervous system also plays an important role in transmitting messages for erections, ejaculation, and bladder function. Diabetic men with autonomic neuropathy become impotent, are unable to ejaculate, and may even have trouble emptying their bladders completely when they urinate.

Inadequate autonomic nervous system function can also occur in older nondiabetic men. Idiopathic autonomic insufficiency produces similar symptoms of inability to stand upright without feeling faint, loss of the ability to empty the bladder, impotence, and inability to ejaculate.

In terms of sexual potency, men with diabetes mellitus have to contend with two problems—altered nerve function and diminished blood flow due to diabetes-induced damage to blood vessels. In addition to causing nerve damage, diabetes attacks the blood vessels that must dilate and enlarge to pump blood into the penis for an erection to develop.

Symptoms suggesting diabetic nerve damage include loss of sensation at the tip of the penis, numbness of the lower extremities, and spasms or unexplained pain in the legs. The regularity with which impotence occurs in diabetics is striking. Young diabetics have no more sexual dysfunction than their nondiabetic contemporaries do. But they can anticipate a progressive decline in sexual function. Ten years after the onset of diabetes, 50 percent of diabetic men will be impotent. By age seventy, more than 95 percent are impotent. We do not yet know how to repair diabetic nerve damage, although there are treatments for the impotence it causes. Penile implants (see Chapter 18) and penile injections (see Chapter 19) and on occasion Viagra have been used to help restore potency in men suffering from diabetic neuropathy.

Chronic Kidney Disease

The kidney filters waste products from the bloodstream to be excreted in the urine. When the kidney can no longer accomplish this task, waste products build up in the bloodstream and cause a condition known as uremia. In the past, uremic men and women had a limited life expectancy, and sexual function was not a primary concern. However, with the availability of dialysis therapy and kidney transplants, life expectancy for uremic people has been greatly extended.

As chronic renal disease persists and dialysis becomes a way of life, two systems vital for normal male potency fail. For reasons that are still unclear, dialysis patients experience nerve damage. When this extends to the nerves required for normal erections, impotence develops.

Kidney disease can also disrupt the endocrine system. Production of testosterone declines, and secretion of prolactin, a sexually inhibiting hormone, increases. Low serum testosterone and high serum prolactin levels individually or together can cause impotence. Treatment aimed at normalizing serum prolactin and testosterone values can help restore sexual function.

TREATMENT OF NEUROGENIC IMPOTENCE

Men with neurogenic impotence have several options. They can adopt a fatalistic view and live with their impotence, choose to have penile implant surgery, or learn to inject a drug like alprostadil, papaverine, or phentolamine or a combination of all three (Tri-Mix) into their penis to achieve an erection. Unfortunately, it is these men who are most susceptible to priapism, a prolonged painful erection, the most worrisome side effect of penile injection therapy. The benefits and risks of penile injections as a treatment for impotence are reviewed in Chapter 19.

Prior to the introduction of this novel therapy, many men with neurogenic impotence relied on penile implants (or prostheses) as the only treatment that would provide the penis with sufficient rigidity for intercourse. Penile prostheses have been inserted with variable success. Impotent diabetic men have a higher rate of complications from such surgery than do men with other forms of neurogenic impotence. This is most likely because diabetic men are unusually prone to infection, and following surgery, the development of an infection, especially in the area of the penile implant, can threaten the survival of the prosthesis. This is discussed in more detail in Chapter 18.

Recent evidence suggests that a select group of men with neurogenic impotence as a result of spinal-cord injury may have improved erections with sildenafil (Viagra). See Chapter 11 for more details.

Men who have experienced spinal-cord injuries have some penile swelling and tumescence after vibratory stimulation of the penis. With vibration alone, the penis rarely becomes firm enough for vaginal penetration. However, spinal-cord injured men who respond partially to vibration are capable of having significantly improved erections with sildenafil (Viagra). If vibratory stimulation does not cause any penile response, then Viagra is not likely to be beneficial.

Men with spinal-cord injuries and their partners often have many questions about sexuality after injury. *Sexuality After Spinal Cord Injury* by Stanley Duchane and Catherine Gill offers thoughtful responses to the most commonly asked questions and is an excellent source book.

THE FLOW OF BLOOD: ARTERIES AND VEINS

What Is Normal?

The transformation of a man's penis from a limp to an erect state depends first on the neural trigger to sexual arousal and then on the unrestricted flow of blood into specialized cylinders in the penis (the corpora cavernosae and the corpus spongiosum). It is the unusual architecture of these cylinders that makes it possible for a man to develop an erection. The erectile tissue is in reality an elaborate spongy honeycomb designed to trap blood. In the early stages of an erection, blood is diverted into these spongy spaces. As they absorb more blood, the penis becomes fully erect. When a maximum erection is achieved, blood does not flow out of the penis because the draining veins are choked off (or compressed).

The penis remains erect until ejaculation. Then the spongy cylinders discharge their captured blood back into the bloodstream, and the penis reverts to its normal flaccid state. When the arterial inflow and venous outflow systems break down, vasculogenic impotence develops.

If a man's penile erectile cylinders do not fill with blood, he will be unable to initiate an erection. If blood trapped and stored in the penis leaks out prior to ejaculation, he will be unable to maintain his erection. Thus, vascular problems causing impotence have been defined as either "failure to fill" or "failure to store."

Failure to Fill

Blood released from the heart is pumped through arteries to provide oxygen to the heart as well as to the lungs, brain, kidney, and other tissues. The aorta is the main conduit for transfer of blood from the heart to the rest of the body. It can be thought of as a large tree with branches emerging at different junctions to supply blood to individual sectors of the body. The main branch bringing blood to the pelvis is the iliac artery. The iliac artery spawns its own subdivisions. Some branches supply blood to the lower extremities as well as the buttocks. Another tributary, the internal pudendal artery, is responsible for ferrying blood to the six small arteries nourishing the penis and its corporal erectile cylinder bodies. (See Figure 10.7.) For most of the day, blood bypasses the erectile cylinders and serves only the needs of the penis.

Impotence due to a failure to fill is the result of sluggish blood flow to the penis. Problems restricting the flow of blood can originate at any level of the arterial tree: Large, medium-size, and tiny arteries can be blocked.

When obstruction is present in a large artery such as the iliac artery, a limited amount of oxygenated blood is available for the muscles of the lower extremities as well as the pelvic arteries. In addition to impotence, other symptoms reflecting the inadequate blood supply to a man's leg muscles are cramps in the calf muscles after long walks. If, on the other hand, vascular disease is confined to the small blood vessels in and around the area of the penis and the sinusoids, impotence will be the only symptom.

Two basic problems, atherosclerosis (hardening of the arteries) and arteriolarsclerosis (scarring of the smaller blood vessels called arterioles) can re-

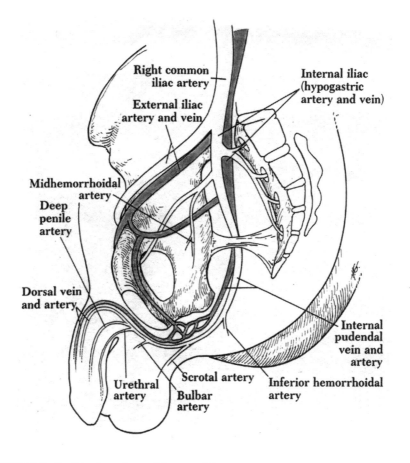

FIGURE 10.7 The branches of the arterial tree carrying blood to a man's penis.

strict blood flow to the penile area. Men with high serum cholesterol levels and high blood pressure are particularly susceptible to atherosclerosis. Cholesterol can lodge in and clog arteries, creating a narrow channel impeding the blood supply to the pelvis and genital area. Inadequate blood flow to the penile arteries prevents the full and uninterrupted transfer of blood into the penile erectile cylinders. Men who are heavy smokers or are diabetic often experience local arterial inflammation and scarring. This, too, restricts blood flow to the penis.

Some men are more likely than others to develop impotence due to a failure to fill. They can be recognized early in their adult life because of the presence of four arterial risk factors (ARFs):

The ARFs that increase a man's chance of becoming impotent include:

1. High blood pressure (hypertension)
2. Cigarette smoking

3. High serum cholesterol levels
4. Diabetes mellitus

In one study, evidence of hypertension, diabetes mellitus, heavy cigarette smoking, or high cholesterol levels was found in 79 percent of men with failure to fill. The chance of developing this type of impotence increases as the number of ARFs mount up. The man with high blood pressure and high cholesterol levels who smokes has about a 50 percent chance of developing impotence due to a failure to fill as early as age fifty-five.

The number and type of ARFs also have implications for treatment options. For men suffering from atherosclerosis and selective narrowing of larger arteries due to high serum cholesterol levels and high blood pressure, the area of arterial obstruction can be removed or bypassed by a vascular surgeon so that blood flows more freely to the pelvis, allowing sexual function to be restored. Diabetic men and smokers are more likely to develop scarring of the small blood vessels in and around the penis. This is not amenable to surgery.

Symptoms of Poor Blood Flow: Vasculogenic Impotence

Impotence caused by failure to fill due to hardening of the arteries is a reflection of inadequate blood flow to the penis. (See Figure 10.8.) Only rarely is this process confined to just the arteries carrying blood to the genitals. An inadequate supply of oxygenated blood anywhere in the body creates its own set of distinctive symptoms.

Deprived of oxygen, the brain cannot think well, the kidneys stop making urine, and muscles cry out in pain. Angina pectoris is the term used to describe oxygen deprivation to the heart muscles. Claudication describes insufficient blood flow to other muscles.

Oxygen demand is activity dependent. A muscle at rest requires a minimal blood supply, whereas an active muscle demands a rich supply of oxygenated arterial blood. Muscles cramp when they do not receive adequate oxygen. This may be apparent only when the muscle is challenged by exercise. Consider what happened to Warren.

Warren at age sixty-eight was no longer able to achieve an erection. He maintained that he was physically fit and cited as proof the fact that he played eighteen holes of golf two to three times a week. When pressed, he did admit that his actual exercise was limited because a motorized golf cart, rather than his legs, was his source of transportation on the course. Only when he sliced a shot into the woods did he extend his exercise. Unfortunately, the last few times he prowled around the woods, he developed such severe leg cramps that he was forced to sit down and rest. Symptoms of claudication reflecting inadequate

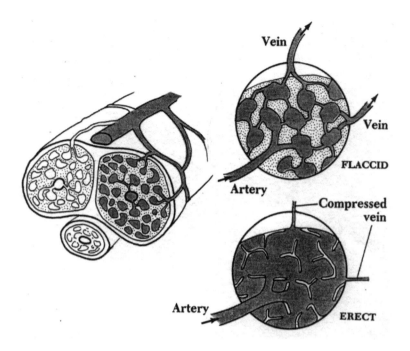

FIGURE 10.8   Patterns of blood flow to and into the penile erectile tissue when the penis is at rest and during an erection. Inflow of blood expands minute chambers (sinusoids) in the penile cylinders. The expanded chambers compress the small veins against the tunica albuginea, preventing blood from draining out of the penis so that an erection can be maintained.

blood flow became manifest only when Warren was forced to expand his range of activity.

Similar information can be obtained from nongolfers by simply asking them how far they actually walk each day and whether they can push themselves and extend that activity without experiencing any discomfort in their legs or buttocks.

When impotence and muscular cramps in the legs coincide, it is likely that an artery that supplies oxygenated blood to the legs and pelvis is obstructed. Men suffering from these obstructions not only experience an inability to achieve an erection but also find that they cannot walk as far as they used to. Walking for any duration causes the muscles of their legs or buttocks to cramp. When the man notices the association between cramps and vigorous walking, he will gradually, almost imperceptibly, adjust his activity. Once he restricts his walking, leg cramps and pains no longer trouble him. When questioned, he can say honestly that he does not now have pain when he walks. A physician trying to make a diagnosis must often pursue this issue with some diligence.

Symptoms of claudication are invariably associated with extensive narrowing or obstruction in the major arterial supply of blood to the pelvis and lower extremities. More selective areas of narrowing do occur and produce their own unusual set of symptoms, such as the pelvic steal syndrome.

Pelvic Steal Syndrome

The pelvic steal syndrome (also called the iliac steal syndrome) is a consequence of the competition between muscles of the lower legs and the penis for a marginal blood supply. In such a competition, the penis is destined to lose.

A man with pelvic steal syndrome can acquire an erection. Problems develop after penetration. When he attempts to thrust his hips, the erection deflates. Increased activity of the pelvic and lower leg muscles creates a demand for additional oxygenated blood. First, cramping in the buttocks and legs occurs, then, as blood is diverted away from the penis to the buttocks and legs, the erection fades.

Men with this sort of vasculogenic impotence usually have a significant narrowing in one or both iliac arteries—the major branches of the aorta that carry blood to the pelvis. Surgical reopening of the artery restores potency.

Medium-Size and Small Arteries

Injury to small arterial tributaries out of the main artery may cause impotence without compromising blood flow to the lower extremities. In this case, cholesterol deposits obstructing these penile arteries stifle penile blood flow.

It is easy to see how major pelvic injury, pelvic X rays, and injury to the penis can lead to vasculogenic impotence either by directly interrupting blood supply to the penis or by injuring the linings of the artery, which eventually encourages the accumulation of cholesterol. But less dramatic forms of pelvic trauma may also be responsible for impotence.

Cycling and Sex

Men who are competitive long-distance bicyclists sit on hard bicycle seats and can compress and damage both cavernosal and pudendal nerves. Anecdotes regarding sexual problems occurring after long-distance cycling have been around for years, but no systematic survey of the problem was available until 1997. Then after an annual 540-km bicycle-touring race, 160 male cyclists were surveyed. Thirty-five of the 160 men (22 percent) said they had a numb penis after the race. Impotence occurred in 21 (13 percent) and in 11 lasted for more than a week. Pressure on the pudendal and cavernosal nerves resulting from long stints sitting on the narrow bicycle seat was blamed for the penile numbness and impotence. The genital arteries supplying blood to the penis can also be injured during high-intensity long-distance cycling.

Sexual problems after cycling are much in the news lately and are often discussed in cycling magazines, where concern has generated enthusiasm for design of new seats less likely to cause pressure on a man's genital nerves and blood supply. But cyclists I have spoken to are concerned that the newer seats compromise their competitive edge. Penile numbness and erectile dysfunction is primarily a problem for the competitive cross-country bicycle racers. Weekend and recreational cyclists rarely experience sexual problems after moderate or short-distance bicycle jaunts.

This symptom of penile pain occurs in 10 to 50 percent of men who participate in long-distance bicycling. Bicycle-seat-induced pressure restricting penile blood flow has even been incriminated as a specific cause of impotence in men whose pedaling is restricted to a stationary bike. The height and positioning of the nose of the bicycle seat are critical in determining whether penile blood flow and local nerve transmission to the head of the penis are compromised. Frequently, blood flow is restored and pressure on genital nerves alleviated by simply adjusting the height of the bicycle seat. In normal men, bicycle-seat-induced decreases in penile-artery blood flow are temporary; within thirty minutes, normal blood flow is restored.

Failure to Store

If the flow of blood into a man's penis is inadequate because of arterial (inflow) problems he will never achieve a fully rigid erection. This sequence of events is responsible for the partial erection experienced by many older men; it is still considered a failure-to-fill problem.

Other men, however, have adequate erections initially but cannot maintain them long enough for intercourse. The penis fills, swells with blood, and becomes erect, but like a balloon with a slow leak, it deflates due to a progressive flow of blood out of the penile erectile cylinders. The rate at which blood squirts out of a man's penile erectile chambers is what determines whether a man will hold onto or lose his erection.

It remains unclear what causes this failure-to-store problem, but because the penile veins or emissary veins provide the only channel through which blood can leave the penis, the diagnosis of penile venous incompetence has found favor among urologists.

The amount of blood that must be transferred to the penis to create an erection in the first place is prodigious. Normal men acquire a firm erection when about two ounces of blood per hour are pumped with sufficient force into the penile erectile bodies. Impotent men with venous incompetence can achieve an erection, but only if twice as much blood is pumped into the penis. Nevertheless, they cannot sustain the erection even if the flow of blood is maintained at a rate of *four* ounces per hour.

Today we know much more about the factors that inhibit blood flow to the penis than what causes the premature leakage of blood and loss of an erection. Researchers have been unable as yet to associate venous insufficiency elsewhere in the body with penile venous incompetence. Only a history of prompt acquisition and rapid loss of a rigid erection suggests a diagnosis of penile venous incompetence.

Diagnostic Tests

A diagnosis of vasculogenic impotence requires a demonstration that blood flow into or out of the penile erectile cylinders is not normal.

Doppler Ultrasound Recording.   The arteries that bring blood to the penis, like arteries elsewhere in the body, emit a characteristic pulse. A machine called a Doppler ultrasound uses a process similar to sonar to measure the pulse wave with some accuracy. Blood flowing freely in the penile arteries produces a vigorous pulse pattern; restricted blood flow produces a sluggish pattern.

In addition to estimating the strength with which blood pulses through the arteries in the penis, physicians can make an actual measurement of penile-artery blood pressure. Blood pressure is usually recorded in two phases. The first number (systolic) measures the pressure when the heart contracts and pumps blood into the arteries. The second number (diastolic) measures the pressure when the heart is at rest between contractions. (The Doppler ultrasound records only the systolic blood pressure.)

Penile systolic blood pressure must be related to the blood pressure in the arm (brachial blood pressure). This relationship is the penile brachial index (PBI).

Normally, blood pressure in the penis is slightly lower than blood pressure in the arm. An evaluation of blood flow to the penis can be determined by comparing systolic penile artery blood pressure to brachial systolic blood pressure: PBI = the ratio of penile systolic blood pressure divided by brachial systolic blood pressure.

A PBI of 0.9 or greater is considered normal; a PBI of 0.7 or less indicates compromised blood flow to the penis. PBI values between 0.7 and 0.9 fall into a gray zone, with lower values more strongly suggesting vascular problems.

Pharmacologically Induced Erections.   The muscle relaxant papaverine, when injected directly into the penis, causes a loosening or dilation of the smooth muscles around the tiny intrapenile blood vessels and allows an erection to occur by encouraging increased intrapenile blood flow. If no erection occurs, physicians assume that the tiny blood vessels in the penis are too scarred to relax and expand to allow an onrush of blood (failure to fill). If, on the other hand, a full erection is acquired but not sustained, consideration must be given to the diagnosis of failure to store.

A physician performs the diagnostic intrapenile papaverine injection, first placing a rubber band around the base of the penis to ensure that the injected papaverine will be confined to the penis. Then a small amount of papaverine is injected into one of the erectile bodies (corpus cavernosum). Within minutes, the penis should start to swell and become erect. If the erection appears to be full and turgid, it is presumed that the patient does not have any impairment in arterial inflow to the penis.

When a papaverine injection does not stimulate an erection, a blood-flow problem is strongly suspected as the cause of impotence. If, on the other hand, the penis achieves some degree of swelling but not enough to qualify as a normal erection, the diagnosis of venous leakage can be considered.

Like papaverine, intrapenile prostaglandin E1 (Caverject) injections have been used to segregate men with vasculogenic impotence from men with other forms of impotence. Men with vasculogenic impotence do not experience an erection following prostaglandin E1 injections, whereas men whose impotence is caused by nerve damage and emotional problems do. It is possible that prostaglandin E1 (Caverject) is more sensitive and specific than papaverine in identifying men with vasculogenic impotence.

Arteriography.   Arteriography is a specialized X ray used to define the anatomy of arteries transporting blood to the penis. An artery in the groin is punctured with a hollow needle. A small plastic tube (catheter) is threaded through the hollow of the needle and then pointed in the direction of arteries that supply blood to the pelvic area. X-ray dye injected through the catheter travels down the arteries to provide a graphic illustration of how arteries look as blood (dye) flows to the pelvis and penile erectile cylinders. Arteriography locates the site or sites of arterial blockage, narrowing, or damage for the surgeon.

Treatment of Vasculogenic Impotence

Impotence due to a failure to fill is treated by isolating and identifying the site or sites obstructing the vigorous flow of blood to the penis. Vascular surgeons have become remarkably successful in creating new channels in arteries or bypassing areas of obstruction so that free flow of blood to the pelvic arteries can be reestablished.

The best surgical results have been achieved in men with well-defined narrowing in large or medium-size arteries. The surgeon removes the area or areas of obstruction and establishes a new, wide channel to restore a full flow of blood to the penis.

Surgery is successful in about one-third of the cases. Unfortunately, in about one-half of these men, the success is temporary. Impotence returns in six months to a year. In addition, another one-third experience postoperative priapism (persistent painful erections).

Failure to store requires a different approach. Several different methods have been devised to enhance the competence and holding capacity of the intrapenile veins so that they do not allow blood to drain prematurely from the penis during an erection. Sagging veins responsible for venous inadequacy are shored up by urologic surgeons. Sometimes the penile veins are closed or removed to limit the number of channels draining blood.

About 22 percent of men who have venous surgery experience immediate and sustained restoration of potency. About 19 percent remain impotent. An intermediate group of men (15 percent) experience a temporary restoration of potency. The remaining men (44 percent) can achieve an erection with intrapenile papaverine injections. Whether this response is sustained or whether men are willing to continue with a penile injection program has not been reported. (See Chapter 19.)

The reason for the disappointing results of venous surgery is not entirely clear. It is possible that current diagnostic tests lack specificity. Venous insufficiency may be only one factor responsible for sexual dysfunction. One urologist has found that the vast majority of impotent men who have venous insufficiency also have arterial inflow problems. Thus, correction of the venous leakage alone is unlikely to help.

This finding has prompted some urologists to combine arterial and penile venous surgery. Opening and widening the arterial channels bringing blood to the penis while simultaneously closing veins taking blood away from the penis has intrinsic appeal. Initial results have been promising, but it is still too early to know whether this dual surgical approach will be effective in the long term.

Dramatic improvements in sexual potency are apparent in some men following arterial or venous surgery. For many of them, potency is sustained. If there is only a temporary improvement in sexual function, the fault may not be related to the surgery. If high blood pressure, smoking, uncontrolled diabetes mellitus, or other arterial risk factors persist, then results will be less than ideal. More effective regulation of blood pressure and consistent management of blood-sugar levels in diabetic men as well as treatment to stem the tide of advancing hardening of the arteries is feasible. With guidance from his physician, these are the steps a man needs to work on to help restore his sexual capabilities.

11

Male Sexual Chemistry and Viagra

From the moment Viagra came on the market, men, and women, too, have been intrigued by this new "potency pill." In this chapter, you will find answers to many of the commonly asked questions about Viagra.

1. What is so special about Viagra?
2. Understanding male sexual chemistry: What makes Viagra work?
3. How does Viagra differ from other impotence treatments?
4. Is Viagra effective for every impotent man?
5. What are the side effects of Viagra?
6. Is there reason to fear Viagra?
7. Death after sex and/or Viagra: What is the risk?
8. What are the fantasies, fears, and reality of philandering after Viagra?
9. Can Viagra take the worry out of sex?
10. How can Viagra be used for maximum benefit and minimal risk?
11. The politics of male sexuality: Who will pay for Viagra?
12. Does Viagra work for women?
13. What's next after Viagra?

His Cheshire cat smile, renewed vigor in stride, and different gaze—firm, straight-ahead, no longer oblique or downcast—tells me what I want to know before Michael opens his mouth.

"It worked!"

Eager to elaborate, he went on: "I took the pill around 9 P.M., watched a little TV, then in the middle of the 10 o'clock news decided to join my wife on the couch and started in like when we were first dating."

"I'm waiting to hear the weather, she protested."

"This will be more interesting than the weather," I insisted, feeling myself starting to swell."

"What's gotten into you?" she wanted to know."

"I'll tell you later."

"Before long our clothes were off, we were in the bedroom, and my penis was firm. Then the more we played, the firmer it became. I could not remember the last time I was this powerful or excited. The more we played, the harder it got, and when we made love, it was exciting and wonderful, like it was before I had, you know *my problem*. Now I feel like a new man," Michael enthused.

Michael and millions of men just like him, once impotent and fearful of entering into any sexual activity because of lingering doubts about whether they would be able to "perform" during sexual intimacy, can now look forward to enjoying sex once again, all because of a tiny blue pill.

In the past "the Pill" referred only to the oral contraceptive birth control pill. That "Pill" liberated women, allowing them to enjoy sex and be sexually active without fear of pregnancy. The new "Pill" is equally revolutionary because it deciphers the mystique of a man's sexuality.

Maybe it was inevitable. Sooner or later someone had to solve the riddle of a man's unique sexual chemistry. Once doctors knew what controls a man's sexual urges and his ability to have sexual intercourse, they believed they would know all there was to know about men's sexuality. For too many years, everyone, scientists and public included, attributed *all* male behavior to too much or too little *testosterone*. Now we know that testosterone is still important, even vital, for many male directed sexual behaviors. Indeed, today we have a better and much more sophisticated understanding of the promises and perils of this prototype male hormone. (See Chapter 13.) But testosterone alone is not the whole story.

Men's sexual chemistry depends on even more. Once scientists understood the chemical reactions involved in the transformation of a man's penis from limp to erect, they could develop a "designer potency pill." The goal was to recharge a man's sexual batteries and make it possible for a man who, for one reason or another, had lost the ability to have sex to reclaim his manhood. Such a pill would allow a sexually impaired man to feel confident about his ability to have erections and take pleasure in sexual intercourse once again.

Over the years, many pills containing yohimbine, vitamin E, and zinc were hawked as male restoratives (see Chapter 21). Many are still used to bolster a man's sexual appetite and power and continue to enjoy great popularity today. However, none of these oral medications achieved the immediate stardom or instantaneous success of sildenafil (Viagra).

From the beginning, the buzz on Viagra was extraordinary, like that for no other new drug in the history of medicine. Viagra's FDA approval shouldered aside, at least temporarily, the public's obsession with President Clinton and Monica Lewinsky. The prestigious column-one slot in the *New York Times* was devoted to FDA approval of this pill to treat impotence. Every major newspaper and newsmagazine followed suit, and overnight Viagra became a household word.

WHERE DID VIAGRA COME FROM?
UK-92480 SILDENAFIL-VIAGRA

The development of a "potency pill" that is a medication that could actually make it easier for men to have sex was sheer fantasy until scientists stumbled on sildenafil (Viagra). Originally called UK-92480, then given the generic name sildenafil and more recently the brand name Viagra, this new medication was widely heralded as *the pill that could cure impotence.*

Sildenafil (Viagra) was originally developed as a blood-pressure-lowering (antihypertensive) medication. Early studies designed to evaluate exactly how effectively sildenafil lowered blood pressure revealed remarkable and unexpected side effects.[1] Hypertensive men taking sildenafil started to experience a surprising number of frequent firm erections.

WHAT IS SO SPECIAL ABOUT VIAGRA?

Viagra, unlike yohimbine, does not purport to be an aphrodisiac, something that can mysteriously heighten a man's sexual desire. Rather, Viagra has been specifically designed to improve the vigor of a man's erection. It does this by bolstering a man's own natural sexual chemistry to make it easier for his penis to acquire and maintain a firm erection during sex.

To date, we know the following about this medication. Viagra speeds up the rate at which blood flows into the penile erectile bodies, the corpora cavernosae. To understand exactly how Viagra works, you have to know a little about what is rapidly emerging as the new science of *male sexual chemistry.*

MALE SEXUAL CHEMISTRY

The names of the chemicals involved in male sexual chemistry are not particularly erotic, but they are the driving force of men's sexuality. The inter-

---

[1] This was not the first time a pill originally developed to treat high blood pressure caused unanticipated problems. Minoxidil, which also lowers blood pressure, causes *excessive hair growth*, a side effect that made minoxidil unacceptable as an antihypertensive medication. The scientists who developed minoxidil were disappointed but determined to turn their medical sow's ear into a silk purse. They first decided to jettison plans for using minoxidil as a blood pressure lowering pill and reengineered their product's future. Minoxidil lotion is now an approved treatment for baldness. You probably know it as Rogaine.

action of these chemicals is not really that complicated once you know the names of the players.

1. NOS stands for nitric oxide synthase, the enzyme that releases NO (nitric oxide) into the penis.
2. NO starts blood flowing into the penile erectile chambers to start penile swelling, or *tumescence.*
3. cGMP (short for cyclic GMP) accelerates penile blood flow, resulting in penile *rigidity.*
4. PDE-5 (phosphodiesterase-5) inactivates cGMP, causing both cGMP levels and a man's erection to dwindle.
5. Sildenafil (Viagra) blocks PDE-5 and helps maintain cGMP stability as well as the vigor of a man's erection

Here's how it all works.

During sexual excitement, a man's own natural body chemicals diffuse or are *transmitted* into his penis to trigger the release of nitric oxide (NO). Blood starts to flow into the penile erectile chambers so that the penis plumps up. This is known as *tumescence.* But the penis is still not ready for sex. The swollen or tumescent penis must be taken to the next plateau, *penile rigidity.*

Penile rigidity requires a second locally generated chemical called cyclic GMP (cGMP). It is the presence of cGMP that maintains the furious onrush of blood needed for a man's penis to be converted from tumescent to rigid.

As cGMP takes center stage and even more blood flows into the penis, the pent-up pressure caused by accelerated penile blood flow is so intense that the penis looks like a stuffed sausage straining at its casing. As blood pressure within the penis mounts, the tiny draining emissary veins are choked off so that no blood can leave the penis. (See Figure 11.1.)

A man's sexual capability is therefore dependent on a chemical chain reaction beginning with the enzyme NOS, followed by NO, and finally culminating in cGMP to activate the blood flow needed for him to get an erection. The system can break down at any point.

Men who have a substandard quotient of the enzyme NOS within their penile tissue cannot make enough NO to initiate the full and unfettered flow of blood into the penile erectile chambers and as a consequence have difficulty developing a full erection. Lower than normal NOS levels are found in men who are *heavy cigarette smokers* and in those who have *diabetes mellitus* or *low testosterone levels.* This explains, in part, why impotence is so common among long-term smokers, diabetic men, and men with testosterone deficiency.

> **Vasodilation**— (tumescence)
>
> Arginine + 02 + NADPH + NOS ➡ Citrulline + NO ↑
>
>   + Guanyl Cyclase
>
>   c GMP ↑

> **Vasoconstriction**— (detumescence)
>
>   PDE 5 ⟶ c GMP ↓
>
> **sildenafil** blocks PDE 5 ⟶ c GMP ↑ + vasodilation

FIGURE 11.1   The nitric oxide cascade. The chemicals nitric oxide and cGMP create a penile erection and phosphodiesterase-5 (PDE-5) terminates it. Sildenafil (Viagra) blocks PDE-5 metabolism of cGMP to enhance the vigor of a man's erection.

WHY DOES A MAN LOSE HIS ERECTION?

A man's firm and turgid erection persists until he achieves climax and ejaculates. After ejaculation, his erection fades and his penis returns to its limp (flaccid) state. That process, the conversion of the penis from the sexually prepared and erect condition back to its normal resting flaccid state is also under chemical control. Another intrapenile chemical, an enzyme, called phosphodiesterase 5 (PDE-5) determines whether an erection will stand or collapse.

Enzymes work to either activate or inactivate proteins, and in this case, what is inactivated by PDE-5 is cGMP, the chemical that helped the penis remain erect. As levels of intrapenile cyclic GMP levels fall, so does a man's erection.

Sildenafil (Viagra) inhibits PDE-5 and allows a man's cGMP levels to remain elevated. When cGMP levels remain high, a man's erection persists.

This is good news for men who suffer from impotence or erectile dysfunction.

As long as Viagra helps maintain high intrapenile cGMP levels, a man's erectile vigor is sustained. With Viagra treatment, between 65 percent and 80 percent of impotent men are able to acquire and maintain erections satisfactory for sexual intercourse. (See Table 11.1.)

TABLE 11.1   Male Sexual Chemistry

Body Chemical	Does What?
Nitric Oxide Synthase (NOS)	Releases Nitric Oxide (NO)
Nitric Oxide	Starts blood flowing into penis causing swelling (tumescence)
Cyclic GMP (cGMP)	Increases blood flow so that penis becomes firm and rigid
Phophodiesterase 5 (PDE-5)	Metabolizes cGMP causing loss of erection
Sildenafil (Viagra)	Inhibits PDE-5 allowing cGMP levels and a man's erection to be sustained

HOW DOES VIAGRA DIFFER FROM OTHER IMPOTENCE TREATMENTS?

Viagra Is Not an Aphrodisiac

Currently available impotence treatments all work in different ways to help man acquire an erection. For example, yohimbine (Yocon, Yohimex) has been thought of as an *aphrodisiac*, a medication that increases a man's libido or sexual desire. Viagra does not increase sexual desire.

Sexual Stimulation Required

Some impotence treatments like intrapenile papaverine, alprostadil (Caverject) injection, or MUSE (medicated urethral suppository) (see Chapter 19) will allow a man to have an erection in the absence of any sexual stimulation. Indeed, men who opt for penile injection or MUSE therapy can experience penile swelling and a full erection within twenty to thirty minutes after their first treatment in the asexual, antiseptic environment of a doctor's office. It is likely that both intrapenile injections and MUSE work by increasing levels of intrapenile NO and cGMP, directly bypassing the normal mechanisms involved in a sexually stimulated erection. There is, however, a difference between the erections men have after Viagra and sexual stimulation and intrapenile injection or MUSE therapy.

Priapism Is Uncommon After Viagra

The erection triggered by both intrapenile injections and MUSE does not always fade spontaneously after ejaculation. This results in a serious medical problem: a persistent painful erection called priapism. Unfortunately, *priapism* occurs with distressing frequency in men using penile injection or MUSE. Priapism is less common but can occur in a handful of Viagra-treated men. Priapism, whether caused by intrapenile injection, MUSE, or after Viagra use, is considered a medical emergency. Men whose erection lasts for more than four hours require immediate medical treatment. Fortunately, for the majority of men the effect of Viagra is not sustained beyond the moment of ejaculation.

Thus, because of Viagra's gentle action *in turning on* and *allowing nature to turn off* male sexual chemistry, Viagra seemed to be an ideal medication to use for men with erectile dysfunction.

EARLY EXPERIENCE WITH VIAGRA

At first, doctors used Viagra only in impotent men with psychogenic impotence who had "erectile dysfunction of no known organic cause." The very first studies were done to determine:

1. The frequency and vigor of a man's erectile response to erotic videotapes before and after treatment with different doses of Viagra or an inactive placebo pill.
2. The ability of men who had complaints of impotence to have erections after placebo or Viagra.
3. How often men with sexual problems were able to have sexual intercourse after treatment with placebo or different doses of Viagra.
4. Side effects of Viagra.

Effect of Viagra on Men's Erections After Viewing Erotic Films

In one small study, a dozen impotent men with psychogenic (emotionally based) impotence were evaluated. These twelve men were shown sexually explicit erotic videos to see if their response to this sexual stimulus was different before and after treatment. Participants first received either one of three doses of sildenafil or placebo and then viewed two hours of erotic films (visual sexual stimulation). While they were watching the films, the number and strength of their erections was measured. With placebo treatment, men who viewed the erotic films had only minimal penile swelling and no fully rigid erections. Then when they received progressively increasing doses of Viagra and viewed the same sexually stimulating films, they had fully rigid erections, with the most improvement seen with the 50-mg (milligram) Viagra dose. After participating in this phase of the study, all twelve men had the opportunity to use Viagra or placebo at home with their sexual partners. In that more normal sexual setting, two of ten placebo-treated men and ten of twelve Viagra-treated men were able to acquire erections good enough for sexual intercourse.

How Often Do Impotent Men Recover
Erectile Function After Placebo or Viagra?

Several investigators have asked this question and have had slightly different responses. In another large study, 351 generally healthy men with psychogenic impotence were questioned before and after treatment with placebo or Viagra about whether treatment improved erections. A surprisingly large number, 38 percent, of *placebo-treated men* were convinced that the pills they were taking improved their erectile function. In contrast, 65 percent of men on the lowest and 89 percent of men on the highest Viagra doses reported better and stronger erections.

Reports of Erections Satisfactory for
Sexual Intercourse After Treatment with
Placebo or Different Doses of Viagra

The results of an American study of 416 men treated with placebo or 5, 25, 50, or 100 mg of sildenafil (Viagra) are shown in Table 11.1. Participating men were asked two types of questions:

1. Was overall sexual function improved with treatment?
2. On a scale of 1 to 4 (with 1 indicating "inadequate" and 4 indicating "maximal" erection), how would you rate your ability to acquire and maintain an erection with treatment?

As is evident from Table 11.1, the numbers of men who said their sexual function was "better" with treatment ranged from 28 percent with placebo to 78 percent with the highest 100-mg dose of sildenafil.

To assess the effectiveness of treatment, impotent men in this study were asked:

1. During sex are you able to achieve an erection that is firm enough to penetrate your partner? (Penetration requires that the tip and base of the penis remain rigid for several minutes [see Figure 11.2].)
2. Once you have penetrated, are you able to maintain your erection until you reach orgasm?

Fundamentally, the investigators wanted to know how often men could enjoy sex before and after treatment with Viagra or placebo.

More than one-fourth (28 percent), of placebo-treated impotent men reported that they had improved sexual function. However, the number of men who recaptured the ability to have and enjoy sex with Viagra dwarfed the numbers of men who responded to placebo. The majority of men expe-

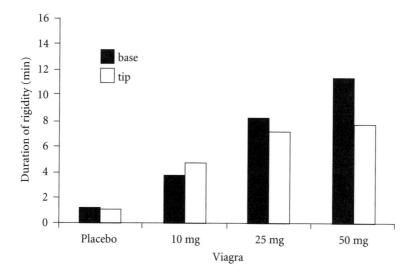

FIGURE 11.2   Average duration of nighttime erections' penile rigidity at base and tip of penis in men treated with placebo or different doses of sildenafil (Viagra). SOURCE: Adapted from M. Boolell, S. Gepi-Atee, G. C. Gingell, M. J. Allen, "Sildenafil: A Novel Effective Oral Therapy for Male Erectile Dysfunction," *Br. J. Urology* 78 (1996): 257–261.

TABLE 11.2   Responses of 416 Men Reporting Improvement from Treatment with Placebo or Escalating Doses of Viagra

Responses of 416 men	Placebo	5 mg Viagra	25 mg Viagra	50 mg Viagra	100 mg Viagra
% Better	28 %	48 %	61 %	72 %	78 %
Acquire (scored 1–4)	2.0	2.7	2.9	3.2	3.3
Maintain (scored 1–4)	2.0	2.4	2.9	3.3	3.6

rienced stronger, more lasting, and more useful erections following Viagra. Doses as low as 25 mg produced a significant improvement over the placebo responses (Table 11.2).

Eventually Viagra was used to treat not just men with psychogenic impotence but others whose sexual problems were caused by both psychologic and physical (organic) problems, including those with high blood pressure, diabetes mellitus, heart disease, high cholesterol levels, or prostate cancer.

Data adapted from the multicenter study reported by Dr. Irwin Goldstein and his colleagues in the May 14, 1998, *New England Journal of Medicine* are itemized in Table 11.3.

TABLE 11.3   Characteristics of impotent men treated with Viagra and placebo

Characteristic	Dose Response Study		Dose Escalation Study	
	Placebo	Viagra	Placebo	Viagra
Average Age	57 years	58 years	59 years	60 years
Range of Ages	20–79 years	24–87 years	31–81 years	26–79 years
Average duration of erectile dysfunction	3.2 years	3.2 years	4.7 years	5.0 years
Cause of erectile dysfunction (% men)				
Organic	77 %	78 %	63 %	55 %
Psychogenic	10 %	9 %	16 %	14 %
Mixed	13 %	13 %	22 %	31 %
Concomitant conditions (% of men)				
Hypertension	26 %	30 %	28 %	24 %
Ischemic heart disease (past or present)	8 %	8 %	8 %	15 %
Hyperlipidemia	16 %	19 %	14 %	15 %
After prostatectomy	10 %	12 %	11 %	9 %
Diabetes mellitus	15 %	13 %	11 %	8 %

Once again, some of the impotent men (in this study about 24 percent) did say that they had improved sexual function when they were taking placebo pills. However, more improved with Viagra and the degree of improvement seemed to be related to the dose of Viagra. With the 25-mg Viagra dose, 67 percent improve compared to 78 percent with 50 mg, and 82 percent achieve increased erectile vigor and sexual success with the 100-mg Viagra dose. (Figure 11.3.)

Men participating in this study were asked rather pointed questions to determine whether with Viagra treatment there was:

1. An improvement in erections.
2. Change in orgasms.
3. Overall sexual satisfaction.
4. Any change in sexual desire.

These issues—erections, orgasms, sexual satisfaction, and sexual desire—are referred to as *domains* of normal male sexual function.

Several currently available questionnaires allow doctors to gauge the level of men's sexual desire. Viagra-treated men notice an improvement in their ability to acquire and maintain their erections, indicating that with Viagra, erectile function was significantly improved. As a result, men's contentment with their ability to have sexual intercourse was also enhanced (Figure 11.4) and pleasure with orgasms intensified (Figure 11.5), but surprisingly, even with this remarkable improvement in sexual functioning, their level of sexual desire did not increase (Figure 11.6).

Thus, one domain of normal male sexual function, *sexual desire, or libido, does not improve* with Viagra. This indicates that Viagra alone may not be effective when decreased sexual interest or diminished libido is the primary sexual problem.

WHY DOES A MAN LOSE INTEREST IN SEX AND HAVE DECREASED LIBIDO?

Depression and testosterone insufficiency are the two most common causes of decreased libido. Providing treatment to alleviate depression or normalize blood testosterone levels may be all that is needed to restore sexual function in these men.

DOES VIAGRA WORK FOR EVERY IMPOTENT MAN?

While Viagra improves sexual function for men whose impotence is caused by a wide variety of physical and emotional problems, it does not work as well for every man every time. Much has been made of the fact that follow-

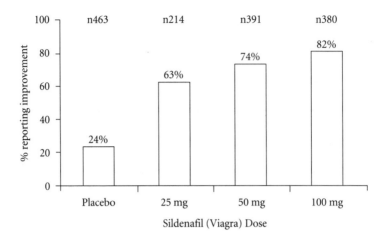

FIGURE 11.3   Men's reports of penile erections occurring with placebo and after increasing doses of sildenafil (Viagra). SOURCE: Adapted from Pfizer sildenafil-Viagra package insert.

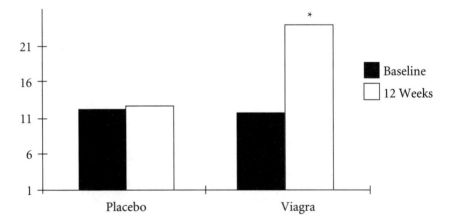

FIGURE 11.4   Men's erectile function before and during 12 weeks of treatment with either placebo or Viagra. SOURCE: Adapted from I. Goldstein, T. F. Lue, H. Padma-Nathan, R. C. Rosen, W. D. Steers, P. A. Wicker, and the Sildenafil Study Group, "Oral Sildenafil in the Treatment of Erectile Dysfunction," *N. Engl. J. Med.* 338 (1998): 1397–1404.

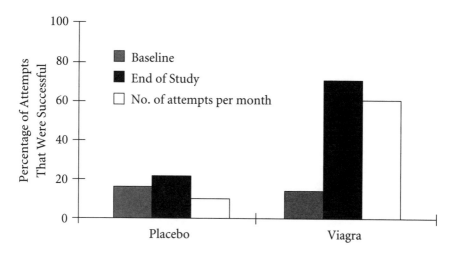

FIGURE 11.5   Sexual intercourse attempts before and during 12 weeks of treatment with either placebo or Viagra. SOURCE: Adapted from I. Goldstein, T. F. Lue, H. Padma-Nathan, R. C. Rosen, W. D. Steers, P. A. Wicker, and the Sildenafil Study Group, "Oral Sildenafil in the Treatment of Erectile Dysfunction," *N. Engl. J. Med.* 338 (1998): 1397–1404.

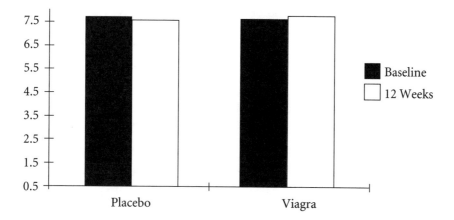

FIGURE 11.6   Sexual desire (libido) before and during 12 weeks of treatment with either placebo or Viagra. SOURCE: Adapted from I. Goldstein, T. F. Lue, H. Padma-Nathan, R. C. Rosen, W. D. Steers, P. A. Wicker, and the Sildenafil Study Group, "Oral Sildenafil in the Treatment of Erectile Dysfunction," *N. Engl. J. Med.* 338 (1998): 1397–1404.

ing his prostate cancer surgery, former senator Bob Dole participated in one of the early Viagra trials. He was so pleased with the result that he went on the *Larry King Live* show touting the benefits of this new medication for men with erectile dysfunction. Not all men who have had prostate cancer surgery do as well as former senator Dole. After prostate cancer surgery, less than 50 percent of Viagra-treated men are able to have sexual intercourse. This is especially true in men who have had the more aggressive prostate cancer surgery called radical retropubic prostatectomy (RRP), which cuts into neurovascular bundles vital for normal erectile function. (See Chapter 24.) Other coexistent medical problems such as diabetes mellitus and spinal-cord injury may also limit Viagra's efficacy.

DIABETIC MEN

Impotence is common and a distressing problem for men with diabetes mellitus. A combination of factors including diabetes-induced damage to blood vessels and nerves contribute to the sexual dysfunction experienced by men with diabetes. In placebo-controlled studies, impotent diabetic men did benefit from Viagra, but not quite as well as men without diabetes. In one study, a little more than half (56 percent) of impotent diabetic men taking a 50-mg dose of Viagra reported improved erections. Sixty-one percent were able to have sexual intercourse on at least one occasion. Twenty-two percent of impotent diabetic men reported successful sexual intercourse with placebo treatment.

My experience and that reported by others who treat men with impotence and diabetes mellitus is in line with the results reported above. A little over 50 percent of impotent diabetic men have improved erections and are able to have sexual intercourse with Viagra treatment.

VIAGRA TREATMENT OF MEN WHO
BECOME IMPOTENT AFTER SPINAL-CORD INJURY

An intact spinal cord is critical for normal erections. The thoracolumbar erection center, located in the mid-spinal cord, is responsible for relating the neurologic signals associated with psychogenic erections, whereas another center located in the lower spinal cord controls reflex erections. (See Chapter 10 for more details.) Spinal-cord injury commonly interrupts the neural impulses a man needs for both psychogenic and reflex erections. Men with erectile dysfunction caused by spinal-cord injury have been treated with Viagra with encouraging results. In one short-term twenty-eight-day study of men rendered impotent as a result of spinal-cord injury, nine of twelve (75 percent) Viagra-treated and one of fourteen (7 percent) placebo-treated men reported improved erectile function. Eight of twelve (67 percent)

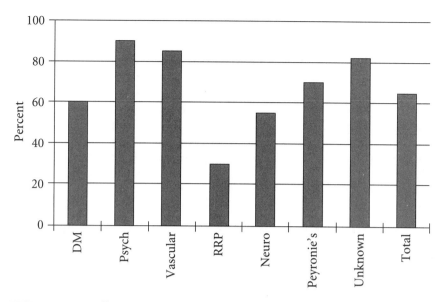

FIGURE 11.7   Effectiveness of Viagra in restoring erectile function in men whose impotence was caused by diabetes mellitus, psychologic or vascular factors, radical retropubic prostatectomy (RRP), neurologic factors, Peyronie's disease, or unknown causes. SOURCE: Adapted from J. P. Jarow, A. L. Burnett, and A. M. Geringer, "Efficacy of Sildenafil Citrate Based upon Diagnosis or Response to Previous Therapy," Abstract 21, presented at the Twenty-Fourth Annual Meeting of the American Society of Andrology, Louisville, Kentucky, April 10–13, 1999.

Viagra-treated and two of thirteen placebo-treated men were so satisfied with treatment that they wished to continue their respective treatment. The sexual partners of these men were not as impressed. A more detailed study evaluating the long-term effectiveness of Viagra in men with spinal-cord injury and resulting erectile dysfunction is in progress.

The chance of having improved erections with Viagra treatment is determined in part by the specific cause of the sexual problem. Men with psychogenic impotence respond best, whereas a smaller percentage of those who have had prostate cancer surgery with radical retropubic prostatectomy are likely to benefit from Viagra (Figure 11.7).

Other coexistent medical problems that may result in a less than ideal or suboptimal Viagra response are listed in Table 11.4.

WHAT ELSE IS IMPORTANT?

Viagra improves chances of acquiring and maintaining an erection by working to enhance penile biochemistry. We often forget that although the

TABLE 11.4 Medical Conditions Associated with Suboptimal Viagra Response

Medical Problem	Viagra ineffective because:
Decreased Sex Drive (libido)	Does not increase sex drive
Depression	Low Sex Drive Common
Low testosterone level	Decreased Libido and low NOS
Diabetes mellitus	Low NOS, neuropathy, vascular disease
Cigarette smoking	Low NOS, vascular disease
Nitrate medication*	Low blood pressure
No sexual stimulation	Sexual stimulation essential
Angina*	Increased angina with sex
Sickle cell, leukemia, myeloma	Priapism risk
Peyronie's disease	Penile distortion

* Men who have heart disease or angina or are taking nitrates should not take Viagra.

penis is the instrument of sexual pleasure, it is not a self-governing organ but rather is attached to a thinking, worrying, feeling human male body. If something is disrupting a man's emotional equilibrium or if concerns about business activities, financial troubles, or the health of beloved friends and family members preys on his mind and intrudes into the bedroom, sexual responsivity to Viagra or any other treatment designed to trigger an erection will be impaired. There are some impotent men for whom Viagra would be effective, but these men are simply too timid or too frightened to try this medication (see "Fear of Viagra" below).

SIDE EFFECTS OF VIAGRA

Now, in order to get a true sense of what Viagra's side effects are, it is necessary to compare problems reported by men taking Viagra and men taking placebo pills. If Viagra-treated men have headaches more often than those men who received placebo pills, then headaches are considered a Viagra side effect. Symptoms that occur with equal frequency in both Viagra- and placebo-treated men cannot be considered to be Viagra side effects (Table 11.5).

From this type of survey, we can determine that certain side effects, headache and facial flushing, for example, are more common with Viagra, whereas other problems like dizziness and stuffy nose occur about as often with Viagra as with placebo. A handful of men do have Viagra-triggered headaches or flushing. Even fewer have visual distortions and see blue images for a period of time.

Only a handful of men chose to discontinue treatment because of Viagra-induced side effects. In one recent study, 31 of 316 men receiving Viagra stopped treatment because of side effects. In the same study, 36 of 217

TABLE 11.5   Adverse Effects Reported by Impotent Men Who Took Viagra or Placebo

Adverse Effect	On Viagra	On Placebo
Headache	16%	4%
Flushing	10%	1%
Indigestion	7%	2%
Dizziness	2%	1%
Stuffy nose	4%	2%
Visual distortion	3%	0%
Diarrhea	3%	1%

placebo-treated men also decided to stop treatment because of "side effects."

This is in striking contrast to other impotence therapies like penile injection, where many men experience erections initially but despite this favorable response do not continue with treatment. For penile injection, the dropout rate often approaches 70 percent.

Notably missing from this list of adverse effects are life-threatening or serious adverse events. Why? Was Pfizer, the drug company that developed and marketed Viagra, trying to cover up something? Apparently not.

From the beginning, Pfizer was concerned that its product might be used inappropriately and was fierce in advising physicians to screen patients carefully before prescribing Viagra. Men who routinely use a class of medication called nitrates like nitroglycerin or isosorbide (Isordil), commonly prescribed to prevent or alleviate a form of heart pain called angina pectoris, should not take Viagra. No ifs, ands, or buts.

IF YOU TAKE NITRATES, YOU MUST NOT TAKE VIAGRA!

Pfizer was quite adamant about this from the beginning.

Not only did they tell *doctors* about the dangers of mixing nitrates with Viagra, but they alerted *pharmacists* to this drug interaction. So, when patients went to fill their prescription, most pharmacists checked their computers to see if the man for whom Viagra was prescribed had in the past also filled prescriptions for nitrates. If so, pharmacists were supposed to indicate to these men that the two prescriptions were incompatible. Pharmacists could then *warn a man* of the dangers of taking Viagra if he was also taking nitrates.

As if that were not enough, the *package insert* accompanying the bottle of Viagra tablets also informed men of the hazards of taking Viagra if they were also using nitrates.

Male Sexual Chemistry and Viagra

Even those entrepreneurs who were hawking Viagra over the Internet were careful to make sure that their *on-line clientele* had answered "no" to the question "Are you taking nitrates such as nitroglycerin, isosorbide, or Isordil?" Only then would they ask for the customer's credit card number and address to send both the Viagra tablets and a bill. (The cost for on-line Viagra is about $10.00 per pill, plus shipping and handling, and for the on-line "consultation" about $85.00—caveat cyber emptor!)

Warnings from the doctor's office, at the pharmacy, and even on-line were not sufficient. Men who should not have taken Viagra still did, and unfortunately some of them died.

Why?

Just before Viagra was released, I had the opportunity to speak before a group of Pfizer representatives and indicated that no matter how many warnings they put in place, men being men would always want to "stretch the sexual envelope" in the hopes of recapturing their lost sexual brio.

I had anticipated the following scenario:

An impotent man with known heart disease, taking nitroglycerin or isosorbide or both, is nonetheless eager to have sex. So one day he does not take Isordil. That evening he takes Viagra, gets an erection, has sex, and sometime during the middle of, or after completing, the sex act he develops heart pain (angina pectoris). Automatically, he reaches into his pocket for a nitroglycerin tablet, puts the tablet under his tongue, has a sudden fall in blood pressure and collapses.

This sequence of events or something similar seems to have been responsible for many of the deaths attributable to Viagra. It was primarily those Viagra-treated men with severe preexisting heart conditions or those taking inappropriate medications who succumbed after sexual intercourse. *But was it the Viagra or the sexual intercourse that was responsible for their demise?*

Before this question could be answered, the newspapers and television news stations were filled with reports of men who used Viagra, had sex, and then died. This created a new problem: *fear of Viagra.*

FEAR OF VIAGRA

"I didn't use the pills," confessed Walter, a cherubic sixty-five-year-old pipe smoking academic, when I asked him how the Viagra samples I had given him had worked out.

"My wife wouldn't let me," he said in explanation.

"But it was your wife who was most concerned about your impotence." (Walter and his wife had not had sex for three years.)

"In fact, she was the one who called to set up your appointment. What happened?" I wanted to know.

SEXUAL HEALTH FOR MEN

"She decided that living with sexual frustration was better than living as a widow." Walter heaved a regretful sigh, then went on. "It's in the papers, you know, and on TV, and on radio, about all those men who drop dead right after they used Viagra."

At this time, late November 1998, just months after this new medication had come on the market, newspaper reports indicated that 130 men died sometime after taking Viagra. Almost all were known to have severe heart problems. Many were taking nitrate medications like nitroglycerin and isosorbide (Isordil) and should not have used Viagra in the first place. I was aware of that, but I also knew that the majority of men who used Viagra successfully experienced no, or only trivial, side effects. Thus, millions of impotent men had had their sexual potency restored with Viagra. The small number of unfortunate men who expired sometime after they used Viagra paled in comparison to the overwhelming majority of men who had used Viagra, achieved erections, had satisfactory sexual intercourse, and had experienced no ill effects.

"More than 6 million men have used Viagra safely and with only positive results," I explained to Walter. "Those few men who died all had serious cardiac disease. Many were taking medications that were not safe to use with Viagra. Walter, you do not take any of those medications and you have never had any heart problems. For men like you, Viagra can be both safe and effective."

I double-checked his record yet again to ensure that he had none of the coexistent medical problems and was not taking any of the inappropriate medications that were part of the profile of the unfortunate men who had expired after taking Viagra. Walter simply could not be reassured.

"If you are not comfortable with Viagra, would you be willing to try . . . ?" I listed other treatments to help correct his impotence, but his wife's concerns had so rattled him that he had lost interest in his own sexuality. If he were forced to choose, as he believed he was, between living and dying, he would of course choose living. By rejecting all treatments to retrieve his ability to enjoy sexual intercourse again, Walter made a definitive decision. He opted for what he anticipated would be a long, albeit celibate, life.

"I guess you could say that having life without sex is better than no life at all" was how he put it, before he shook my hand. "Thank you so much for trying to help."

Then this once ebullient, now dejected, professor dropped his chin to his chest and left so quietly I barely heard the door close behind him.

Evan was next.

A short, balding, beefy-faced retired engineer, Evan was both the father of two grown daughters and a proud grandfather. He had been plagued by years of sexual failures and was as sexually insecure as Walter. Unlike Walter, Evan had actually used the Viagra samples and couldn't wait to tell me how well they had worked.

"Twice in one night, Doc, I'm telling you, twice in one night! One right after the other! Mary was stunned. She called me her *stud*. I'm telling you I haven't been that virile since I was in my twenties." He beamed.

Glistening perspiration gathering on the dome of his scalp migrated toward his eyes, circumvented the detour created by his plump eyebrows, then coalesced into parallel streams to trickle like cascading sideburns down his face. As a salacious grin split his seventy-four-year-old ruddy and wrinkled face, he leaned across the desk. Like a teenager energized after his first sexual experience, he continued excitedly, determined to elaborate about his further adventures with Viagra.

"Listen to this, listen to this," he said, barely able to contain himself.

"Mary and I went to the monthly condo meeting the next night, and everyone was talking about Viagra, mainly what they read or the latest Jay Leno Viagra joke. I didn't say anything at first, but then Myra, this red-headed widow from 12C, started sounding off. She thought it was terrible that there was so much interest in this *sex drug* and not enough attention paid to more important medical problems like prostate cancer, which had taken her Morrie from her when he was only fifty-nine."

"Well, that was the night *after* Mary and I had our double-header, you know what I mean, Doc. I wanted to say something but held my tongue for a while, but then Myra she just kept going on and on, yammering about how the medical profession is interested only in men's sexual problems but is not paying enough attention to other health issues, and she just wouldn't shut up, so I finally said, 'It certainly could help some men who need it.'"

"How would you know?" she challenged.

"Well, you know, just what I read about."

"Have you ever tried Viagra?" Myra was dogged and persistent.

"Yes," I admitted, "I guess you could say that I am the Man from Viagra."

"Really?" she pulled her chair closer. "How does it work?"

"Very well, I would say."

"How well?" Myra wanted to know. "She was determined to get details, and I was wondering how I would avoid telling her any more, when . . . 'Myra, how nice to see you,' Mary boomed. 'I couldn't help noticing you've been having such a nice long chat with *my husband*. Whatever did *the two of you* find to talk about for so long?'"

A week later, Evan called to say that his wife Mary thought they would both be better off if he stopped taking Viagra.

What transpired after the condo meeting was that Evan, the self-proclaimed Man from Viagra, and his wife Mary were now, thanks to the talkative Myra, unwilling condominium celebrities. Neighbors who barely spoke to them all year were now seeking them out. Mary was invited to a series of coffees, and Evan, who had always been something of a loner, was now in demand as a companion. Suddenly, extra sports-event tickets materialized for Evan, and Mary was suddenly in demand as a bridge partner. At the time, Viagra was so new that both the men and women wanted more information from "experts." But their curiosity was gender-specific.

The men were more interested in process and mechanics—*How long did it take to kick in? Was it really guaranteed to work? Did Evan wake up with a headache . . . or indigestion . . . or see blue?*

The women were more interested in feelings and wanted to know what it was like for Mary *after all these years.* She told them that she was surprised at the sudden rekindling of Evan's interest in her as a sex partner. They had of course been faithful to one another for years, and even without sex, each had been totally committed to and dependent on the other. Mary was actually quite pleased at how things had turned out. Then, the others, women who were widowed like Myra, told Mary over and over again how fortunate she was and wondered whether Evan, who was, after all, so handy, could come over and fix a faucet, help with their taxes, or just drop by. All of this sudden attention and the news reports started Mary wondering.

1. Can Viagra cause otherwise healthy men to keel over and drop dead after sex?
2. Will impotent men who become potent after taking Viagra turn into senior citizen Lotharios and, as Mary feared, menace the condominium subculture and disrupt the fabric of every elderly couple's otherwise tranquil life? See "Philandering After Viagra: Fantasy, Fears, and Reality" below.

Concerns about Viagra's safety surface at both the doctor's and the patient's level.

1. Doctors are concerned that the patient for whom Viagra is prescribed be an appropriate candidate for this medication. Always cautious, doctors avoid giving a Viagra prescription if there is a high probability of a medication-induced side effect. They have been advised not to prescribe Viagra to any man with severe heart disease, particularly if he is taking medications like nitroglycerin or isosorbide (Isordil). Others for whom the use of Viagra would be unwise include those men with very high or very low blood pressure or those with an inherited eye disorder called retinitis pigmentosa.
2. Men with sexual problems are understandably troubled by reports of sudden death occurring in men shortly after they take Viagra.

The disquiet of physicians and their patients is ultimately translated into the number of men who actually walk out of the doctor's office with a Viagra prescription. One of my colleagues, Dr. Andre Guay, who is director of the Sexual Dysfunction Program at the Lahey Clinic in Peabody, Massachusetts, has kept a running tabulation of the numbers of men he has seen in consultation in the first six months after Viagra was approved by the FDA (Table 11.6).

TABLE 11.6   Number of Men with Complaints of Erectile Dysfunction for Whom Viagra Was and Was Not Appropriate

Evaluated	551 patients
Medically unsuitable	44 (8.6%)
Fear of Viagra	65 (12.8%)
Lost to follow-up	13 (2.6%)
Total not using Viagra	122 (24%)
Using Viagra	429 (76%)

SOURCE: Andre Guay, M.D., F.A.C.E.

Even when doctors try to identify only those men who are appropriate candidates for Viagra and weed out others for whom Viagra might pose a substantial health risk, a third group surfaces. They are the men who are so frightened by the press reports of death after Viagra that they refuse Viagra treatment on their own. Indeed, at the Lahey Clinic more men opted out of Viagra treatment on their own than were disqualified because of any known risk to their health.

Why would impotent men reject a treatment that might allow them to have sex once again? Which is more perilous, sexual intercourse or Viagra?

DEATH AFTER SEX AND/OR VIAGRA:
WHAT IS THE RISK?

Along with its obvious pleasures, sexual intercourse poses a definite risk to a man's health. We have known for some time that *the heart works harder* to keep pace with the excitement and passion of sexual intercourse. Under normal circumstances, when healthy men have sexual intercourse their heart rate and blood pressure increase. When men with heart disease have sexual intercourse, their damaged hearts cannot always keep pace. Often, men with heart problems can neither muster the pulse increase nor blood pressure elevation their bodies expect. The act of sexual intercourse demands a physiologic response that is sometimes beyond what the damaged heart can supply.

In the *pre-Viagra era*, for example, men questioned after they had heart attacks (myocardial infarctions) recalled that chest pain was the first clue to their impending heart attack. They can often relate the onset of their chest pain to some physical or emotional stress. Sometimes that stress is physical, like the exertion required to lift a heavy object or shovel snow. Sometimes the physical exertion is the act of sexual intercourse.

- Men who die immediately after having had sexual intercourse (also known as coitus) are said to have experienced a "coital death." Heart attacks are what kill most men. Occasionally, doctors are curious enough to inquire into the events preceding a man's fatal heart attack and want to know if he was:
    1. Sleeping quietly in bed and never woke up the following morning.
    2. Rushing to catch a train when he had chest pain and then collapsed on the rail station platform.
    3. Embroiled in a fractious argument with a business colleague or competitor or with a rebellious child, wife, or lover.
    4. Lifting weights or shoveling snow.
    5. Having sex sometime during the twenty-four hours before he expired. If so, then he would be classified as having had a *coital death*.

In 1963, *thirty-five years before Viagra*, we knew that among men who die suddenly very few (0.6 percent) have coital deaths. Some men have their fatal heart attack during or immediately after sexual intercourse. Subsequently, other reports told us that:

- Twelve percent of men admitted to the hospital with *nonfatal heart attacks* will admit that they have had sexual intercourse two to twenty-four hours prior to the onset of their chest pain.
- The heart's response to sexual intercourse has actually been studied in some detail. In the interest of science, some men with known heart disease have agreed to have their pulse, blood pressure, and heart strain measured during sexual intercourse. After being hooked up to wires that record their heart rate and change in cardiogram pattern, they have sex in the privacy of their own bedrooms. The next day, their records are analyzed. The men also keep a log of any cardiac symptoms (chest pain, palpitations, and so on) they might have experienced during sex.

These reports told us that almost one-third (31 percent) of men had cardiogram patterns suggesting heart strain (called coronary ischemia). Only 7 percent had chest pain during sex. The majority (24 percent) of those with heart strain during sex had no discomfort and were classified as having "silent coronary ischemia."

WHO WILL AND WILL NOT HAVE HEART STRAIN DURING SEX?

Men who have decreased cardiac blood flow during sexual intercourse are the same men who have decreased heart blood flow with any sort of exercise. When doctors want to know exactly how much exercise a man can tolerate, they do an exercise stress test and ask the man to walk on a treadmill. While he is walking, his heart rate and blood flow can be measured. During the exercise stress test, the man is encouraged to do as much as possible to establish his "cardiac reserve" to define how much activity his heart can tolerate.

As a man walks faster and faster on a treadmill, his heart rate (the number of beats per minute) increases. Men with the least damage to their hearts can reach peak heart rates of about 150 without showing evidence of heart strain. During sexual intercourse, their peak heart rate reaches 117 and shows no signs of heart strain. Contrast this to men with cardiac problems who develop chest pain during sexual intercourse. The peak heart rate they can muster is 113 during exercise. But when the strain of sexual intercourse pushes their heart rate beyond this limit to 122, their hearts cry out in pain. Men with less severe heart disease can achieve higher heart rates and may have no discomfort during sexual intercourse, yet their cardiograms still show evidence of heart strain (Table 11.7).

TABLE 11.7 Maximum Heart Rate Achieved by Men with Moderate and Severe Heart Disease During Cardiac Stress (Treadmill) Test and Sex

	Chest Pain	Maximum Heart Rate (bpm)	Heart Strain
Moderate Heart Disease			
Treadmill	No	150	No
Sex	No	117	No
Severe Heart Disease			
Treadmill	Yes	113	Yes
Sex	Yes	122	Yes
Treadmill	No	136	Yes
Sex	No	114	Yes

- Heart attacks develop when the heart does not receive enough oxygen due to low coronary artery blood flow. Viagra lowers blood pressure, and when combined with other medications like nitrates, which also lower blood pressure, it can diminish coronary blood flow, setting the stage for a heart attack.

- Two other unexpected problems, *unrelated to nitrate use*, may occur. One affects men with a predilection for another type of heart problem called an arrhythmia, or irregular heartbeat, which means not just any skipped heartbeat but a dangerously irregular heartbeat called *ventricular tachycardia*. Men who develop this irregular and chaotic heart rhythm usually have major heart damage as a result of prior attacks. It appears that when such men use Viagra to enable them to have sexual intercourse, they may also increase their chances of developing ventricular tachycardia.

Ventricular tachycardia is a life-threatening irregularity of the heartbeat. Often, men who develop ventricular tachycardias require cardiac shock therapy to *jolt their hearts back to a normal heartbeat*. It may be that men with such severe heart disease with a known predisposition for ventricular arrhythmias should also be discouraged from using Viagra.

- The other unanticipated problem *affects female sex partners of men who use Viagra*. Bladder infections called cystitis develop in about 15 percent of women who have had sexual intercourse with Viagra-treated men. It has been known for some time that there are some women who often develop bladder infections after sexual intercourse. The term "postcoital cystitis" has been used for those women who develop bladder infections after sexual intercourse. In severe cases, antibiotics are necessary to treat the bladder infection. On most occasions, all that is required to prevent postcoital cystitis is adequate hydration and urinating immediately after sexual intercourse.

WHO DIES AFTER SEX?

Earlier on, I referred to the fact that 0.6 percent of men experience a "coital death." That means they die sometime after they have had sex. We have this remarkable information because an enterprising pathologist in Tokyo decided to look into the details of over 5,000 sudden unexpected deaths. Of 5,559 individuals who died suddenly in Tokyo, a total of thirty-four (28 men and 6 women) expired during or shortly after sexual intercourse. Heart attacks were the cause of death in men, whereas strokes were responsible for the demise of women who died after sex. Twenty-three of the 34 deaths occurred outside the home in hotels or in the beds of mistresses or prostitutes. Thus, the events that favor a coital death are quite specific.

Male Sexual Chemistry and Viagra   125

TABLE 11.8   Cause of Death in Men Who Expired After Using Viagra (From FDA 11/24/98)

Cause of Death	Number of Men
Murder	1
Drowning	1
Heart Attack	77
Cardiac Arrest	27
Stroke	3
Unknown	48

1. Extramarital relationship.
2. Younger sexual partner.
3. Sex in an unfamiliar environment.

This implies that in Japan, spontaneous coital deaths are most likely to occur in a hotel, a lover's boudoir, or a bordello.

WHAT CAUSES DEATH IN MEN WHO TAKE VIAGRA?

In November, 1998, just six months after Viagra was approved, 6 million prescriptions had been written for this medication and 50 million Viagra tablets had been dispensed. In this interval, 130 men died sometime after they took Viagra. We know this because of what is called post-marketing surveillance.

Once a medication has been approved for use and is available by prescription, doctors continue to look for an unexpectedly high number of their patients developing one problem or another.

The close relationship that most doctors have with their patients allows for a frank discussion of treatment results and adverse effects of any new medication. Most patients do not hesitate to tell their doctors when a medication has caused a particular problem. Doctors all over the country then gather this information and report back to the drug company—in this case Pfizer—or the FDA, which is obliged to survey and keep accurate records of problems that were not apparent before but surface only after a new drug is released. The official term for this data collection is "post-marketing surveillance."

As a result of post-marketing surveillance, we know that abnormal liver function tests may occur with some common cholesterol-lowering medications. Thus, doctors prescribing these medications periodically do special blood tests to see if their patients have had any disruption in their liver-function tests, and if so, they stop the medication so that that liver function returns to normal.

SEXUAL HEALTH FOR MEN

TABLE 11.9   Hours Elapsed Between Sex and Fatal Symptom, Usually Chest Pain*

Chest Pain	Number of men
During sex	27
4–5 hours	44
More than 5 hours	6
More than 24 hours	8
More than 48 hours	5
3–7 days later	4

* Most (70%) of the men who died had one or more risk factors for heart disease including high blood pressure, elevated cholesterol levels, cigarette smoking, diabetes mellitus, obesity or a known cardiac history. Some even had vials of nitroglycerin tablets in their pockets at the time of death. Only twelve men had no cardiac history, but for them the interval between the use of Viagra and the onset of their symptoms was so prolonged that it seemed unlikely that Viagra actually contributed to their deaths. Nonetheless, they are included in the survey.

For Viagra, post-marketing surveillance provided valuable information on the number of men who died after using this medication and also provided more information on those men for whom Viagra was risky (Table 11.8).

Details leading up to the deaths were varied. For example, one man was murdered and another drowned. Three expired after suffering strokes, and 77 had heart problems. Forty-one of those 77 had definite or suspected heart attacks, and 27 men died because their heart stopped beating (cardiac arrest).

Excluding the 2 men who were murdered or drowned, we know that 44 (34 percent) of the 128 men who died had the onset of heart symptoms, usually chest pain, four to five hours after they took Viagra. Twenty-seven had their symptoms during or immediately after sexual intercourse. Six experienced heart pain much later on that same day (Table 11.9). In others, the association between Viagra use and onset of symptoms was more tenuous, with 8 noticing chest pain more than twenty-four hours later, 5 forty-eight hours later, and 4 three to seven days after Viagra use.

As a result of these findings as well as other post-marketing surveillance problems such as painful prolonged erection (priapism), a new set of warnings regarding safe use of Viagra was issued. *Men should not take Viagra if they have*:

1. Had a heart attack, stroke, or irregular heartbeat (arrhythmia) within the last six months.
2. Very high (> 170/110 mmHg) or very low (<90/50 mmHg) blood pressure.
3. Severe heart disease and chest pain from angina pectoris.

4. Retinitis pigmentosa.
5. A prior history of painful prolonged erections.
6. Liver failure.
7. Severe kidney disease.

WHY IS IT NECESSARY TO WORRY ABOUT LIVER AND KIDNEY DISEASE?

The liver and the kidney clear waste products as well as medications from a man's system. When the liver and kidney are not functioning properly, Viagra is not metabolized efficiently; some otherwise innocuous medications like the antibiotic erythromycin disrupt and slow down Viagra's metabolism. During erythromycin treatment, blood Viagra levels build up and remain unusually high for a prolonged period of time. Whenever liver or kidney disease or erythromycin allows blood Viagra levels to remain high, opportunities for developing a Viagra-related side effect increase.

Using the seven guidelines listed above, along with a generous sprinkling of common sense, will allow for the safe and effective use of Viagra.

HOW WILL SILDENAFIL (VIAGRA) BE USED?

Once men with preexisting heart problems and those using nitrate medications are excluded, there remain millions of impotent men for whom Viagra treatment is both useful and appropriate. Those men should know how to use Viagra to achieve maximum benefit.

- The usual starting dose of Viagra is 50 mg, taken one hour before planned sexual activity.

- Men over age sixty-five are advised to start with a 25-mg dose, again one hour before planned sexual activity.

- Men who have no adverse effects from taking one dose of Viagra but do not achieve an ideal erectile response at that dose may take the next-higher dose, up to a total single dose of 100 mg.

Men who have side effects such as light-headedness, dizziness, or headache at any dose are encouraged to "step down" and try a lower dose to minimize or eliminate these adverse effects. Some men who are able to tolerate the 50-mg dose but feel they have not had a fully satisfactory dose may do better on the higher 100-mg dose of sildenafil.

WHY WAIT ONE HOUR AFTER
TAKING VIAGRA BEFORE HAVING SEX?

Once the Viagra tablet is swallowed, the medication passes through the stomach and into the bloodstream. It takes about forty minutes to one hour before sufficient Viagra has built up in the body to be effective, but a man's penis does not automatically become erect and stiffen at this time. Viagra works only in a setting of sexual stimulation such as the standard embraces and genital stimulation and caressing that is a normal component of healthy lovemaking. In this way, Viagra more closely mimics the normal pattern of sexual interaction between couples than does penile injection therapy, penile prosthesis, or MUSE.

PHILANDERING AFTER VIAGRA:
FANTASY, FEARS, AND REALITY

The potentially dangerous interaction of Viagra with medications commonly used to treat heart conditions was anticipated, whereas the sudden empowerment of once impotent men with a new sense of sexual security was seen as a benefit, not as a threat. No one envisioned that anyone could interpret the availability of this new medication otherwise. Somebody did. What happened?

TAKING THE WORRY OUT OF SEX

There is a natural tendency to fret whenever new medications make it easier for men and women to have trouble-free sexual intercourse. Certainly when birth control pills became available, women who had previously shied away from intimate relations could feel more comfortable and less frightened about becoming pregnant. The birth control pills were introduced just before the 1960s sexual revolution and no doubt played a role in contributing to the sexual freedom and perhaps the promiscuity of that era. Women who took their birth control pills daily could and did engage in sexual intercourse more often than they had before the availability of this medication. However, other powerful forces were afoot shaping this turbulent decade, and the birth control pill is probably best viewed as a "facilitator" rather than an instigator of a more relaxed attitude toward sexual behavior. Not all medical advances that made it easier to have sex have had a comparable impact on sexual mores.

When penile prosthesis surgery was introduced a decade earlier, some worried that when impotent men were suddenly equipped with a device that allowed them to have an "on-demand" erection, their sexual behavior would

---

change. They would no longer confine their sexual activities to the privacy of their bedroom but would be inclined to stray and seek out new and varied sexual partners. Some may have, but all of the currently available data indicate that the majority of impotent men who had penile prosthesis surgery were pleased to be able to have sexual intercourse again with their spouses alone.

WHAT DRUGS CAN AND CANNOT
BE USED SAFELY WITH VIAGRA?

Some drugs classified as vasodilators, commonly used to treat symptoms of heart disease such as the chest pain of angina pectoris, tend to lower blood pressure. Medications like nitroglycerin and isosorbide are classified as nitrates. Because these medications, as well as some others known as alpha blockers like prazosin (Hytrin), lower blood pressure the same way that Viagra lowers blood pressure, the combined use of the two types of medications is discouraged. If blood pressure drops too much, as it may when the nitrates and Viagra are taken together, there is insufficient blood flow to the brain and in that case, a man will black out and faint. It is possible that other unfavorable drug interactions will be discovered in the future, but for the moment, it is the combined use of Viagra and nitrates that is most worrisome. This may create a hardship for millions of men with heart disease who have relied on nitrates to ward off or control the cardiac pain of angina pectoris.

PRESCRIPTIONS WITHOUT PROPER DIAGNOSIS

Men eager to get their hands on and doctors willing to prescribe Viagra may do so without pursuing the standard diagnostic evaluation accorded to all men with erectile dysfunction.

What has emerged is a worrisome phenomenon of *prescribing without diagnosing.* This has resulted in a sequence of events in which a man suffering from impotence or erectile dysfunction builds up the courage to discuss this with his doctor. The harried doctor hears the term "erectile dysfunction" and without either exam or diagnostic evaluation scribbles a prescription for Viagra and hustles the man out of his office. This all-too-common practice has allowed men with serious conditions such as pituitary tumors to go undiagnosed. This is an unfortunate consequence for men with prolactin-secreting pituitary tumors, where delay in diagnosis allows further pituitary tumor growth and poor prognosis.

The man with erectile dysfunction deserves something more than a prescription. Asking about standard medical history, conducting a physical exam, reviewing possible risk factors, and taking hormone measurements as outlined elsewhere in this book are essential procedures. Once the physician is confident there are no other sexual impediments such as depression, cigarette smoking, diabetes mellitus, low testosterone, or high prolactin levels and no cardiac history, then a prescription for Viagra is in order.

TIPS ON USING VIAGRA FOR
MAXIMUM BENEFIT AND MINIMAL RISK

A Viagra tablet is not like an aspirin. If you have a headache and take two aspirin you will start to feel better within about twenty to thirty minutes. Viagra takes a little longer to work. A man planning to have sex should take his Viagra tablet about one hour earlier. Then enough Viagra will be in his system to work effectively. However, it would be unwise for a man to swallow a blue Viagra tablet at 8 P.M., then stare at the clock and have the sense that he must rush into the bedroom at precisely 9 P.M. before the effect of the Viagra wears off. We know now that the effect of this medication is *first apparent* within an hour, but Viagra *continues to be effective* for several more hours. Twenty-four hours later, it is almost completely washed out of a man's system. The effectiveness of Viagra, with its rapid onset of action and prompt clearance from the body, has made this medication very useful for the treatment of men with erectile dysfunction.

THE POLITICS OF MALE SEXUALITY:
WHO WILL PAY FOR VIAGRA?

As soon as it became apparent that Viagra was effective and allowed sexually impaired men to enjoy sexual intercourse once again, there was an overwhelming lust for this new medication. Demand for Viagra skyrocketed, and within six months after it had been released and made available in drugstores, Viagra sales exceeded *$5 hundred million.* First-year projections were expected to top *$1 billion,* making Viagra the most successful drug ever launched in the history of medicine.

- Pfizer, the drug company that developed and was marketing Viagra, was overjoyed at the success of its new medication.
- Impotent men, no longer sexually impaired, now enjoying sex again were thrilled.
- HMOs and managed care organizations, however, were frantic.

Shortly after Viagra was released, almost all managed-care organizations panicked and, perceiving Viagra as a threat to their bottom line, circled the wagons. Surely, they reasoned, a medication this effective will be sought after by every male and some females. If we, as insurers, allow reimbursement for this medication by anyone who wants it, we will surely suffer. So HMOs decided that they would either not pay for any, or *severely restrict, the numbers of Viagra pills* their subscribers could receive.

Their tactics were simple.

- Demonize Viagra as a frivolous "sex pill."
- Point out that Viagra was not a lifesaving medication.
- Equate Viagra with other sexually related products like birth-control devices.
- Blame pharmacies for charging $10.00 per pill for Viagra.
- Make it difficult for doctors to prescribe Viagra.

Here is what happened.

Before HMOs had any true sense of what the demand for Viagra would be, HMO executives in this country and the National Health Service in Great Britain projected what it would cost them to cover the cost of providing Viagra. When they calculated anticipated demand and multiplied this number by the wholesale per-pill cost, they choked.

Proclaiming everything from imminent fiscal doom to a need to raise premiums to keep up with demand, they blitzed the media. Dr. David Eddy, a prominent health-care economist, talked about making choices, and the choice he made, on behalf of Kaiser Foundation Health Plan, was *not to provide* this "sex pill" for any of Kaiser's millions of male subscribers. Impotence was, he reasoned, not life-threatening, and therefore he felt under no obligation to provide this medication. Curiously, impotence was the only non-life-threatening health condition treated this way. Other "quality of life" non-life-threatening conditions like acne, for example, were still deemed important enough to be covered in Kaiser's "comprehensive" care. Many health plans followed Kaiser's lead, and at first neither Aetna US Health Care nor any of the Prudential health insurance plans were willing to cover the cost of a single Viagra tablet.[2]

Different insurers proved to be less miserly and grudgingly agreed to cover the cost of Viagra, but only in limited quantity. Tufts Health Plan, a popular Massachusetts insurer, will pay for four Viagra tablets per month, figuring that no man in his right mind would want to have sexual intercourse more than once a week. Each health plan scrambled to cope, and within months after Viagra was available, all had settled on ways to "deal with the Viagra problem." Strategies were hastily devised as each HMO crafted an individual policy on its willingness to pay for Viagra. (See Table 11.10.)

---

[2]Concern for cost was contagious and spread overseas. On Sept 14, 1998, *one day before* Viagra was approved in the United Kingdom; the British Government's Department of Health issued an edict urging doctors not to prescribe Viagra. The widespread availability of Viagra on the Internet pointed out the folly of this edict.

TABLE 11.10   HMO's Policies on covering the cost of Viagra. (Plans vary according to state.)

HMO/ Insurer	Number Viagra Tabs allowed per month.
Kaiser, Prudential, Aetna US Health Care	None (until 12/31/98)
Tufts	4
Cigna	6
Harvard Pilgrim Health Care	4 initially then 2
Blue Cross (various)	4–6
Medicaid	4**

** Maximum allowed by Medicaid in Massachusetts. Some states like New York allow none.

No other medication, including even the most expensive prescription products for lowering high cholesterol levels and any of the other erectile dysfunction treatments, has been so severely restricted. The limitations imposed on Viagra did not, at first, also apply to other approved impotence treatments like Caverject and MUSE. Many insurers even willingly covered the cost of vacuum devices if prescribed by a physician. Why then were HMOs so restrictive when it came to Viagra?

Cost.

Reasons may have differed for each insurer, but in the final analysis, it was not concern for their subscribers' welfare but rather preoccupation *with HMO profitability* that compelled HMOs to either avoid paying for or severely restrict Viagra's availability to their subscribers. Further, they found that they could trivialize the value of this medication by demonizing Viagra as a "sex drug" that would benefit only some sexually obsessed men. Finally, they maintained that Viagra's cost would be a financial burden that would force HMOs to charge more for their annual health-care premiums. Threatening to raise the amount they would have to charge their subscribers, the HMOs were confident they could avoid a customer backlash.

All of this was played out in newspapers and on television news programs. Media watchdogs raised no objection and were perfectly willing to accept the HMOs' explanation that drawing the line with Viagra was just another one of their clever cost-control maneuvers designed to squelch ever-escalating health-care expenses.

Then, when no one objected to their singling out male sexual problems as frivolous concerns, they learned that they could also limit their payments for all erectile dysfunction treatments. In Massachusetts, for example, Blue Cross will cover the cost of Viagra, MUSE, Caverject, or vacuum erection devices only if the patient's private physician discloses intimate details of each man's sexual inadequacies. Prying into patients' lives to this degree is unique to the treatment of erectile dysfunction. In essence, HMOs had made the unilateral decision to single out one medical problem for derision and by so doing ignored the plight and rights of 30 million American men.

Doctors were appalled, patients bewildered, and they collectively contrived new strategies for providing Viagra to men with erectile dysfunction. Some men discovered that the pharmacies in large chain stores like Wal-Mart and K-Mart were, for a while, selling Viagra for about $8.00 per pill rather than the $10.00-per-pill price that prevailed at large chain pharmacies. (The wholesale price to all was about $7.50 per pill.) Those who made this discovery passed the word on to their doctors, who, in turn, encouraged their patients to shop at the less expensive Viagra vendor. Some of my patients who were pleased with the results they achieved with Viagra did not want to limit their sexual activity to the once-a-week schedule ordained by their HMO, which would pay for only four Viagra tablets each month. So they requested two prescriptions, one for the four tablets that would be covered by their insurance and a second one for another four to six, which they would take to another pharmacy, paying cash for the additional pills. This gave these men and their partners the freedom to have sexual intercourse more often than was sanctioned by their HMO.

For a while, some insurers like Harvard Pilgrim Health Care (HPHC) were paying for a few Viagra tablets no matter what the dose. "Aha!" thought doctors prescribing Viagra. Now we can outwit the stingy HMOs. We know that most men can have erections and sexual intercourse after they take a 50-mg Viagra tablet. If we write a prescription for *four 100-mg* Viagra tablets and give the patient a pill splitter, we can effectively provide him with eight 50-mg doses, twice as much Viagra as the HMO is willing to pay for. For example, Harvard Pilgrim Health Care, one of the big insurers in the New England area, set out precisely those guidelines, indicating that it would cover the cost of four Viagra tablets per month. Doctors started writing prescriptions for "Viagra 100 mg, 4 tablets." It did not take the HMOs long to discover the doctors' subterfuge. Within a few months, HPHC had rewritten its guidelines to stipulate that it would only cover the cost of *two Viagra pills* each month.

The politics of Viagra is always in flux. For example, California-based Kaiser Foundation Health Plan, which had dug in its heels refusing to pay for any Viagra, was rebuked by the State of California and ordered to provide for this medication for its subscribers. Kaiser does not plan to appeal this decision, an unusually submissive response considering its strident opposition to providing this drug benefit in the past.

VIAGRA FOR WOMEN?

The phenomenal success of Viagra in men has led some to wonder if Viagra would enhance sexual responsiveness in women. Sexuality in women has several components, including desire (libido), arousal, and orgasm. Not all women are equally enthusiastic about sex. For many, inhibited desire is the primary impediment to pleasure, whereas others have normal desire but just do not get aroused during sex. It is this second group of women with inhibited arousal who are most likely to benefit from Viagra. A woman's clitoris, like a man's penis, is highly vascular and normally becomes engorged with blood during sexual arousal. Some women seem to have difficulty becoming aroused, possibly because of inadequate blood flow to their clitoris. Viagra should be effective for those women. It is less likely to help women with inhibited sexual desire.

Early studies of Viagra in women conducted in Europe were at first disappointing, possibly because the women enrolled in these studies had a mixed bag of sexual problems, including many with inhibited sexual desire who would not improve with Viagra. Only those with arousal phase disorders could be expected to respond to Viagra. When more definitive placebo-controlled studies restricted to women with arousal phase disorder are completed, we will know for sure whether the medication that works wonders in impotent men will be as effective in those women who currently derive little satisfaction from sex.

WHAT'S NEXT AFTER VIAGRA?

IC351

Eli Lilly Corporation, a pharmaceutical company known for its insulin products, the antidepressant Prozac, and many commonly used medications, has established a joint venture with ICOS Corporation to develop a PDE-5 inhibitor currently known only by the designation IC351. Preliminary reports have been encouraging. Men with mild to moderate impotence took IC351 or a placebo and then viewed an erotic video. Increased erectile strength and vigor and duration of erections was evident from RigiScan recordings during IC351 treatment but not with placebo. Additional IC351 studies will have to be performed to determine the long-term safety and efficacy of this new medication. Inevitably, IC351 will be pitted against Viagra to determine the differences, if any, in patient satisfaction as well as the side effects of both medications.

Vasomax

Shortly after Viagra was approved, news of other pills specifically designed to make it easier for men to have erections started to appear in the popular press. The one that seems to have created the greatest buzz was a medication called Vasomax, a pill containing phentolamine. Urologists were very familiar with this medication, for they had been injecting phentolamine directly into the penis to stimulate erections in impotent men for years. When injected alone, phentolamine was only marginally effective in inducing erections, but like a gasoline additive, it did improve the efficiency and minimized noxious side effects of the more powerful penile erection medications. Used as a fusion "cocktail"—that is, a sprinkling of phentolamine, along with a dash of papaverine and a pinch of alprostadil—the combination known as Tri-Mix enjoyed some popularity as a kinder, gentler intrapenile injection regimen. It was alleged that bundling the three medications worked best, as Tri-Mix erections were more consistent and side effects less apparent than when either papaverine or alprostadil was used alone.

Like many other medications, phentolamine had been around for decades, approved by the FDA as a blood-pressure-lowering medication for both men and women whose high blood pressure was caused by a rare condition of an adrenaline-producing tumor of the adrenal gland called a pheochromocytoma (Pheo). Phentolamine can counteract the adrenaline effect by blunting propensity to cause blood vessels to narrow (constrict) and drive blood pressure up. Phentolamine allows vascular spaces to relax, dilate, or widen, specifically what is needed to allow blood to flow into the penile erectile chambers, and precisely what is needed to encourage the development of an erection.

Although business pages have been trumpeting the arrival of this new pill to treat impotence, which is said to be as effective "as Viagra, but with fewer side effects," very little information has been available for scientists to analyze.

The first published report of the use of phentolamine pills to treat erectile dysfunction came in 1988. Dr. Grant Gwinup, who had some experience with phentolamine because he had used it to treat men and women with pheochromocytomas, learned that urologists had started using intrapenile phentolamine injections to stimulate an erection. Dr. Gwinup rounded up eight men with erectile dysfunction and gave them either placebo pills or phentolamine tablets to see if they had any improvement in their erections. He decided to give some men either placebo or phentolamine first and then in phase two reversed the order of pills. When placebo was given first, two of eight men had erections, whereas when phentolamine was first, erections occurred in five of eight men. Two men who did not have erections with phentolamine had erections with placebo. The results were so confusing that no further research with phentolamine pills was done for another decade.

Then, in April 1998, one month after the FDA approved Viagra, another article evaluating the effectiveness of oral phentolamine appeared. By this time phentolamine had a new name, Vasomax. This time forty impotent men had their erectile function evaluated after they took placebo pills or different doses of Vasomax (Table 11.11).

TABLE 11.11   Effect of Placebo and Vasomax (Oral Phentolamine pills) on erectile function in impotent men

Medication & dose	Number of Men	Full erections
Placebo	10	2
Vaomax 10 mg	10	3
Vasomax 40 mg	10	5
Vasomax 60 mg	10	4

The results are presented in Table 11.11 above but can be summarized as follows. The men studied were considered to have impotence for at least three years and were treated with placebo pills or three different doses of Vasomax. Twenty percent of placebo-treated men said they achieved full erections with placebo, whereas full erections were reported by 30 percent of men after 10 mg, 50 percent of men after 40 mg, and 40 percent of men after the 60-mg dose of Vasomax.

The 20 percent of men who had erectile function restored after placebo is similar to the 24 percent of placebo responders in the earlier Viagra trials. However, unlike those studies that demonstrated 70–80 percent responses with escalating Viagra doses, no more than 50 percent of Vasomax-treated men had improved erectile function; and surprisingly, in this small study, an increasing dose was not associated with increased response. It is possible that larger studies may reveal increased effectiveness of Vasomax, but for the moment, the available data indicate that this medication is considerably less effective than Viagra.

12

Hormones and Sexuality

Hormones course through your bloodstream every moment of every day, yet you usually remain oblivious to their presence. Only when production exceeds or fails to keep pace with your daily needs are you obliged to acknowledge the existence of hormones. Some hormones *enhance*, and others *inhibit*, normal male sexual function. For example, testosterone is the hormone all men and some women need to become and remain sexually active. Prolactin, on the other hand, is a sexually inhibiting hormone for men as well as women. This chapter describes which hormones do and do not boost a man's sexuality.

The word "hormone" comes from the Greek word *horman*, which means "to urge on." Testosterone is the hormone responsible for urging on a man's sexual function.

Other critical testosterone-dependent actions are:

- Development of normal male genital anatomy
- Activation and maintenance of adult male sex drive
- Preservation of normal sperm production and fertility
- Maintenance of strong bones
- To help maximize muscle and minimize fat mass

WHAT IS NORMAL?

Testosterone in the Womb and the Normal Infant Male

The impact of testosterone is apparent very early in life. Immediately before conception, a swarm of sperm circle the ovum. Only one will inseminate. All others will be rebuffed. If the inseminating sperm carries a Y chromosome, the fetus will be genetically destined to develop as a boy. Then the developing infant's gonad is programmed to develop as a testicle. Thereafter, hormones take over. Surprisingly, all of the hormonal activity required to define a child as a male takes place in his mother's womb within a relatively narrow time frame.

The developing boy's fetal testicle begins to secrete testosterone as early as the twelfth week of pregnancy. From this point on, *testosterone* and its metabolic offspring, the powerful male hormone *dihydrotestosterone* (DHT), help sculpt the appearance of the normal baby boy's genitals. The period of fetal testosterone-dihydrotestosterone production is fleeting, extending only from the twelfth to the twenty-fourth week of pregnancy. After the twenty-fourth week of pregnancy, the testicles enter a state of hormonal hibernation and are dormant. By this time, the short-lived intrauterine exposure to testosterone and dihydrotestosterone have properly defined the genital anatomy of the male fetus. Weeks later, when the child emerges from the womb to be born, all eyes will be riveted on the area between the newborn's thighs. Then, seeing a penis and a well-developed scrotum swaddling two tiny testicles, the doctor, midwife, or mother will proclaim with some glee, "It's a boy!"

The Transition from Boy to Man and the Activation of Male Sexual Desire

A young boy's gonadal hormone production is restrained and held in check during his preadolescent period. Only a trickle of testosterone leaks out from the testicle in these formative years. Then, at about age thirteen or fourteen, an extraordinary event occurs. The dormant testicle suddenly starts manufacturing and releasing large amounts of testosterone into the bloodstream. This surge of testosterone provokes a series of dramatic and well-recognized events.

In response to the sudden surge in blood testosterone levels, the young boy/man notices that:

- Glands in his skin increase the production of sebum; acne often follows.
- His vocal cords thicken; his voice first cracks, then deepens.
- His muscles grow.
- He has a midadolescent growth spurt and his height increases dramatically as bone growth centers (epiphyses) elongate. When testosterone closes epiphyses at age sixteen to eighteen, his growth ceases.
- His mustache hair and beard whiskers begin to appear.
- His sweat glands pump out secretions with a distinctly musky odor.
- His penis becomes longer and wider.
- His scrotum becomes wrinkled with ridges.
- His testicles start growing and enlarge to fill the scrotal sac.
- He may note that he is starting to experience stiffening of his penis in the middle of the night. This is the onset of nocturnal erections.

- He may also be befuddled to discover that he has had a nocturnal emission, or "wet dream."
- Equally perplexing is the sudden shift in attitude toward the girls in his class, who are, inexplicably, no longer insufferable but actually desirable.

All these startling transformations are due to one hormone, and that hormone is testosterone. Tethered and restrained during his preteen years, testosterone production is quite suddenly cut loose and set free to wreak havoc with his body.

What Causes the Sudden Increase in Testosterone Production During Adolescence?

Spontaneous testosterone secretion does not occur. The testicle requires a go-ahead signal from the youngster's brain, which somehow knows that it is time to make the transition from boy to man. The pituitary gland, a tiny pea-sized structure tucked away at the base of the brain, is pressed into service. The pituitary hormone responsible for overseeing testosterone production is luteinizing hormone (LH). Under the influence of LH, the testicle starts siphoning cholesterol from the bloodstream. Enzymes in the testicle gnaw away at the unwieldy cholesterol molecule to manufacture and release testosterone.

Anything that interferes with normal testosterone production or action causes a decrease in libido and ultimately impotence. Some men have suboptimal testosterone production as a consequence of inadequate pituitary stimulation of the testicle. Without LH to stimulate it, the testicle does not manufacture testosterone. But it is not only the mere availability of LH but also the manner in which LH is delivered to a man's gonads that determines the testicle's ability to make testosterone.

The testicle is finicky. It will not respond to a steady stream of LH. The testicle produces testosterone only when periodic bursts or pulses of LH appear in the bloodstream. This is precisely what occurs at the onset of adolescence when there is a sudden shift in activity in the hypothalamus. (See Figure 12.1.)

The hypothalamus, pituitary, and testicle remain in a state of suspended animation until adolescence. Then, for reasons not fully understood, the hypothalamus acquires the ability to release bursts of a hormone that triggers the pulsatile secretion of pituitary LH. Pulses of LH released from the pituitary travel through the bloodstream to activate testosterone production.

LH is referred to as a *gonadotropin* because it stimulates the male *gonad* (testicle). The hypothalamic hormone, called gonadotropin-releasing hor-

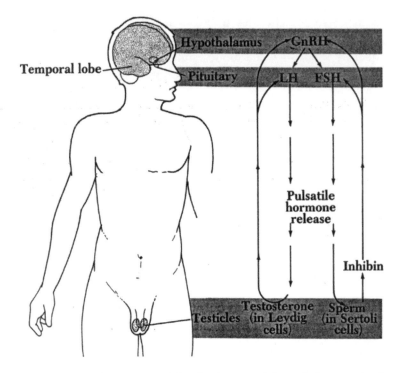

FIGURE 12.1   How hormones originating in a man's hypothalamus stimulate the pituitary to activate testosterone secretion from his testicles.

mone (GnRH), provides the hypothalamic stimulus for pulsatile release of LH from the pituitary.

The hormonal interaction among the hypothalamus, the pituitary, and the testicles is a bond that persists throughout a man's life. This entire system, referred to as the hypothalamic-pituitary-testicular axis, is responsible for creating and maintaining a man's libido, sexual potency, and fertility.

Sperm Maturation and Fertility

Male fertility demands an output of hundreds of millions of sperm from the testicle every day. Two hormones—testosterone and a second pituitary gonadotropin, known as follicle-stimulating hormone (FSH)—are charged with the responsibility of ensuring that the testicle meets its quota for sperm production every day. FSH is yet another pituitary hormone released from the pituitary in tandem with LH. Both LH and FSH levels increase in response to episodic pulses of GnRH. Both speed through the body to activate designated cells in the testicle.

SEXUAL HEALTH FOR MEN

TABLE 12.1   Causes of inadequate testosterone production in man

Problem	Possible Causes	Testosterone- LH
Primary Hypogonadism	Klinefelter's syndrome, mumps other viruses, radiation,trauma, chemotherapy	Low-High
Secondary	Pituitary-hypothalamic tumors, hyperprolactinemia	Low-Low
Miscellaneous	Aging, Obesity, Alcoholism	Low- Normal

FSH affects sperm production, whereas LH initiates testosterone production. The abundant supply of testosterone within the testicle is required for sperm to mature and attain full fertilizing capability. (See Chapter 25.)

WHAT CAN GO WRONG? SPECIFIC HORMONE PROBLEMS

Low Testosterone Production

If a man loses his ability to maintain adequate testosterone production, blood testosterone levels will decline and he will suffer a diminution in sex drive and become impotent.

Conditions responsible for low testosterone output are designated as primary hypogonadism and secondary hypogonadism. When the testicle itself does not function properly, the diagnosis is *primary hypogonadism*. In contrast, *secondary hypogonadism* occurs when normal testicles cannot manufacture testosterone because the stimulating hormones of the pituitary or hypothalamus are missing or inadequate.

Primary Hypogonadism

Primary hypogonadism may be congenital (present at birth), like Klinefelter's syndrome, acquired as the result of a virus that lodges in the testicles, or caused by external assaults such as testicular injury, radiation treatment, and chemotherapy. (See Table 12.1.)

Occasionally, failure of the gonads is ordained at conception. Instead of the normal complement of forty-six chromosomes—*46 XY*—some men are born with one extra X chromosome. This results in an unusual chromosomal pattern *47 XXY*. The condition is called Klinefelter's syndrome, after the physician who first recognized and described the characteristic physical features of this disorder.

As children, boys with the 47 XXY group of chromosomes are indistinguishable from other boys. The first signs of Klinefelter's syndrome surface during adolescence. Although the pulsating rhythms of the hypothalamus and pituitary start on schedule, the testicles of the boy afflicted with this syndrome are unable to respond.

Some youngsters with Klinefelter's syndrome produce no testosterone at all. They retain a youthful appearance, but without testosterone to signal an end to their adolescent growth spurt, they continue to grow and often become very tall. Under the continuous influence of growth hormone, boys grow taller, tower over their classmates, and often bring a twinkle to the eye of the high-school basketball coach. Despite their height, young boys with Klinefelter's syndrome do not make good basketball players because without adequate testosterone, their muscles remain unstimulated and undeveloped. This is yet another legacy of their testosterone deficiency.

Not all young men with Klinefelter's have such severe defects. Some boys make some testosterone early in their adolescence, do not grow to unusual heights, and become virilized. Their testicles produce testosterone briefly, then sputter, and thereafter fail. Men with the milder form of Klinefelter's syndrome have low sexual desire but may enjoy brief intervals of potency. They eventually suffer the same fate as their more severely affected counterparts. As their testicles fail, testosterone and sperm production cannot proceed and they are left impotent and infertile.

Mumps and Other Viruses

The cells that produce testosterone contribute very little to testicular size. Sperm-producing cells make up the bulk of testicular tissue. Often the same process that destroys the testicle's testosterone-producing capability also attacks the sperm-producing cells. When this happens, the testicle shrinks (or atrophies). This is often the fate of men who develop mumps as adults.

Childhood mumps generally spares the testicle. But when mumps strikes an adult male, the virus may spread through the bloodstream and attack his testicles. Initially, the testicles swell and feel extremely tender. As the infection subsides, the testicles decrease in size. What follows is a predictable sequence of events.

First, sperm-producing cells and later testosterone-secreting cells are damaged, compromising fertility and eventually sex drive and potency.

Raymond had two children, both in their twenties, both adopted. He had come to terms with his infertility and even joked that his low sperm count allowed him to save a fortune on birth control. Now, at fifty-seven, Raymond was impotent, and he had run out of jokes. The cause of his current impotence and prior infertility were traced to a common event. Thirty years earlier, while an elementary schoolteacher, he contracted mumps, which caused pain and swelling in both testicles. The pain was so severe that he could not bear to have his testicles touched and was obliged to wear an athletic supporter for two weeks. He and his wife resumed normal sexual activity when the swelling subsided, but she did not become pregnant. A semen analysis revealed that he had a low sperm count. That was when he and his wife decided to adopt. He remained potent for more than two decades. Then he noticed a gradual decline in his interest in sex and ability to acquire and sustain an erection. Hormone studies now revealed low serum testosterone levels. The infection that had destroyed his testicles' sperm-producing cells had left sufficient residual damage to compromise testosterone secretion. Testosterone treatment restored potency.

Other viruses that lodge in the testicles produce symptoms that are less dramatic than those of mumps, but the net effect is the same.

Secondary Hypogonadism

Men with *normal testicles* may still be incapable of producing testosterone if the stimulus to testosterone production is absent or blunted. The causes of secondary hypogonadism include benign tumors (adenomas) of the pituitary and the hypothalamus.

Pituitary Adenomas

The pituitary gland is responsible for regulating thyroid, adrenal, and testicular hormone secretion. When the pituitary becomes tumorous, these functions cannot be sustained. It is still capable of low-level hormone production, but it does not respond adequately to the pulsating hypothalamic GnRH hormone. As a result, pituitary hormones seep out, rather than burst out, into the bloodstream. The testicle will not respond to pituitary LH if it is not delivered in pulsatile bursts. Without LH pulses, the testicle cannot manufacture sufficient testosterone, and blood testosterone levels decline.

Tumors that destroy the pituitary's LH-secreting capability can also compromise other pituitary functions. It is in the pituitary gland that adrenocorticotropin (ACTH) and thyroid stimulating hormone (TSH) are made and released into the bloodstream to activate adrenal and thyroid hormone secretion, respectively. Inadequate secretion of all pituitary hormones causes a severe illness, *panhypopituitarism*. In addition to impotence, patients suffer low blood pressure, weakness, fatigue, and other symptoms of adrenal and thyroid hormone deficiency. The majority of these symptoms are relieved by adrenal and thyroid hormone medications. But treatment with testosterone restores potency to only 50 percent of the affected men; those who remain impotent have pituitary tumors that produce excessive amounts of the hormone prolactin. Men with pituitary tumors who regained potency with

---

testosterone injections had low serum prolactin levels. Those who remained impotent had high serum prolactin levels (hyperprolactinemia).

What Is Prolactin and Why Does It Disrupt Male Sexual Function?

We frankly do not know why men have prolactin-producing capability at all. Prolactin serves an important function in women, but only at a specific moment in their reproductive lives. At the end of a woman's pregnancy, her pituitary produces and releases generous amounts of prolactin into the bloodstream to stimulate breast-milk production. Nursing mothers usually have no menstrual periods because prolactin levels, when elevated, extinguish the pulses of pituitary hormones required to activate the normal menstrual cycle. When a woman stops nursing, prolactin levels decrease, pulsatile pituitary hormone secretion resumes, and menstrual function returns.

How does this relate to impotence in men? The same hormonal events that cause hyperprolactinemic women to stop menstruating while they are nursing also causes hyperprolactinemic men to become impotent.

Elevated serum prolactin levels create two problems that are inimical to sexual potency. With high serum prolactin levels, normal pulsatile GnRH and LH secretion does not proceed. This is why nursing mothers stop menstruating. Without pulsatile LH release, a man's testicle is stranded without adequate stimulation and cannot produce its full ration of testosterone. Serum testosterone levels then fall. But giving more testosterone is not the remedy because elevated serum prolactin levels also prevent the body from responding normally to testosterone.

Two treatments—one surgical, the other medical—curtail excessive prolactin secretion by the pituitary.

Surgical removal of the prolactin-secreting pituitary tumor eliminates the source of excessive prolactin. Unfortunately, excision of only the pituitary tumor, while desirable, is not always feasible. Whittling away at the pituitary mass does make a significant dent in prolactin secretion but rarely decreases it to the normal range. In these cases, impotence persists.

Doctors have discovered that a chemical in the body called *dopamine* normally reins in pituitary prolactin secretion in men. Without dopamine, prolactin levels increase. A selective dopamine deficiency in the hypothalamus is therefore presumed to be responsible for hyperprolactinemia in men. By restoring dopamine levels to normal, pituitary prolactin production is suppressed.

Three medications, bromocriptine (Parlodel), pergolide (Permax), and cabergoline (Dostinex) have dopaminelike properties, and any of them can be an effective dopamine surrogate. When hyperprolactinemic men or women are treated with bromocriptine (Parlodel), pergolide (Permax) or cabergoline (Dostinex), serum prolactin levels promptly return to normal. Continued treatment is required to keep prolactin levels fully suppressed.

This treatment has been effective in two respects. Lowering serum prolactin levels to normal restores sensitivity to the sexual effects of testosterone. *As serum prolactin levels fall, serum testosterone levels increase and potency returns.* Bromocriptine (Parlodel) or cabergoline (Dostinex) treatment also decreases pituitary tumor size and shrinks prolactin-secreting tumor tissue.

In some impotent hyperprolactinemic men, bromocriptine (Parlodel) or cabergoline (Dostinex) treatment alone suffices. Men with recent onset of impotence and small pituitary tumors are more likely to respond. Other men, especially those with large pituitary tumors, are not able to revitalize their own testosterone-producing capability without the additional help of testosterone injections or patches. Once serum prolactin levels are normalized, these impotent men regain their responsiveness to the sexually stimulating effects of testosterone.

Vincent was forty-one, weak, fatigued, impotent, about to lose his business and maybe his wife. His doctor noted that Vincent had unusually low blood pressure and small testicles. X-rays disclosed an enlarged pituitary, and blood tests established that—as a consequence of inadequate stimulation from his pituitary—adrenal, thyroid, and testicular hormone production were subnormal. Treatment with adrenal and thyroid hormones so invigorated Vincent that he was able to return to work, and his business prospered. Testosterone injections normalized serum testosterone levels, but he remained impotent. Ordinarily, testosterone-deficient men experience a brisk increase in sexual desire and potency with testosterone therapy. Treatment failures occur in men who have, in addition to their testosterone deficiency, other problems such as neuropathy, vascular disease, depression, or hyperprolactinemia. In Vincent's case, hyperprolactinemia was the culprit. His large pituitary gland, incapable of supporting function of his adrenal, thyroid, or testicle, was not totally inert, for it continued to produce prolactin in exorbitant amounts. Only when bromocriptine treatment normalized serum prolactin levels were testosterone injections effective in restoring Vincent's sexual drive and potency.

Bromocriptine was the treatment of choice once it was established that Vincent's sexual problems were linked with his high serum prolactin level. At that time, bromocriptine was the only medication available to normalize his serum prolactin level.

Subsequently another prolactin-lowering medication, pergolide (Permax), was made available. Both bromocriptine and pergolide will lower prolactin production, but to be effective, they must be taken every day. Cabergoline (Dostinex) also lowers prolactin production but differs from bromocriptine and pergolide because of its long duration of action. Taken once a week, or at most twice weekly, cabergoline is all that is needed to normalize serum prolactin and testosterone levels in the majority of hyperprolactinemic men and women.

Pituitary tumors are not the only causes of hyperprolactinemia. Many drugs used to treat high blood pressure, emotional problems, and gastric problems can compromise the action of dopamine and allow prolactin levels to increase. These problem drugs include reserpine (Serpasil), methyldopa (Aldomet), chlorpromazine (Thorazine), trifluoperazine (Stelazine), thioridazine (Mellaril), haloperidol (Haldol), prochlorperazine (Compazine), and metoclopramide (Reglan).[1]

Tumors of the Hypothalamus

Although the hormones responsible for triggering testicular hormone secretions are based in the pituitary, hormones released by an area of the brain called the hypothalamus govern the fate of these pituitary hormones. Tumors of the hypothalamus severely limit the pulsatile release of hormones.

Hormone pulses must occur with sufficient frequency and reach sufficient amplitude to be effective. If the pulses occur infrequently, or with too little vigor, testosterone levels fall and men become impotent.

Time takes a toll on the intensity of the hypothalamic-pituitary signal to the testicle. With aging, the hypothalamus slows down and pulses with less strength. This may be one of the explanations for the fall in testosterone levels in men as they age.

Hypogonadism, Cause Unknown

One group of men with no visible hypothalamic or pituitary abnormality is incapable of launching pulsatile GnRH secretion at adolescence. Their LH pulses are totally absent, causing impotence and infertility. The condition, called idiopathic hypogonadotropic hypogonadism, can be corrected by re-instituting normal GnRH pulses.

[1]Although medication-induced elevations in serum prolactin level disrupt man's sexual function, this side effect can benefit some women. One *prolactin-stimulating* medication, metoclopramide (Reglan), has been used to help mothers of premature infants produce more breast milk. Ordinarily as a woman proceeds through a full pregnancy, her body produces progressively increasing amounts of estrogen and prolactin to stimulate breast-milk production. With shortened pregnancies, peak prolactin production does not occur naturally and breast-milk output is often inadequate. Metoclopramide (Reglan) stimulates pituitary prolactin output and can augment breast-milk production to the satisfaction of both the nursing mother and her baby.

Thyroid Hormone Disorders

The thyroid hormone thyroxine stabilizes the body's metabolism and allows us to proceed on an even keel from day to day. Both excessive and inadequate thyroxine production (hyperthyroidism and hypothyroidism) can interfere with normal male sexual function.

The diagnosis of thyroid hormone disorders is usually not difficult in young men. Nervousness, palpitations, weight loss, tremor, and anxiety are manifestations of excessive thyroid hormone secretion. Fatigue, lethargy, slowness of thought, constipation, dry skin, cold intolerance, and a deepening voice are indications of hypothyroidism.

In the older man, symptoms are more subtle. An irregular heartbeat or unexplained weight loss may be a clue to an overactive thyroid. Memory loss can reflect inadequate thyroid production. In the middle-aged or older male, impotence may be the only obvious evidence of either condition.

Daniel, a fifty-two-year-old scientist, became impotent shortly after his divorce. His impotence was thought to be related to depression, and he had been seeing a psychiatrist for about one year. He had made some progress coping with his postdivorce depression, but his impotence persisted. Now he had a new problem—his left breast seemed to be growing.

Physical examination revealed a rapid pulse and a slightly enlarged thyroid. Daniel's left breast was indeed large and glandular. His hands trembled. The thyroid enlargement, increased breast size, rapid pulse, and tremor suggested the possibility of an overactive thyroid. Blood tests provided confirmation. With treatment, thyroid hormone levels normalized, breast tissue receded, and potency was restored.

Disorders of thyroid function are generally not considered in the evaluation of impotence despite the fact that loss of libido (in about 70 percent of cases), impotence (in about 55 percent of cases), and breast enlargement (incidence unknown) are prominent in hyperthyroid men. It remains unclear exactly how hyperthyroidism predisposes men to these sexual problems. The hyperthyroid state does create several associated hormonal abnormalities. Testosterone production is adequate, but the body converts an inordinate amount of the testosterone into an estrogen hormone (estradiol). Correction of the hyperthyroidism diminishes the stimulus for excessive estrogen production and coincides with a return of libido and potency.

Men with underactive thyroids tend to have low serum testosterone levels. Correction of the hypothyroidism usually allows serum testosterone levels to return to normal, and sexual function resumes. Unfortunately, some hypothyroid patients experience failure of both thyroid and testicular hormone secretion. For those men, treatment with thyroid hormone and testosterone together is necessary to restore metabolic, and then sexual, health.

Men with hypothyroidism have one other hormone abnormality that contributes to their sexual dysfunction. Their serum prolactin levels are often elevated. For them, bromocriptine treatment is unnecessary; thyroid hormone alone will normalize prolactin levels. Once prolactin levels normalize, sexual function resumes.

TREATMENTS TO INCREASE
A MAN'S TESTOSTERONE LEVELS

Testosterone Pills and Injections

Hormone therapy returns sexual function to the vast majority of men with specific disturbances in their body chemistry. The basic principle of any hormone therapy is to re-create a state of hormonal equilibrium. For men with thyroid or adrenal hormone disorders, this can be accomplished with hormone pills. Unfortunately, such is not the case for impotent men with testosterone deficiency.

Testosterone pills are available, but they are less effective than testosterone given by injection. Testosterone pills are not well absorbed from the stomach, and blood testosterone does not always reach useful therapeutic levels. The pills also have a serious side effect—liver damage.

Giving testosterone injections once a week, every two weeks, or even once a month, although effective, causes wide fluctuations in serum testosterone levels, with highest values occurring shortly after injection. Then, with normal metabolism, levels fall until the next injection. This results in a variable sexual response. Adjusting the dose or frequency of testosterone injections smoothes out testosterone levels and maintains a steady state of sexual function.

Testosterone Skin Patches

Prescribing testosterone has, until recently, been fairly prosaic, for doctors had only to choose between the daily administration of a testosterone pill or periodic testosterone injections to maintain normal testosterone levels in the bloodstream of testosterone-deficient men. Testosterone pills had been under a cloud because they were burdened by a legacy of liver toxicity. No comparable problem plagued testosterone injections, but even though they were safe, their effectiveness depended on their being given as deep intramuscular injections every two to three weeks. Although both testosterone

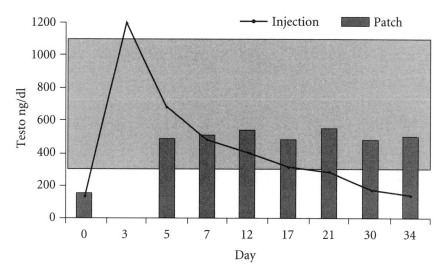

FIGURE 12.2   Blood testosterone levels after a single injection of long-acting testosterone on day 0 or daily application of a testosterone patch.

pills and injections worked, they were considered to be far from ideal, and scientists started looking for new, less toxic and more convenient ways to provide a man with the testosterone he needed. That is what spurred the development of the testosterone skin patch.

Doctors have been rubbing medications on the skin surface for years with good results, for they knew that blood circulating under the skin and nourishing it would absorb and transport medicine from the skin into the bloodstream. Cigarette smokers eager to stop can go into any drug store and pick up a set of nicotine-impregnated skin patches programmed to deliver progressively decreasing amounts of that drug to help them kick the nicotine habit.

Today postmenopausal women have, at their disposal, a variety of estrogen-containing pills and at least two different types of estrogen skin patches to overcome their diminished estrogen production, but until recently, the production of a testosterone patch seemed to stymie scientists. However, the technical problems that plagued early efforts of testosterone-patch development have been overcome. Today, there are three testosterone skin patches available. They are marketed under the names Testoderm, Androderm, and Testoderm TTS.

All three patches provide a steady supply of testosterone, helping to stabilize serum testosterone levels in testosterone-deficient men, and they avoid the dramatic swings in serum testosterone levels that occur with testosterone injections. (See Figure 12.2.) However, to maintain their effectiveness, patches must be changed daily and applied properly.

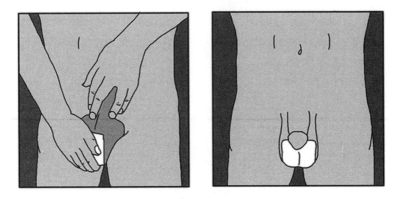

FIGURE 12.3   Proper placement of Testoderm scrotal patch

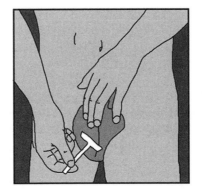

FIGURE 12.4   Dry shaving of
scrotal hair prior to placement of
Testoderm scrotal patch.

- The original Testoderm patch is only effective when placed on the thin skin of the scrotum. (See Figure 12.3.) To maximize adherence to this sensitive area, it is necessary to "dry shave" the fine hairs in this area. (See Figure 12.4.) Then the patch must be heated with a hair dryer to activate testosterone embedded within the patch to expedite hormone release after the patch is applied to the scrotum.
- The Androderm patch, on the other hand, can be worn on any portion of the body. The most common sites of application are the arms, back, and buttocks. No shaving or heating is required. However, two 2.5-mg

TABLE 12.2   Current Treatments Used to Increase Man's Testosterone Levels

Type	Route	Example	Problems
Pill	by mouth	Android	Liver damage
Injection	Intra-muscular	Depo-T	Pain
Patch 1	Scrotum	Testoderm	Shave scrotal hairs
Patch 2	Arms, Legs, Torso	Androderm	Rash
Patch 3	Arms, Legs, Torso	Testoderm TTS	Rash

> patches or a single larger 5-mg Androderm body patch must be used to achieve the same effect as a single 6-mg scrotal Testoderm patch.
>
> • The manufacturers of the original scrotal Testoderm patch have developed a newer Testoderm TTS patch that is also effective when affixed to a man's torso or extremities.

All three patches can help normalize a man's testosterone level without causing the variations in the testosterone levels that are so common with testosterone injection therapy (Table 12.2).

Problems with Testosterone Patch Therapy

To be effective in transferring testosterone from the patch into a man's bloodstream, patches must remain in close proximity to the skin. The adhesive in the patch usually takes care of this, but the bond between the adhesive and skin breaks down when men sweat. None of the patches are effective when wet. Men who like to go to the gym to exercise learn this very quickly and will often remove their patch and store it on a shelf in their lockers just before starting their workout. Then they can work up a sweat during exercise or plunge into a pool or hot tub without compromising the effectiveness of their patch. When they have concluded their workout they can shower and towel off, and once dry, can safely reaffix the testosterone patch to maintain its effectiveness.

It is not just those men who exercise at the gym who must follow these guidelines. Men who sweat copiously while gardening or doing heavy labor or perspire during periods of increased stress must be aware that sweating will limit the effectiveness of their testosterone-impregnated patches and take similar precautions.

Skin Reactions with Testosterone Patches

The key element needed for the patches to work is a substance called a chemical "enhancer." It is the enhancer that makes it possible for testosterone to get out of the patch, go through the skin, and enter the bloodstream. Differences in enhancer properties define both effectiveness and toxicity, with Testoderm's enhancer working only when applied to thin scrotal skin, whereas the enhancer in the Androderm and Testoderm TTS patches is significantly stronger, permitting diffusion of testosterone across all skin surfaces, but not without extracting a toll. Skin irritation, rashes, itching, and occasionally blisters and hives are among the reactions commonly associated with the use of the Androderm and Testoderm TTS patches. (Curiously, skin irritation is less common with the scrotal Testoderm patch.) Some men have no skin irritation at all with either the Androderm or Testoderm TTS body patch, whereas others do. Men who have fairer skin seem to be more likely to develop these skin reactions and rashes. Those who are susceptible to skin reactions can minimize or totally prevent the occurrence of the rash by pretreating the skin with a pea-sized dollop of a cortisone-like cream called triamcinolone. (I usually offer a prescription for triamcinolone cream whenever I write a prescription for either Androderm or Testoderm TTS patches.)

Newer Testosterone Delivery Systems

In addition to the testosterone patches, other products are just now being developed for testosterone-deficient men. One company is developing a sublingual (under the tongue) testosterone pill that allows testosterone to be absorbed through the mouth, bypassing the stomach and thereby avoiding the liver toxicity associated with currently available testosterone tablets. Another pharmaceutical firm is investigating testosterone and dihydrotestosterone gels that are rubbed directly on the skin and absorbed into the bloodstream. These gels will be sold as "single-dose sachets." The sachets will look like the ketchup packets currently available at local fast-food chains. Men will tear the top off the sachet and rub the gel on the surface of their skin. Absorption is rapid, and blood testosterone levels increase within a few minutes to an hour after the gel is applied. In early studies, rashes have not been a problem. A new drug application for the testosterone gel is currently pending before the FDA.

Others are working on the development of very long-acting testosterone implants to provide a stable source of testosterone for several months. The impetus for the development of this wide array of testosterone products may relate to the perceived needs of the increasing numbers of healthy older men in whom advancing years and retreating testosterone production coincide. (See Chapter 27.)

What Else Can Be Done to Enhance a Man's Testosterone Output?

Three techniques, one old and two new, have been developed to allow men to increase the testosterone output of their testicles.

---

1. Human chorionic gonadotropin as an LH surrogate.
2. Pulsatile GnRH release via implantable pump.
3. Clomiphene.

Human Chorionic Gonadotropin is an LH surrogate.   The testicles of men with secondary hypogonadism are inherently normal but lack the appropriate stimulus to make testosterone. If that stimulus can be provided, the testicles should be able to function once again.

Produced by women during pregnancy, human chorionic gonadotropin (hCG) acts directly on a man's testicular Leydig cells to stimulate testosterone production. Synthetic hCG is available and when injected into the muscle of the shoulder or buttocks enters the bloodstream and acts just like LH to provoke a brisk increase in serum testosterone levels. Unfortunately, the effect of a single hCG injection is short-lived; twice-weekly injections are needed. This is more troublesome than a testosterone injection once a month. Today, hCG treatment is reserved for infertile men with low sperm counts.

HCG acts directly on the testicle, bypassing the hypothalamus and pituitary. The two new treatment methods increase testosterone production by activating a man's hypothalamus or pituitary.

GnRH Pump Therapy.   Dr. William Crowley of Massachusetts General Hospital has developed a small battery-powered pump that is loaded with the hypothalamic hormone GnRH. The patient wears the device on his hip. A thin tube extending from the pump ends in a needle that is placed under the skin of impotent men with GnRH deficiency (idiopathic hypogonadotropic hypogonadism). The pump is programmed to release pulses of GnRH to stimulate pulsatile release of both pituitary LH and FSH. Exposed to LH pulses, the testicle starts manufacturing testosterone, and potency is restored. Pulsatile FSH release is also activated so that sperm production increases gradually. This enables a group of men previously thought to be hopelessly impotent and infertile to have a normal sex life and become fathers. (See Chapter 25.)

Clomiphene.   Clomiphene, a medication commonly used to treat infertile women, can also stimulate testosterone production in some men with secondary hypogonadism. Clomiphene is effective in men because it increases pulsatile pituitary LH stimulation of the testicle. Early pilot studies have been encouraging. One clomiphene tablet every other day can maintain normal testosterone levels. This avoids the peaks and valleys of blood testosterone values resulting from testosterone injections. We know this about clomiphene because several investigators, my own group included, have performed clinical investigations to determine how this medication activates and enhances testosterone secretion in men. Clomiphene therapy for men is still considered an experimental or investigational treatment. Clomiphene is currently an FDA-approved medication only for the treatment of infertility in women.

Which Is the Best Test to Assess a Man's Testosterone Level?

While it is convenient to think of testosterone as "the male hormone," there is still more to the story. When testosterone leaves the testicles, it is immediately seized upon and yoked to a blood protein called sex hormone binding globulin (SHBG). The SHBG + Testosterone complex is what the standard testosterone test measures. But when testosterone is linked this way to SHBG, it is ineffective as a male hormone. Only when testosterone is "free" can it work properly. Most often, doctors measure total testosterone levels, not the "free" testosterone. This works out well for younger men.

However, for men past the age of fifty, the "free" testosterone measurement provides a more accurate reflection of their male hormone output, as does another test referred to as "bioavailable testosterone" (BT). (See Figure 12.5.)

Finding Hormone Problems in Impotent Men

All the necessary hormone measurements needed to detect hormone abnormalities can be performed on a single blood sample. Hormone levels normally vary throughout the day but generally fall within a range that is bracketed by an upper and lower limit called the reference range. When a *man's blood hormone levels fall within the reference range*, both physician and patient can safely assume that *sexual dysfunction is due to some problem other than hormone malfunction.*

Hormone values do have a tendency to bob up and down throughout the day. Bear in mind: Slight increases in serum prolactin levels above and modest decreases in testosterone below the accepted ranges may occur in perfectly normal potent men. Men whose impotence is truly caused by disorders of hormone production *have sustained and persistently subnormal blood testosterone, elevated prolactin*, or *abnormal thyroid hormone levels.*

Physicians should routinely measure serum testosterone, free testosterone, and prolactin values in impotent patients; thyroid hormone evaluation is usually reserved for those men who have symptoms or show physical signs compatible with disordered thyroid function.

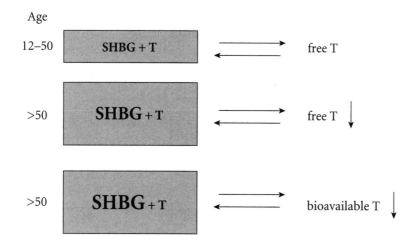

FIGURE 12.5   Most blood testosterone assays measure total testosterone, i.e., testosterone circulating in a man's bloodstream bound to a protein called sex hormone binding globulin (SHBG), but a man's body only responds to testosterone that has shed the shackles of SHBG and is measured as "free" or bioavailable testosterone.

How Common Are
Hormone Problems in Impotent Men?

Hormone abnormalities, once thought to be a rare cause of impotence, are now recognized with increasing frequency. In one study of 422 impotent men at a Veterans Administration hospital, disorders of hormone secretion were detected in 29 percent. Primary hypogonadism and secondary hypogonadism dominated (19 percent), while 4 percent had hyperprolactinemia and 6 percent had disorders of thyroid hormone production.

This coincided with our prior experience. In our 1980 study of 135 impotent men, evidence of hormone dysfunction was found in 34 percent, although we tended to see more hyperprolactinemic patients than our colleagues at the Veterans Administration hospital.

A 1989 survey evaluated hormone function in 600 impotent men in Florida. Thirty-two percent (192 of 600) were found to have disorders of hormone secretion including testosterone deficiency (26 percent), hypothyroidism (6 percent), and hyperprolactinemia (3 percent).

Who Does and Does Not Benefit
from Hormone Therapy?

Hormone treatment is effective only in impotent men with bona fide hormone abnormalities. Indiscriminate use of testosterone, bromocriptine, or thyroid hormone is neither warranted nor effective; the practice

---

of arbitrary administration of testosterone therapy to "boost" testosterone levels is similarly of no value. Testosterone increases libido and improves erectile function only in men with proven low testosterone production.

Adverse effects of hormone therapy are uncommon. Muscular discomfort from an injection can be minimized by rotating the site of injection. Skin irritation from testosterone patches can be minimized by pretreatment of the skin area with a pea-sized dollop of triamcinolone cream. Concern that long-term administration of testosterone by injection or patch might accelerate prostate growth or activate cancer in many testosterone-deficient men has not proven to be a significant problem to date.

Bromocriptine (Parlodel), pergolide (Permax), and cabergoline (Dostinex) can cause nausea and lightheadedness. Symptoms usually can be avoided by taking the drug with food or at bedtime and starting with low doses. For bromocriptine, the initial recommended dosage is half a tablet (1.25 mg), taken at bedtime with a snack, and then the dosage is gradually increased until serum prolactin levels are normal. With cabergoline (Dostinex), 0.5 mg once a week is the starting dose. If serum prolactin levels do not normalize, then twice-weekly cabergoline is recommended (Sunday and Thursday is what my patients prefer). Thyroid hormone administration is relatively free of side effects when dosages are monitored by appropriate blood tests.

If, in addition to hormone abnormalities other problems such as psychologic conflicts exist, the response to hormone therapy will be less than ideal. For this reason, a careful and comprehensive evaluation looking for all possible causes of impotence is recommended before embarking on a course of hormone therapy.

Hormones, Impotence, and the Temporal Lobe

Our understanding of the hormonal interplay necessary for normal male sexual function continues to evolve. Medical professionals used to consider the pituitary the master gland, the agent that doled out specific instructions to regulate the function of the other endocrine glands—thyroid, adrenals, and testicles. Twenty years ago, it became clear that the pituitary could not discharge this important regulatory function on its own but was beholden to a higher hormonal power located in the hypothalamus. The pituitary was then more properly recognized as an intermediary existing to fulfill the hormone directives issued by the hypothalamus.

Just as we became comfortable with this concept, another area of the brain, the temporal lobe, entered the playing field. The role of the temporal lobe in hormone secretion appears to be more meddlesome than regulatory. This is especially true when viewing the effect of temporal lobe influences on male sexual function.

Scientists studying the temporal lobe in humans were fully aware of its critical role in the reproductive and sexual function of animals. Experimental destruction of a specific portion of the temporal lobe (the amygdala) caused testicular degeneration in male rats and cats. Implants of estrogen in rabbits' amygdalae provoked hyperprolactinemia. But how do these animal experiments relate to humans?

As mentioned, some men suffer from a temporal lobe disorder called temporal lobe epilepsy (TLE). They have decreased libido and are often impotent. Some of these men have low serum testosterone levels; others have increased blood levels of prolactin.

TLE is different from other forms of epilepsy. Early symptoms are subtle and are characterized by a series of "spells." Sudden attacks of abdominal pain, dizziness, fugue states, bed-wetting, and rage as well as auditory hallucinations may be clues to the presence of a temporal lobe disorder. The coexistence of a form of epilepsy and a hormone disorder initially created a dilemma for the physician. Which condition should be treated first?

Experience provided the answer. Patients with TLE and hypogonadism are, at first, unresponsive to testosterone injections, and those with TLE and hyperprolactinema do not benefit from bromocriptine. (This distinguishes them from other hypogonadal or hyperprolactinemic men.) Antiseizure medications such as phenytoin (Dilantin) or carbamazepine (Tegretol) must be the first line of treatment. Then conventional hormone therapy is beneficial. (Frequently, the antiseizure medications not only control TLE symptoms but also allow serum hormone levels to return to normal.)

The diagnosis of TLE requires specialized testing. An unusual type of brain-wave test, the sleep-deprived electroencephalogram (EEG), detects subtle disturbances in temporal lobe electrical activity. A new diagnostic probe, single photon emission computerized tomography (SPECT scan), may also help. The SPECT scan registers different colors in relation to blood flow. Areas of greatest blood flow in the brain show up with the whitest colors. Since increased blood flow is one characteristic of seizure-prone brain tissue, these areas light up on SPECT scan.

Hormone disorders are perhaps the most easily diagnosed causes of impotence, and hormone measurements should be an integral part of the early evaluation of the impotent man. Hormone abnormalities, once detected, can be treated with some dispatch and considerable success.

13

The Testosterone Renaissance

Testosterone has spawned its own myths and legends. This chapter deals with the role of testosterone in maintaining a man's health and vitality. The muscle-building properties of testosterone have attracted considerable attention and have created a culture of testosterone abuse. This quintessential male hormone is needed to maintain every man's sexuality and fertility and is more important than previously believed in sustaining a woman's sexuality. In Chapter 14, we will discuss why and when eliminating testosterone can be of benefit to some men and society. Then Chapter 15 will examine the role of the powerful new male hormone dihydrotestosterone. Here, you will find discussions on the following:

1. What does testosterone do to maintain a man's health?
2. The athlete-doctor schism: Does testosterone increase muscle and decrease fat?
3. Athletes, bodybuilders, and male hormone supplements
4. The "array" to counter side effects of male hormone supplements
5. Mortal men and testosterone
6. Testosterone and sex: Who needs testosterone, anyway?
7. Testosterone's role in women's sexuality
8. Trouble with testosterone: The problem of delayed premature (precocious) puberty
9. Using testosterone to jump-start delayed puberty

Two grown men, a seventeen-year-old boy, and a woman want testosterone.

Glenn at 28 already looks like he has had more than his share of testosterone. Fully dressed, there is every reason to believe him when he tells me he is a competitive bodybuilder. His gray "big and tall" men's suit jacket can barely contain arms that are the size of an average man's thighs. During the day, he works at his job selling electronics, but at night he pursues his passion. In every spare moment, he is at the gym working to further define his muscle groups to impress the judges when he oils up and steps on the stage to "display." He has not yet won any major competition but is hopeful that someday he will. It is his belief that with just the right dose of testosterone his chances will improve.

Glenn may be correct, but in order to achieve his goals, he will need massive doses of testosterone as well as other muscle-building (anabolic) male hormone (androgenic) steroids (AAS). (See the section "How Do Athletes and Body-builders Use AAS?" later in this chapter.) Their use may cause side effects (breast enlargement, acne, edema, and balding), requiring yet an additional array of medications. Glenn must also be willing to skirt the law, for testosterone supplement use is approved only for hypogonadal men and in wasting states such as occur with cancer or AIDS.

Abner, age fifty-seven, is no bodybuilder but would like a better body. He, too, works out at a place across town from Glenn's gym. Even though he is there five nights a week and occasionally on Saturday, Abner still does not have the brawn he desires. He envies Burton, who has the immediately adjacent locker and has become more heavily muscled. Abner is at a loss to explain why. Like Burton, he takes Mega-Man vitamins, in addition to vitamin E, creatine, saw palmetto, selenium, and zinc. Abner was sure he was doing everything in his power to protect his health. But he wasn't taking testosterone. Burton was. So Abner was wondering if testosterone would do as much for him as he reckoned it had done for Burton. Then one night, his wife mentioned that Abner's erection was not as strong as it had once been. First thing the following morning, Abner called for an appointment, started reading everything he could, and came to the office armed with fully highlighted and underlined books on testosterone.

Abner may qualify for testosterone treatment since he is at the age when a man's testosterone output starts to wane. If he has a below-normal testosterone level, his doctor will have no qualms about providing him with a testosterone prescription. This may be all he needs to catch up with Burton at the gym. He has to be careful that the testosterone prescribed is safe and is not likely to cause any liver damage. (See the Appendix in Chapter 17.)

Steven, who says he is seventeen but looks closer to twelve, just wants to be normal so the other kids in his class will stop their teasing and using him for a punching bag. A tall, awkward youngster struggling to pitch his still soprano voice to a lower key, he feels like an alien adolescent, more milquetoast than manly. Would he benefit from a touch of testosterone?

Actually a little testosterone would be very helpful for Steven. There is fundamentally nothing wrong with this youngster other than a condition called delayed puberty. In time, his own body will provide the testosterone he needs, but that will not help him cope now. This is a controversial area, and some doctors are willing to sit back and let nature do the job. Others, sensing the youngster's anguish, would be inclined to treat him with a little testosterone now and let him "catch up" to his classmates and then stop treatment when his body is ready to make its own testosterone. (See the section on "Trouble with Testosterone" later in this chapter.)

Then there is Linda, now age fifty-five, who says, "I have no sexual desire . . . absolutely none!" And she insists, "It wasn't always like this."

But when her fibroid-loaded uterus kept gushing blood, her doctors told her she had to have a hysterectomy. To be on the safe side and so she would never have to worry about ovarian cancer, they took out her ovaries along with her uterus in one operation when she was fifty-one. She has never been the same.

"There's nothing wrong with my husband's libido, and he's starting to wonder why I'm never interested. My girlfriend who had the same problem no longer does because her gynecologist gave her something—she says it's testosterone. Can that be right?"

Yes, it can be. We are just starting to learn how important testosterone is to a woman's sex drive, mood, and desire. Testosterone provided in pills and patches has been used with considerable success recently in improving the sexual desire, mood, and well-being of women who, like Linda, are now postmenopausal and have lost the capacity to generate their own small but vital ration of testosterone. (See the section "Testosterone for Postmenopausal Women" later in this chapter.)

THE MALE HORMONE (ANDROGEN) MYSTIQUE

Testosterone!

Before Viagra, everybody was talking about testosterone.

Newsweek's cover story on testosterone, coupled with a feature on another male hormone called DHEA, antedated that same weekly magazine's different, but equally enthusiastic, cover story on Viagra. Both testosterone and DHEA were also featured in prominent stories in the *Wall Street Journal*, and on the *CBS Evening News*. Male hormones were then and still are one hot topic.

Testosterone, we are told, will give men of all ages massive muscles, invigorate aging men, spice up the sexual desire of menopausal women. Further, this special male hormone is said to work wonders to improve flagging muscle strength and is being touted as a panacea to resolve many of the problems currently plaguing both young and older men and women today. Could all this hype really be true, and if so, why aren't more men taking testosterone supplements?

THE CLOUD OVER TESTOSTERONE

All is not wine and roses; testosterone also has a dark side because it is a *steroid*. The word "steroid" refers to the peculiar chicken-wire structure of this hormone. Other vital hormones made in the adrenal glands and the ovaries also have a steroid configuration. These steroid hormones course innocently through our bloodstreams every moment of every day. Neither the ovary's *estrogens* nor the adrenal gland's cortisone shares testosterone's nefarious legacy.

- When you read in the paper that an athlete has been disqualified from competition because he or she *"tested positive for steroids,"* testosterone or one of its close androgenic (male hormone) relatives is the steroid they are referring to.
- Rival industries, one devoted to *promoting*, the other to *detecting*, illegal male hormone use among athletes are now firmly in place.
- Androgen enthusiasts have amassed enough information to publish their own *Anabolic Steroid Hormone Users Bible* with surprisingly accurate descriptions of individual anabolic steroids and tips on how to cope with common problems linked with steroid use. This information is considered so valuable that it is printed in blue ink on thin paper so that it cannot be photocopied.
- The anabolic steroid watchdogs, on the other hand, have been busy devising methods to detect inappropriate and illegal use of male hormone supplements in athletes and bodybuilders. It is now possible to distinguish between a competitive athlete's own naturally occurring male hormones and illegal male hormone supplements just by examining athletes' urine samples to look for the telltale disruptions in the testosterone-epitestosterone ratios.
- To bedevil those intent on rooting out inappropriate anabolic steroid use, an equally ardent counterindustry has conjured up means to avoid detection by spiking the urine with a few drops of alcohol to foil test results.
- When lawyers seek to find extenuating circumstances to explain what motivated their client to commit some violent act, they frequently invoke *"steroid rage"* defense. They use this strategy to plead that the "accused should be excused" because at the time of the crime while in the grip of these *mighty male hormones*, he was powerless to control his aggression.

- In Europe, Israel, and California, men convicted of repeated sexual offenses for molesting children are offered the opportunity to avoid, or have a more lenient, prison sentence if they agree to a chemical castration to nullify the impact of testosterone as one means of discouraging further deviant sexual behavior.
- Does this mean that testosterone turns men into sexual deviants? No, but men who are inclined to a pattern of aberrant sexual behavior need testosterone to fuel their misdirected sexual urges. Take away their testosterone, and they stop preying on children.

What is it about testosterone that inspires so much passion? How much of what they say is true? We are just starting to get answers to these questions.

TABLE 13.1   Impact of Testosterone on Different Parts of the Man's Body

Body Part	Testosterone Effect	Why?
Brain	Increases sexual desire	Activates sexual centers controlling libido
Penis	Allows erections to occur	Increases enzymes in penile erectile chambers
Testicle	Enhances sperm production	Stimulates sperm maturity
Skin	Increases acne	Enhances sebum production
Growth	Defines Ultimate Height	Absence permits growth.
Bone Marrow	Increases blood count	Encourages red blood cell production
Bones	Prevents osteoporosis	Maintains bone calcium content and bone density
Prostate	Stimulates prostate growth	Converts testosterone (T) to dihydrotestosterone (DHT)
Scalp Hair	Male pattern widow's peak and balding	DHT receptors in hair follicles
Larynx	Deep voice	Thickens vocal cords
Breasts	Enlargement of glandular breast tissue	Excess testosterone converted to estrogen
Body Hair	Increases	Stimulatory effect on body hair follicles
Muscle and Fat	Increases muscle and decreases fat mass	Activates protein synthesis in muscle

WHAT DOES TESTOSTERONE DO TO MAINTAIN A MAN'S HEALTH?

Testosterone made in the testicles is released into a man's bloodstream to transform cells scattered throughout the body. As an androgen (a male hormone), testosterone can only work on *androgen receptors*. Cells without androgen receptors would not be expected to, and do not, respond to testosterone. However, androgen receptors are widespread. So this male hormone can accelerate, slow down, or wreak havoc with a remarkably diverse array of individual and uniquely male physical responses. (See Table 13.1.)

As one would expect, testosterone is vital for normal male sexual behavior. Testosterone has other functions—some advantageous, others less savory, and still others downright harmful. Listed below are some of the ways testosterone makes its presence known in different parts of the body. Testosterone interacts with androgen receptors on muscle to increase muscle mass and seeks out bone marrow androgen receptors to stimulate bone marrow to make more red blood cells. Other consequences of testosterone-androgen receptor interplay force the kidney to hold on to more sodium, stimulate the skin to develop acne, help build strong bones, increase body hair while simultaneously accelerating the loss of scalp hair, and thicken a man's vocal cords, giving him a deep voice.

Testosterone's power in bringing about all of these remarkable physical changes is well documented, but when most men think of testosterone, they tend to focus primarily on the *muscle-building* and *sexuality-enhancing* properties of this male hormone. Other, more subtle issues like the important role of testosterone in maintaining a woman's sex drive and the invigorating impact of testosterone on a man's overall quality of life have only recently come into focus.

TESTOSTERONE INCREASES MUSCLE AND DECREASES FAT: THE ATHLETE-DOCTOR SCHISM

Although men and women who compete in sports routinely depend on testosterone to increase muscle bulk, tone, and function, doctors have had a hard time accepting what for athletes is a matter of faith. This is because those who do use supplemental male hormones also train vigorously. It has been impossible to sort out how much improvement in a man or woman's athletic performance is due to obsessive and diligent training and how much to testosterone.

Doctors' experience with hypogonadal men—that is, men with lower than normal testosterone levels—has been instructive. When *testosterone-deficient men* are given just enough hormone to regularize their blood testosterone levels, they have an unequivocal 11-percent increase in lean body (muscle) mass. Further, individual muscle groups such as upper arm and thigh muscle mass expanded by 21 percent and 11 percent, respectively, with proper hormone treatment. This impressive augmentation of muscle bulk can occur after just ten weeks of testosterone therapy.

But these were not normal men, for *below-normal testosterone* levels had left them with *below-normal muscle mass*. The testosterone treatment merely brought them back to their predetermined baseline, and no further. For men who already have normal male hormone levels, the advantages of further testosterone supplementation are less clear.

Designing a study to answer a question as apparently straightforward as "Does testosterone use increase a man's strength?" has proven to be a remarkably challenging task.

Much of our current thinking about anabolic steroids changed on July 4, 1996. On that date, Dr. Shalender Bhasin and his colleagues in California and Oregon reconciled the differences between skeptical physicians and steroid-conscious athletes.

In a carefully controlled study, Dr. Bhasin demonstrated for the first time that *massive doses of androgens,* in this case 600 mg of testosterone weekly (*roughly fifteen times the normal man's testosterone output of 42 mg per week*), did increase weight, muscle mass, and strength.

The greatest gains in muscle mass and strength were observed in trained athletes who received testosterone and also participated in a supervised exercise program. Athletes in the testosterone plus exercise group who weighed 167 pounds at baseline weighed 180 pounds after ten weeks of high-dose testosterone. Their bench-press strength—213 pounds before— was 261 pounds at week ten.

Trained athletes who exercised regularly but received placebo injections had no significant weight gain (188 at start, and 190 pounds at ten weeks). Their bench-press strength was 240 pounds before and 261 pounds after ten weeks of supervised training.

Thus, compared to placebo-treated men, testosterone-treated athletes gained thirteen more pounds (most of it muscle) and could lift more weight than they could at the outset. The eleven-pound weight gain and the ability to bench press twenty-seven more pounds than the placebo-treated men was significant, proving that massive doses of testosterone did increase weight, muscle mass, and muscle strength.

But what about the average man or the proverbial "couch potato" who does not have the time, energy, or inclination to commit himself to a lengthy and intensive program of physical conditioning? Will he also experience an increase in body weight and improved muscle strength after receiving enormous amounts of testosterone? The answer is "yes," but to a significantly lesser degree.

For example, placebo-treated untrained men had no increase in body weight and could bench press the same amount of weight before and at week ten of the study. With testosterone, their weight increased from 181 to 189 pounds. Their bench-press prowess, 213 pounds at baseline, was up to 231 pounds after ten weeks of high-dose testosterone therapy, once again

TABLE 13.2   Effect of Massive Doses of Testosterone and Placebo Injections on Body Weight and Bench-Press Muscle Strength in Untrained Men (Couch) and Trained Athletes (Trained) Who Do and Do Not Exercise

Variable	Couch + Placebo	Couch + Testosterone	Trained + Placebo	Trained + Testosterone
Body Weight—Baseline	174.9	181	188	167
Body Weight—10 wks.	178	189	190	180
Bench Press Baseline	194	212	239.8	213
Bench Lbs —10 wks.	194	231	262	262

demonstrating the profound impact of very large doses of testosterone on both muscle mass and muscle strength. (See Table 13.2.)

To achieve these striking results, doctors had to give deep intramuscular injections of extraordinary doses of testosterone. Blood testosterone levels increased to values a man would never be able to achieve on his own. Those who volunteered to take part in this study had entirely normal serum testosterone values between 430 and 550 ng/dl. (The normal serum testosterone range is 300–1,000 ng/dl.) The amount of testosterone administered left men so awash in testosterone that *one week after the last testosterone injection, serum testosterone levels were 3,244 ng/dl,* or 300 percent higher than the highest serum testosterone level a man could hope to achieve naturally.

Because serum testosterone levels reached such extraordinary heights, far greater than would be possible under normal physiologic conditions, the dose of testosterone administered is said to be "supraphysiologic," that is, more than the body is programmed to make or cope with. During ten weeks of supraphysiologic testosterone treatment, men noted some increased acne, but not much else in the way of adverse effects. Tests designed to test their level of aggression before and during the onslaught of testosterone did not uncover any heightened tendency toward aggressive or antisocial behavior. But this was only a short-term study. The adverse effects of large doses of testosterone are more readily apparent with long-term high-dose testosterone use.

SIDE EFFECTS OF TESTOSTERONE SUPPLEMENTS

High-dose testosterone does not linger unchanged in a man's bloodstream and must be processed (metabolized) by the body. Some testosterone wends its way through a man's bloodstream unaltered, but a portion is transformed to other active products like the powerful male hormone *dihydrotestosterone* or the female hormone *estradiol* or is alternatively transformed into inert hormone by-products. (See Figure 13.1)

Testosterone, when it is unaltered, acts directly on male hormone—androgen—receptors, not just to help build muscle but also to activate andro-

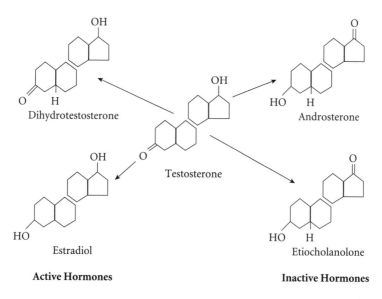

Active Hormones   **Inactive Hormones**

FIGURE 13.1   Once in a man's bloodstream, testosterone can be metabolized to other active hormones like dihydrotestosterone and estradiol or to inactive steroid hormones.

gen receptors in the skin. The skin responds by cranking out more and more of an oily skin secretion called sebum. Acne blossoms when skin sebum levels are high. On the other hand, that portion of testosterone that is metabolized to dihydrotestosterone (DHT) has an entirely different effect. DHT build-up in scalp hair follicles contributes to male-pattern baldness. Men who overstock their body with testosterone supplements often have abundant chest hair (due to testosterone) but sparse scalp hair (caused by high DHT levels). Minimizing the transformation of testosterone to DHT with a medication like finasteride (Propecia) lowers blood DHT levels and helps reverse the process of balding in men. (See Chapter 15 for more on DHT.)

The fraction of testosterone transformed to estradiol sets the stage for another problem. When a man's blood estradiol is high enough, the glut in this female hormone can cause him to have embarrassing breast enlargement. The technical term for breast enlargement occurring in the male is "gynecomastia."

MALE BREAST ENLARGEMENT (GYNECOMASTIA)

Men may first notice embarrassing breast enlargement during their teenage years. The sudden surge in adolescent testosterone and its metabolic spillover seems to overwhelm the body at first. The temporary torrent of estradiol distorts the balance of power, altering the young teenager's testosterone-estradiol (T/E) ratio. For a brief period of time, the relative excess of female hormones in the young teenager's bloodstream stimulates his breasts to start growing. Gradually, the T/E ratio tilts again in favor of testosterone. Then as estradiol levels dwindle, the stimulus to further breast growth first attenuates, then ceases. Occasionally, breast enlargement (gynecomastia) lingers into adulthood, causing significant chagrin. Grown men with large breasts may have to resort to surgery to reduce breast size. Innovative hormone treatments with dihydrotestosterone (DHT) may provide a nonsurgical alternative to restore normal breast size without resorting to surgery. (See Chapter 15).

HOW DO ATHLETES AND BODYBUILDERS USE TESTOSTERONE AND OTHER ANABOLIC ANDROGENIC STEROIDS (AAS)?

The carefully crafted and meticulously executed Bhasin study cited above used a single consistent very high dose of testosterone. Its conclusions will most likely satisfy both scientists and athletes. But those who endorse and promote "off-label" AAS use view most scientific studies with disdain because these reports failed to replicate the complex sequencing of steroid administration preferred by those who rely on AAS to gain a competitive edge. Athletes tend not to take medication in the strictly controlled amounts required for credible research studies. Rather, they cycle AAS use to maximize benefit and decrease the risk of detection in urine assays. A practice known as "stacking," the ritual sequencing of more than one steroid, is common. Athletes believe that by using more than one AAS they will be able to activate more and different types of androgen activity (androgen receptors). There is no scientific proof that this practice actually works, for there is only one androgen receptor and it is already filled to maximum capacity by the doses of AAS routinely used by athletes. Some also believe that optimum benefit cannot be achieved with any single AAS schedule. To avoid a "plateau," they scramble the order of AAS administration, often beginning their cycle with low doses, then building with sequentially higher doses before tapering down just prior to competition, constructing in essence an AAS "pyramid."

Androgens are known to be potent stimuli to prostate growth. Anxiety over the impact of unfettered, relentless androgen stimulation on prostate size has been a cause of considerable anxiety among physicians but has apparently not been one for athletes preoccupied with long-term consequences of "off-label" AAS use. Rather, it is the expectation of *short-term gain, not long-term consequences,* that is of paramount concern to the current crop of AAS aficionados. They tend to equate prostate problems with the remote destination of advanced age, which is not a primary concern of young competitive athletes.

AAS users believe they are clever enough to manipulate drug treatment to fend off the short-term adverse effects of AAS use and are cocky enough to believe they will have the same good fortune in sidestepping the more pernicious long-term consequences of continued androgen bombardment of their bodies. Still, several of the short-term problems—acne, fluid retention, balding, and breast enlargement—caused by high-dose AAS use do require attention. To cope with these bothersome problems, athletes have once again dipped into the pharmacy to concoct "*the array*."

AAS USE AND THE "ARRAY"

Breast enlargement, acne, and edema are undesirable and disadvantageous to athletes and bodybuilders, so AAS users must resort to other medications—anti-estrogens to combat breast enlargement, anti-acne medications to cope with unwanted blemishes, and diuretics to purge the edema from their bodies. The supplemental medications needed to short-circuit the undesirable side effects of AAS are referred to as "the array." Spawned by the latest advantages in pharmacology the "array" takes on each distressing symptom one at a time. To control acne, the antibiotic minocycline (Minocin) is used to blunt the impact of androgen excess on sebum production. Pills like the diuretic furosemide (Lasix), designed to rid the body of unwanted fluid, help control ankle swelling. To fend off breast enlargement, two different medications are called into play. The anti-estrogen tamoxifen helps diminish the male breast response to excessive estrogen in the bloodstream. Testolactone (Teslac)—a pill that disrupts a man's ability to process male hormones like testosterone into female hormones like estradiol—has also found favor among bodybuilders. Dread of balding has created a demand for use of finasteride (Proscar or Propecia). These medications decrease conversion of testosterone to dihydrotestosterone (DHT) and are used to prevent hair loss from the scalp. The medications currently employed in the array are listed below. (See Table 13.3.)

TABLE 13.3   The "Array" used to combat side effects of excessive male hormone use.

Symptom	Treatment
Edema	Furosemide (Lasix)
Acne	Minocycline (Minocin)
Breast enlargement (Gynecomastia)	Tamoxifen, Testolactone (Teslac)
Balding	Finasteride as Proscar or Propecia

ANABOLISM-CATABOLISM AND ANABOLIC ANDROGENIC STEROIDS (AAS)

Anabolism, the building up of muscle, is the opposite of catabolism, the destruction of muscle. Men and women with diseases like cancer and AIDS become weak because of a breakdown of their muscles, a process known as catabolism. Testosterone and its clones reverse catabolism and speed anabolism and are referred to as anabolic (muscle-building) androgenic (male hormone) steroids (AAS).

Healthy men and women who use testosterone or other AAS pills in muscle-building programs are engaging in "off-label" AAS use.

Athletes know that large doses of testosterone or other AAS drugs are needed to help them achieve the bulk, strength, and size they need to be effective in competitive sports. Long-term consequences of male hormones on cholesterol and lipid profile or prostate gland size are of little concern to them when they are struggling to be a split second faster or lift five more pounds. Although most sports organizations have stipulations against the use of "performance-enhancing drugs," few athletes heed these regulations and as role models have fostered an attitude encouraging rampant AAS use.

HOW COMMON IS AAS USE?

In today's culture there is something of an epidemic of AAS use among adolescents and young men and women. One survey of high-school students documented that 5–10 percent of boys and 0.5–2.5 percent of girls admitted to AAS use. Results from another survey indicated that there were more than 1 million former or current AAS users in 1993. Over 50 percent of the lifetime users started at an average age of fifteen. Other surveys of several hundred thousand families have confirmed the appeal of AAS use for both adolescent boys and girls. Enhancement of body image or athletic skills is what draws adolescents and others to AAS drugs.

Over the past decade, there has been an extraordinary increase in the amount of androgens used by both men and women. The Food and Drug Administration, concerned with the burgeoning demand for male hormone supplements, has decided to lump testosterone with another class of powerful agents—narcotics—and insists that when doctors are prescribing testosterone they do so for the proper reasons. The FDA has sanctioned the use of testosterone and other testosterone-like medications for two reasons. One is the treatment of testosterone-deficient men. The other is to help reverse the ravages of other illnesses that cause muscle wasting and frailty.

Most physicians tend to be leery of prescribing testosterone or any other AAS drug for unapproved indications. Yet underground supplies of testosterone pills and other AAS pills are readily available from other sources. Those who do find a supply and are eager to indulge in "off-label" AAS use may be interested in why doctors are uneasy prescribing testosterone pills.

WHY IS OFF-LABEL AAS USE A PROBLEM?

To be useful as a pill, testosterone has to be physically altered. The chemical transformation needed to make testosterone pills *effective* also causes them to be *dangerous*. The most worrisome side effect of testosterone or any other AAS pill is liver damage. Use of testosterone pills can cause a man's liver to become crammed full of blood-filled cysts, a condition known as *peliosis hepatis*. Blood can burst forth from these cysts, causing extensive abdominal bleeding. Fatal liver cancer has also occurred in AAS users. The warning accompanying all AAS pills follows:

> Text of warning for all synthetic anabolic androgenic steroid medications as it appears in the 1999 *Physician's Desk Reference*:
> Peliosis hepatis, a condition in which liver and sometimes splenic tissue is replaced with blood-filled cysts, has been reported in patients receiving androgenic anabolic steroid therapy. These cysts are sometimes present with minimal hepatic dysfunction, but at other times they have been associated with liver failure. They are often not recognized until life-threatening liver failure or intra-abdominal hemorrhage develops. Withdrawal of the drug usually results in complete disappearance of lesions.
> Liver cell tumors are also reported. Most often these tumors are benign and androgen-dependent, but fatal malignant tumors have been reported. Withdrawal of drug often results in regression or cessation of progression of the tumor. However, hepatic tumors associated with androgens or anabolic steroids are much more vascular than other tumors and may be silent until life-threatening intra-abdominal hemorrhage develops.

MORTALS AND TESTOSTERONE

While mortal men and women may marvel at the feats of our athletic heroes and wonder secretly whether their skills are truly natural or androgen enhanced, each one of us may also be curious to know just what this male hormone can or will do for us individually.

TESTOSTERONE AND SEX:
WHO NEEDS TESTOSTERONE, ANYWAY?

Both men and women need testosterone, for this body chemical is essential to both sexes to activate and then maintain normal sexual desire (libido). Different properties of this hormone first allow men to develop an erection for sexual gratification and then allow for normal sperm development to ensure fertility. Women often need testosterone, not as a primary but as an *adjunct hormone,* to help maintain their libido, especially in the years after menopause.

- Libido: Men need testosterone to help them first develop and then focus their sex drive on the object of their desire. The testicles of young boys release only trivial amounts of testosterone before adolescence, years generally notable for sexual apathy. Then with the onset of puberty, the young man's body is besieged by a veritable flood of testosterone to awaken his latent sexual desires.
- Penile erection: In order to translate that sexual desire into sexual action, a man must transform his penis from a limp to a rigid and erect state. The process of acquiring a firm penile erection is yet another sexual activity requiring testosterone. When testosterone levels are low, a man's penis can plump up to some degree; but only when he has an adequate quotient of testosterone in his bloodstream does his penis become fully erect. When a man's testosterone production is very low, he will have virtually no erections. As his testosterone level normalizes, the number and vigor of his erections increases. (See Figure 13.2.)
- Fertility: Finally, a man's ability to father a child relies on a nudge from testosterone. A man can only produce the sperm needed to impregnate a woman if the testosterone-secreting cells in his testicles work in harmony with sperm producing to speed up the transition of cells that are immature sperm wannabes to sperm with maximum fertilizing capacity.
- Testosterone's role in women: Women also rely on testosterone. When they are young, their ovaries produce both estrogen and testosterone. The average female generates only a fraction of a man's testosterone output. Nonetheless, this modest ration of testosterone is vital for her healthy sex drive and libido. The presence of testosterone in the female is but one of the many hormonal influences driving her to seek out a mate, initially for sexual gratification and ultimately to have children. The significance of this hormone is often not apparent, even to the most discerning and perceptive woman, until she reaches menopause. Then both ovarian estrogen and testosterone production grind to a halt. Some believe that it is the loss of ovarian testosterone that is responsible for the diminished libido and sexual satisfaction of menopausal women. If this were true then traditional hormone replacement therapy (HRT) with estrogens alone would be inadequate. Only when a woman's testosterone stores are replenished, they argue, can a menopausal woman be considered to be properly and adequately treated. Despite adequate restocking of *female hormone* stores, her sex drive and sexual

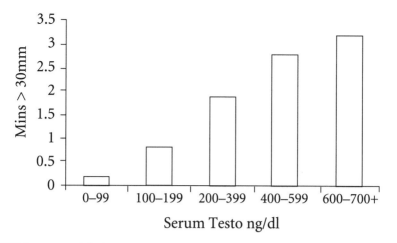

FIGURE 13.2   Nighttime erections in men with low and normal testosterone levels. SOURCE: Adapted from A. R. Granata, V. Rochira, A. Lerchl, P. Marama, and C. Cariani, "Relationship Between Sleep-Related Erections and Testosterone Levels in Men," *J. Androl.* 18 (1997): 522–527.

satisfaction is not what it once was. In that case, a hormone cocktail that includes the *male hormone,* testosterone, as well as the standard female hormones, estrogen and progesterone, may be needed to restore her sexual well-being. However, this is an area of some controversy.

TESTOSTERONE FOR POSTMENOPAUSAL WOMEN

Recognizing that testosterone is the major male hormone and estrogens the hormones of femininity does not mean that gender alone determines exclusive rights to either hormone. Men have small amounts of an estrogen, specifically estradiol, in their bloodstream, and in parallel fashion, women's adrenal glands and ovaries routinely produce small amounts of testosterone. The exact role of the sex hormones of the opposite sex in people has been something of a mystery, but there is increasing evidence that a man's estrogens play a role in stimulating prostate gland growth and that testosterone's presence in a women may be a key factor in maintaining her libido.

Our knowledge of the factors that stimulate or suppress male sexual function, though imperfect, is nonetheless substantially more advanced than our understanding of the hormonal determinants of female sexuality. In adolescent boys, timing of androgen (testosterone) secretion and sexual interest coincide, whereas in young women, androgen secretion and orgasmic capacity are not closely linked. Male hormone production is evident in young girls as early as age ten, when the first wisps of pubic hair appear in response to the increased secretion of the adrenal androgen dehy-droepiandrosterone sulfate (DHEA-S), but orgasms are not evident until later. Further, a woman's androgen levels, both adrenal DHEA and ovarian testosterone, remain fairly constant after the late teens or early twenties, whereas her capacity for orgasms increases steadily.

The best prognosticator of a woman's sexual activity is her free testos-terone level, but this hormone does not appear to influence female sexual behavior as much as cues from peer group women. Adolescent girls tend to be sexually active when their friends are.

Certain androgens such as androstenedione and free testosterone increase just prior to ovulation. This androgen burst coincides with increased sexual activity in all mammals except for the human female, who tends to have an increase in her sexual activity at the conclusion of her menstrual period when her androgens are at their lowest levels.

The pivotal role of testosterone in female libido has not been appreciated until recently and only in those women have had their ovaries surgically re-moved during a total abdominal hysterectomy. It was at this time that women noted a profound diminution in their sex drive. Initially, popular psychologists ascribed this diminution in libido to despondency over the loss of their uterus and inability to bear children. But women who had a simple hysterectomy with their ovaries left intact did not experience the same sexual fate as their sisters who had both their ovaries and uterus re-moved. There was something about their remaining ovarian tissue that al-lowed these women to maintain their libido. Now it appears that that something was testosterone.

Much of our current scientific knowledge about the role of testosterone in female sexuality comes from the extensive studies in Australia and Canada. Only recently has testosterone supplementation for post-menopausal women become popular in this country, and that has been largely due to the efforts of Dr. Susan Rako, a Boston psychiatrist who writes that she became interested in testosterone on her own in 1988 when "her hormones crashed" around the time of her menopause. Traditional HRT to correct her estrogen deficiency, it seems, was not sufficient to correct her "loss of sexual and vital energy." With testosterone supplementation, she felt better and was energized and revitalized.

Eager to share her experience with others, she published a book entitled *The Hormone of Desire: The Truth About Sexuality, Menopause, and Testos-terone*, extolling the benefits and downplaying the adverse effects of bolster-ing testosterone levels in postmenopausal women.

The very first reports of testosterone supplementation had indeed fo-cused on postmenopausal women who, like Dr. Rako, complained of a loss of sexual desire while receiving conventional estrogen and progesterone hormone replacement therapy (HRT).

Studies in Australia and Canada relied on a visual analog scale, asking women "On a scale of 0–100 with 100 being entirely normal, how would you rate your sex drive?" before and during treatment. Women scored themselves low at 20 before and 85 after 6 weeks of estrogen plus testosterone, but were unchanged after estrogen alone.

In Canada, Dr. Barbara Sherwin evaluated not just libido but overall sense of well-being, energy, and appetite in postmenopausal women with no ovaries. She found that compared to placebo or estrogen alone, women who received a combination of estrogen and testosterone, this time by intramuscular injection and not by pellet implantation, had a significant improvement in their well-being, energy level, and appetite. This improvement carries a cost, for all of the testosterone-treated women grew hair on their faces and had a worsening of their cholesterol profile, making them theoretically more susceptible to atherosclerosis. Mindful of the need for safer testosterone delivery systems to activate libido without fostering facial hair growth, new testosterone cremes and lotions are being formulated.

Capitalizing on the recent enthusiasm for providing supplemental testosterone to enhance libido in postmenopausal women, some have started to cautiously explore the potential benefit of a combined estrogen and testosterone pill. Reasoning that unsightly facial hair and disordered lipid profiles are dose related, the manufacturers of Estratest, the most common estrogen and testosterone combination pill, have now come out with Estratest-LD, the LD signifying that the pill contains a lower dose of testosterone than the parent compound. However, the testosterone in both pills is methyltestosterone, one of the 17-alkylated testosterone products known to have significant side effects. We do not yet know the benefits of long-term androgen therapy in women, but we do know of some of the reported risks of this treatment. Most of the currently available testosterone in pills may carry a burden of liver toxicity. (See earlier comments on AAS.)

Doctors are still uneasy about issuing a blanket recommendation for testosterone pills for all postmenopausal women with diminished libido. As additional data emerge from placebo-controlled studies, we should be able to learn whether androgen supplementation is not only effective but also a safe treatment for postmenopausal women with low sexual desire and inhibited sexual arousal.

However, a limited trial of testosterone may be precisely what Linda needs. She may do just as well with either testosterone pills or patches to resurrect her lost libido. For example, to circumvent the liver toxicity of testosterone pills, testosterone patches have been used with some success.

The testosterone patches differ in some respects from those used by men both in dose and use. Men have to change their patches daily, but women seem to be able to go three to four days before changing patches. The use of testosterone patches in women is quite new. We will have a better sense of the value of testosterone patches in postmenopausal women when results of additional research studies are made available.

ARE THERE OTHER LEGITIMATE USES OF ANABOLIC STEROIDS?

In addition to their value as replacement therapy for testosterone-deficient men, testosterone has been invaluable to help "jump-start" the pubertal process in young boys whose onset of adolescence is somewhat behind schedule, a condition known as *delayed puberty*. Today, testosterone has been pressed into service to bolster muscle mass in men with *AIDS wasting syndrome (AWS)*.

AIDS AND TESTOSTERONE

A below-normal serum testosterone level (hypogonadism) is the most common hormone abnormality found in men with acquired immunodeficiency syndrome (AIDS). In some cases, this is the result of viruses or other microorganisms invading and disabling the testicle's testosterone-producing capability. More often, the hypogonadism results from subnormal pituitary signals to the testicle, a condition referred to as secondary hypogonadism. Dr. Adrian Dobs of Johns Hopkins University Medical School was one of the first to note that men with AIDS experience many of the symptoms of hypogonadism. In one of her earlier studies in men with AIDS, she noted that 28 of 42 (67 percent) complained of decreased libido, and 14 of 42 (33 percent) said they were impotent. In addition to the common symptoms immediately attributed to their hypogonadism, men infected with the AIDS virus often experience unexplained decline in weight and loss of muscle mass. This condition is referred to as the AIDS wasting syndrome (AWS) and, in addition to all the other problems AIDS patients have to cope with, AWS is a major cause of morbidity and premature death. We know that in men with spontaneous hypogonadism, loss of weight and muscle mass is common and that for these hypogonadal men, testosterone treatment helps restore weight and strength. Could testosterone treatment work as well in men with AWS?

Preliminary data from Drs. Judith and Richard Rabkin of the College of Physicians and Surgeons, Columbia University, suggest that providing supplemental testosterone or a testosterone analogue, like mesterolone, to men with AIDS who have low serum testosterone levels is beneficial, producing clear improvements in sexual interest, arousal, and overall sense of well-being. Some have even speculated that supplemental testosterone may also have a positive mood-elevating impact similar to that seen with traditional antidepressant therapy.

Men with AIDS were treated with a conventional dose of 100 mg of testosterone per week for eight weeks. They had a significant gain in weight and noted enhanced sexual interest and more energy, suggesting that this form of androgen supplementation is effective in alleviating many of the problems that men with AIDS find so troubling.

As more men with AIDS were subjected to detailed hormonal studies, it became apparent that not all, even those who were suffering from AWS, had below-normal testosterone levels. In June 1996, Dr. Richard Horton of the University of Southern California Medical School found that some men with AWS have normal testosterone levels but are unable to efficiently convert testosterone to a second male hormone, dihydrotestosterone (DHT). He speculated that it was the subnormal DHT levels that were most likely responsible for their inability to gain weight in AWS. (See Chapter 15.)

TROUBLE WITH TESTOSTERONE:
THE PROBLEM OF DELAYED PREMATURE
(PRECOCIOUS) PUBERTY

Some youngsters' testicles start making testosterone earlier than expected, whereas others seem to take forever to turn on their testosterone production. The switch in the brain that starts signaling the activation of testosterone secretion may be held in a state of suspended animation and may not turn on until a boy's late teens or early twenties, as is the case in delayed puberty. Alternatively, when that switch clicks on at an early age, young boys develop precocious puberty. They rush into adolescence by activating testosterone secretion between ages six and eleven instead of the more traditional thirteen or fourteen and are thus unusual and therefore unhappy. These young boys require prompt treatment to shut off testosterone before it does irreparable harm. (See Chapter 14.)

USING TESTOSTERONE TO
JUMP-START DELAYED PUBERTY

For the majority of young men, the transition from boyhood to adolescence passes turbulently but within a relatively narrow time frame. As hypothalamic hormones start pulsating and provoke the pituitary gland to activate testosterone secretion, the anticipated changes in the young man's height, weight, sexual arousal, muscle development, beard growth, and acne

---

are evident. For most, these events tend to start at age thirteen and are complete by age sixteen. Some young men, however, although perfectly normal, lag behind in this process. They find themselves at age fifteen or sixteen looking like they did when they were twelve. This failure to develop normal adult male sexual characteristics by the age of sixteen is referred to as delayed puberty. For most of these pubertal laggards, the only remedy is a little "tincture of time," for they will eventually experience the entire sequence of events that started in their classmates at age thirteen. Knowing this may be reassuring to the concerned parents, but the young man for whom puberty seems to be always "just around the corner" is likely to fuss at being left in what appears to be a perpetually prepubertal state. He is embarrassed in the locker room, teased about his small physical and genital size by not always compassionate classmates. He finds that he is left out of even the most banal conversations comparing the relative merits of shaving with a regular or electric razor and cannot even begin to enter into a conversation on real or imagined sexual conquests. His only advantage, if you can call it that, is his persistent slow but steady increase in height. Whereas most of his male friends reach their peak height and grow no further after they start making adult levels of testosterone, the boy with delayed puberty will continue to grow slowly but steadily each year.

If it is possible to *turn off* hypothalamic hormone secretion to reverse the factors causing precocious puberty, it should also be feasible to *turn on* the hypothalamus to get adolescence started in the young boy with delayed puberty. Indeed it is, but the process is arduous and expensive. A simpler and less costly way to achieve the same goal is to provide the youngster with a brief taste of testosterone therapy. This is an area of considerable controversy. Some ask if there is fundamentally nothing wrong with the young man and he is destined to enter puberty spontaneously at age seventeen, eighteen, or nineteen, why intervene?

The decision to treat is based on what are called psychosocial consideration. Judgment depends on how well the young man can cope with being significantly smaller and more immature looking than his peers. Does he care if he is the only one in his class who has not yet started to experience the tug of testosterone on his libido, beard growth, or penile size? Most young boys do.

A brief course of testosterone treatment can change that, but such therapy can only be considered if the young man, and his parents, have a full appreciation of the consequences and nature of this treatment. He will become more virile. His spindly arms and legs will fill out and become more muscular. Acne, held in abeyance until now, will be unleashed to prey upon his face. His voice will deepen, he will forsake his preadolescent falsetto for a more vibrant resonant tone, and his penis will start to lengthen. The orchestration of this sequence of testosterone treatment must be done with the utmost care and attention in order to provide just enough hormone to bring about the desired changes in physical appearance but not enough to compromise his ultimate height. This is usually achieved by providing the young man's body with a glimpse of some testosterone but only for a brief period of time. Thus, instead of treating him with the full testosterone replacement dose of 100 mg a week, a fraction of that dose, 25–50 mg per week, is administered for 3–6 months and then stopped. During this interval, many of the desired changes in physical appearance will occur, allowing him to be more like the other young boys in his class.

Delayed puberty is precisely what is plaguing Steven. He is tall but in his words still "wimpy looking" and has not yet started to shave or catch up to his classmates in muscular development. More often than not, the systems designed to power his testosterone-secreting apparatus will switch on of their own accord spontaneously *in time,* but patience is not likely to be a virtue of seventeen-year-old boys. At this stage of life, judicious use of small doses of testosterone by injection can be helpful in allowing Steven and other young men like him to start to seem a little bit more manly, just enough so they can start to look and feel better about themselves. This is tricky business, and proper dosing is essential so that these boys' bodies do not hurtle into adolescence too abruptly.

14

Eliminating Testosterone to Benefit Man and Society

Why would you ever want to deprive a man of testosterone? If a full ration of testosterone were so vital to normal male sexual health, muscle mass, and the integrity of a man's skeleton, why would anyone want to deprive an otherwise healthy man of this vital hormone? Doctors only lower serum testosterone levels under unusual circumstances when the presence of persistent testosterone secretion is a threat to the individual man and society's welfare, such as when:

1. Testosterone secretion begins at an inappropriately early age, and causes a premature or precocious puberty.
2. Testosterone is fueling the spread of prostate cancer and decreasing a man's life span.
3. Testosterone allows a sexual predator to continue his pattern of persistent antisocial behavior.

PRECOCIOUS PUBERTY

Boys with precocious puberty are troubled youngsters. Beginning as early as age six, they start making too much testosterone. The surplus testosterone initiates a short-lived growth spurt. For a while, they tower over their classmates. Shaving begins earlier than expected, as does the development of a baritone voice. The penis can become disproportionately enlarged. These young boys are invariably the first to experience nighttime erections and usually experiment with masturbation before anyone else. There are other consequences of their earlier-than-normal testosterone influx. They become more muscular than their classmates do, a phenomenon that impels some to be schoolyard bullies.

The young man whose brain, brawn, and bones are being stimulated by testosterone at an earlier-than-normal age is not normal. His precocious puberty, once recognized, can and should be treated, for if it is left alone, he will not only end up much shorter than everyone in his class but will have to contend with other social pressures as well. Fortunately, by stifling the stimulus for further testosterone secretion, his premature adolescence can be put on hold and temporarily halted. Once the drive to premature testosterone production is disabled, his growth and behavior can be more like that of other boys his own age. With his preadolescent testosterone production held in check, he will continue to grow, but at a more measured pace. As he nears the teenage years, testosterone-restraining treatment is stopped. The stimulus to male hormone production resumes, but this time, he and the other boys in his class are maturing at the same time.

The same treatment regimen—gonadotropin-releasing hormone agonist therapy—that slows down testosterone production and helps the boy with precocious puberty develop normally also helps the man with prostate cancer to live a longer life and, in addition, can allow the man who has become a sexual predator to control his urges. Ultimately, this will permit him to have a less tortured life.

PROSTATE CANCER

Cancer, in particular prostate cancer, requires testosterone to continue its aggressive pattern of malignant growth. Once testosterone production is halted, the advance of prostate cancer slows, and the lives of men with prostate cancer are prolonged. In the past, doctors had to rely on surgical removal of the testicles (castration) to obliterate testosterone production. Today, complete suppression of testosterone production can be achieved without surgery. Rather, an injection given every three months can totally shut down testosterone secretion. This technique is referred to as chemical castration or androgen ablative therapy.

Surgery and chemical castration are equally effective in nullifying men's testosterone production and in slowing the spread of malignant cells and prolonging life for men with metastatic prostate cancer. In some men, another medication—the anti-androgen bicalutamide (Casodex) or flutamide (Eulexin)—is added in an effort to obliterate any vestiges of hormone stimulus to further arrest prostate cancer growth. Without testosterone, men experience all of the symptoms of acute hypogonadism and may even start to have hot flashes. (For more on the role of testosterone in prostate cancer, see Chapter 24.)

CONTROLLING URGES IN SEXUAL PREDATORS

Men for whom young boys and girls are objects of erotic desire are now recognized as sexual predators. Because of their preference for the pediatric population, these men are referred to as pedophiles, often wind up in the criminal justice system, and are incarcerated for a period of time. When released from jail, they often resume their pattern of preying on children. The

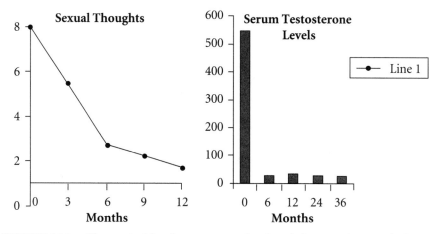

FIGURE 14.1   Change in blood testosterone level and decrease in sexual obsessions in men convicted of sex crimes against children before and after treatment designed to lower their serum testosterone level. SOURCE: Adapted from A. Rosler and T. Witztum, "Treatment of Men with Paraphillia with a Long-Acting Analogue of Gonadotropin-Releasing Hormone," *N. Engl. J. Med.* 338 (1998): 416–422.

reason pedophiles commit antisocial acts is not because they have extraordinarily high serum testosterone levels but rather because they have a *deviant response to perfectly normal male hormone production.*

Psychotherapy and counseling are not effective in defusing or controlling their predatory sexual behavior, but lowering their testosterone level is effective. Surgical castration and the use of an anti-androgen pill have at one time or another been suggested or recommended, as has court-ordered treatment (or punishment) of men convicted of being pedophiles. The same type of treatment used to obliterate testosterone production to save the lives of men with prostate cancer is used to dampen the sexual urges of men known to be sexual predators. With this treatment, they stop making testosterone almost immediately, and as long as testosterone levels remain low, their predatory behavior is held in check. (See Figure 14.1.) Note that testosterone levels become subnormal almost immediately but that testosterone suppression must be sustained for several months before the sexual predators' behavior changes.

15

Dihydrotestosterone (DHT): The Androgen for the Twenty-First Century?

Testosterone may not be numero uno among male hormones for long. One of the by-products of testosterone metabolism, a hormone called dihydrotestosterone (DHT), is already attracting increased attention. Until recently, doctors always thought of DHT as a troublemaker, since it is the hormone most commonly accused as the culprit responsible for two of men's nagging concerns—balding and prostate gland enlargement.

HOW DOES DHT CAUSE BALDING AND PROSTATE GLAND ENLARGEMENT?

DHT can only provoke balding or encourage prostate enlargement in the proper setting. When DHT accumulates within a man's prostate, his prostate gland starts to grow. Similarly, a man requires a generous supply of DHT funneled into his scalp hair follicle to provoke hair loss. How does this happen?

Your prostate gland and hair follicle are equipped to pull testosterone from your bloodstream and then alter it. A unique enzyme called 5-alpha reductase can convert testosterone to DHT. The two absolute prerequisites for balding and prostate gland enlargement are that:

1. Testosterone gets siphoned out of your bloodstream and incorporated into your prostate gland or hair follicle.
2. The 5-alpha reductase enzyme transforms the trapped testosterone to dihydrotestosterone.

Now doctors have known about the importance of testosterone for centuries. Hippocrates taught that "Women and eunuchs do not take the gout or become bald."

What do women and eunuchs have in common? They produce little or no testosterone and therefore have little or no capacity to make DHT.

Several centuries later, doctors at Cornell Medical Center expanded on Hippocrates' observations by noting that *men who make testosterone but not DHT never develop prostate gland enlargement or go bald*, a clear argument in favor of lowering a man's DHT level.

There are reasons to believe that DHT is not just a hormonal nuisance but has a positive role for men. Remember, DHT is the hormone responsible for developing, molding, and lengthening a boy's penis while he is developing within his mother's womb. Further, increasing direct and inferential evidence indicates that DHT plays a critical role in the adult man's sexuality. It is really important for us to understand this curious male hormone.

WHAT IS DIHYDROTESTOSTERONE?

Dihydrotestosterone is created when a man's body decides what to do with all the testosterone he has. By an efficient means of disposal called metabolism, a man's body is equipped to convert testosterone to other sexually active hormones or innocuous inactive hormones. The testosterone that is manufactured in a man's testicles is released into his bloodstream and may do a number of things. It can:

1. Act directly on androgen receptors in the brain, muscle, and bone to maintain libido (sex drive), muscle mass, and bone strength;
2. Become a totally different hormone, either a more powerful male hormone called dihydrotestosterone or a female hormone called estradiol (E2);
3. Be transformed into inactive or inert steroid products that have no known function and simply wash out of a man's system. (See Figure 13.1.)

Whether testosterone will be converted to a female hormone or a more powerful hormone is not a matter of chance. Different enzymes determine the fate of testosterone. The aromatase enzyme, abundant in fat cells, changes testosterone into the female hormone estradiol (E2). A totally different enzyme called 5-alpha reductase is plentiful only in selected parts of the body, including a man's prostate and in those hair follicles that grow hair on his head.

Once testosterone (T) enters a man's prostate gland or his scalp hair follicles, the 5-alpha reductase enzyme goes to work to convert T to DHT, but the rate of transformation of T to DHT may be more aggressive in some men than in others.

Men born without the 5-alpha reductase enzyme cannot convert T to DHT. They seem odd at birth but do grow up to be normal-looking, healthy, well-muscled adult men who have normal T but low DHT levels in their bloodstreams. Men with low DHT levels have a tiny prostate gland as well as a luxuriant head of hair.

They never develop prostate enlargement or go bald!

What would happen if we found a way to lower DHT levels in a normal man? Would his prostate gland shrink? Would he be able to grow more hair on his head? Those were the questions asked by scientists at Merck who went on a diligent search to discover a medication that could allow man to maintain abundant blood testosterone levels while selectively decreasing his DHT. They found finasteride.

Finasteride cross-checks the 5-alpha reductase enzyme and stymies a man's ability to convert testosterone to dihydrotestosterone. Finasteride pills are now approved for two uses, one to prevent or reverse prostate enlargement in older men and the other to increase scalp hair growth in men who are starting to experience male-pattern baldness. Finasteride pills are packaged in different doses. The 5-mg formulation of finasteride is called Proscar. This medication is often prescribed for middle-aged and older men who are known to have enlarged prostate glands, a condition called benign prostatic hyperplasia (BPH). The 1-mg finasteride dose sold as Propecia is used to treat men who have thinning hair, a condition known as male-pattern baldness.

How well does either finasteride pill work to decrease prostate size or reverse male-pattern baldness?

DOES LOWERING DHT LEVELS HELP DECREASE PROSTATE SIZE IN BENIGN PROSTATIC HYPERPLASIA (BPH)?

The very earliest stages of prostate enlargement cause no symptoms. Men are often totally unaware that they have a prostate gland until they have a digital rectal exam (DRE) at their annual physical. When the prostate gland enlarges backward, it bulges into the rectum and will be felt by the doctor as a smooth mass pressing against the lower bowel. If the prostate enlargement creates pressure on a man's bladder, he may start to experience difficulty urinating. (See Chapter 23.)

Here is what was done to find out if lowering a man's blood DHT level decreases his prostate size and makes it easier for him to urinate. Five hundred and ninety-seven men who had BPH and were troubled by symptoms from their enlarged prostate glands participated in a yearlong study to compare the effect of finasteride 5 mg (Proscar) to placebo pills on urinary symptoms and prostate size. Male hormone levels were measured before,

---

during, and after treatment. About one-half of the men (297) received Proscar, and the other 300 were given identical-looking placebo tablets.

Typically, men who have enlarged prostate glands experience problems urinating. They may have a need to run to the bathroom often, wake frequently at night to void, or find it difficult to start the process of urination because of the pressure created by the large prostate bulging up against their bladder. Men can self-rate the severity of their prostate symptoms by filling out a questionnaire. The more difficulty they have urinating, the higher the score. As symptoms subside scores decline.

In this early study comparing Proscar to placebo, the prostate symptom scores before treatment were comparable: 9.8 for the placebo group and 10.2 for the men who were to receive Proscar. Both the Proscar and placebo-treated men had significant difficulty urinating. At the start, neither group was able to urinate freely and vigorously and maximum urinary flow rates were equally impaired. All men had equivalent degrees of BPH, and prostate volume was comparably increased in men destined to receive placebo or Proscar.

With treatment, men who received Proscar had a prompt 80 percent decrease in their blood DHT level. DHT levels were unchanged in men receiving placebo. Blood testosterone levels were either unchanged or increased slightly in the Proscar-treated men. After twelve months, the Proscar-treated men had less trouble urinating, stronger and better urine flow, and smaller prostate glands. Placebo-treated men continued to have difficulty urinating due to their persistently enlarged prostate glands.

From the start, doctors had determined that they would only consider Proscar to be an effective treatment for men with BPH if the medication resulted in both increased urine flow rates and decreased prostate volume. That is precisely what happened to the Proscar-treated men. Urinary flow rate and prostate size were not significantly different from baseline in the men who received placebo. (See Table 15.1.)

Surprisingly, although Proscar did its job well and caused and an 80-percent decrease in serum DHT levels, this dramatic reduction in circulating DHT levels was accompanied by a less impressive but still significant 20-percent overall decrease in prostate size. The decrease has been sufficient for many doctors to continue recommending Proscar treatment for men with urinary symptoms due to an enlarged prostate gland.

If Proscar is that effective in decreasing prostate size and minimizing those pesky symptoms men experience as their prostate enlarges, why don't all men take Proscar routinely as a preventive treatment to maintain prostate health? Unfortunately, there is the problem of sexual side effects associated with Proscar use. (See Table 15.2.)

The sexual side effects noted on page 191 were not expected, because serum testosterone levels remained high during Proscar treatment. Was it

TABLE 15.1   Urine Flow and Prostate Size in Men with BPH After 12 Months of Placebo or Proscar.

Test	Placebo	Proscar
Maximum Urine Flow		
Baseline	9.6 milliliters per second	9.6 milliliters per second
12 Months	9.8 milliliters per second	11.2 milliliters per second
Prostate Volume		
Baseline	61.0	58.6
12 Months	60.0	47

TABLE 15.2   Side Effects During Placebo and Proscar Treatment

Side Effect	Placebo	Proscar
Decreased Libido	1.3%	4.7–6%
Impotence	1.7%	3.4–5%
Ejaculation Problem	1.7%	4.4%

possible that even though testosterone production was unaffected, the lowering of serum DHT levels was somehow a factor in causing sexual side effects? Could DHT have a previously unappreciated role in regulating male sexuality?

PROPECIA FOR MEN WITH MALE-PATTERN BALDNESS

Symptoms of balding are not subtle. Men will note some early hair loss simply by looking in the mirror. Almost all men experience, and accept, some thinning of the hair as they age, but when there is an accelerated hair loss at an early age, men do become concerned. The 1-mg finasteride pill sold under the name of Propecia is prescribed for younger men who are troubled by the distinctive and selective pattern of hair loss, commonly referred to as male-pattern baldness.

The striking observation that scalp hair loss (balding) never occurs in men with low serum DHT levels was the stimulus for this research. Doctors were to determine whether lowering a man's DHT level would reverse or slow down the rate at which he became bald. Only limited studies have been done on this topic, but those that are available indicate that the 1-mg dose of finasteride (Propecia) does lower serum DHT levels by about 65 percent and slows down the rate of hair loss in men with male-pattern baldness. Hair growth resumes with continued use of Propecia and starts to fill in areas that had started to bald. But proving this turned out to be an unusually onerous task.

Balding studies are more difficult to do than studies on urinary flow and prostate size. To give you an example of how demanding this research is, consider the following. In evaluating the effect of finasteride on prostate symptoms, all investigators had to do was ask their patients to fill out a questionnaire on their patterns of urination and arrange for ultrasound studies to determine prostate size before and after treatment.

To do hair-loss studies, doctors had to identify and mark out a single two-inch circular area on the top of a man's scalp as the target area. Then at each visit, they had to count one by one each and every hair in that target area before, during, and after treatment. The results of two combined studies involving more than 1,500 men yielded the following. Men who had 876 hairs in the target area before had on average 983 hairs after treatment, for a net gain of 107 hairs after one year. This does not seem like much but may be enough for those who are distressed by their hair loss. Men with male-pattern baldness age 18–41 years who take Propecia seem to be pleased with the results.

Side effects were similar to what was observed when the 5-mg finasteride (Proscar) dose was used to treat BPH. Sexual side effects, including impotence, loss of sex drive (libido), and ejaculatory problems, occur in about 4 percent of men who take finasteride at this lower 1-mg dose. This once again raises questions about the importance of DHT as a sexually significant male hormone.

IS DHT AN IMPORTANT HORMONAL REGULATOR OF MALE SEXUALITY?

Several lines of reasoning indicate that DHT may be a more important modulator of male sexuality than previously believed. When 100 healthy young male army recruits had baseline hormone measurements and then were asked to record their sexual activity, those with the highest baseline serum DHT level proved to be the most sexually active.

But isn't DHT the hormone that stimulates prostate growth? Wouldn't raising a man's DHT level cause his prostate to enlarge, making it more likely that he would develop BPH? Apparently not.

WHY DOES TESTOSTERONE BUT NOT DIHYDROTESTOSTERONE TREATMENT INCREASE A MAN'S PSA LEVELS?

A man's prostate gland siphons testosterone from his bloodstream. Then an enzyme within the prostate gland converts the trapped testosterone to DHT. It is this DHT made by and retained within the prostate that is one of the factors responsible for prostate gland growth. As far as we know, the prostate gland does not pluck DHT from a man's bloodstream. Further, when blood DHT levels rise, testosterone levels decline, making less testosterone available for the prostate gland to ensnare. With less testosterone to trap, DHT levels within the prostate gland decline; and prostate growth can be held in check. How do we know this?

Older men given testosterone usually have a slight but significant increase in their prostate specific antigen (PSA) levels. But when similarly aged men are given large doses of DHT, their PSA levels do not change. There are probably two reasons for this. When men receive testosterone supplements, their blood testosterone levels increase, making more testosterone available for the prostate to trap and convert to DHT. But when men receive large doses of DHT, their testosterone levels actually decline. There is not as much bloodstream testosterone for the prostate gland to trap, so less is available for conversion to DHT within the prostate gland.

There is a second and more subtle sequence of events that explains why testosterone, but not DHT, stimulates the prostate to generate more PSA. A female hormone, estradiol, is one of the natural by-products of testosterone metabolism. It turns out that estradiol is yet another stimulus to prostate gland growth. Dihydrotestosterone cannot be further metabolized to estradiol or any other prostate-stimulating estrogen. Thus, giving a man more testosterone will raise blood testosterone, estradiol, and dihydrotestosterone levels. The increases in blood testosterone and blood estradiol provide the prostate with two potent hormonal stimuli to prostate growth. Testosterone does this by being trapped by the prostate gland, and after being transformed to DHT, it can increase the growth of the prostate gland. Estradiol then is free to exert a direct stimulatory impact on other prostate cells.

DHT, on the other hand, does not enter the prostate gland and cannot be transformed into another male hormone or estradiol and therefore deprives the prostate of both testosterone and estradiol, nullifying the growth-promoting impact of these two hormones. As a consequence, neither PSA levels nor prostate size increase during DHT treatment.

The ability of DHT to maintain a male hormone presence while simultaneously lowering estradiol levels is what makes DHT an ideal hormone to treat young boys who develop breast enlargement (gynecomastia). DHT has not yet been approved for this use in this country, but in France, where DHT is approved, teenage boys with gynecomastia have benefited from DHT treatment. Published reports indicate that boys' breast size returns to normal with DHT treatment.

WHAT ELSE CAN BE DONE WITH DHT?

Our group has been involved in projects using DHT in gel form to treat two groups of men—those with a condition called AIDS wasting syndrome (AWS) and elderly men with low serum testosterone levels.

We have used DHT gel to reverse some of the ravages of AWS. Men with AWS suffer a progressive weight loss and become disabled and fatigued and are unable to do any meaningful work. In our short-term studies of men with AWS, we found the following.

Prior to treatment, all men with AWS had established a pattern of progressive and intractable weight loss. During only eight weeks of daily DHT treatment, these desperately ill men reclaimed their appetite, put on weight, and increased their strength. Treatment with DHT gel allowed them to reverse course: to eat more heartily and have a significant increase in their total body weight and capacity for physical work. Unlike other AWS treatments, where fluid retention or increased fat accounted for most of the weight gain, the DHT-gel-treated men's weight gain was entirely due to buildup of increased muscle—lean body—mass.

We have been encouraged by our results in men with AWS and along with others are now evaluating DHT gel in elderly men with low testosterone levels.

You will undoubtedly hear more about DHT in the near future.

16

Medications, Chemicals, and Sexual Potency

You depend on your own internal body chemistry to remain sexually interested, active, and fertile. Anything that interferes with the transmission of your body's own internal messages can disrupt your sexual life. External chemicals in the form of prescription medications, alcohol, nicotine, or recreational drugs, alone or collectively, can intrude to disable a man's sex life. This chapter provides a guide to the types of commonly consumed prescription and nonprescription substances that can interfere with a man's libido, erections, ejaculation, and fertility.

Medication-induced impotence is a major problem. In a survey of 1,180 men, medications were recognized as the single most common cause of impotence. The ingredients in many medications cause impotence by disrupting crucial sexual chemistry. In some cases, the medication deadens sex drive or libido. Other chemicals impede a man's ability to have erections; and a few interfere with ejaculation. In most instances, once the relationship between the medication and the sexual dysfunction is recognized and the offending substance is discontinued, sexual function returns to normal.

Medications that can interfere with normal male sexual function are routinely prescribed to treat high blood pressure, heart problems, elevated blood-cholesterol levels, stomach ulcers, anxiety, and depression. These are among the most common medical problems.

Physicians are often aware that the medications they prescribe can impair sexual function. They continue to write prescriptions for these medications for three important reasons:

1. The medication may be more effective than any other available drug.
2. The same medication that produces a sexual side effect in one patient may be benign in the majority of others. (Indeed, only a fraction of men taking the same medication will suffer some impairment in sexual function.)

3. Failure to treat may actually place the man at high risk for the subsequent development of impotence. This is especially true in hypertensive men. (See Table 16.1 for a complete list of drugs and sexual side effects.)

ANTIHYPERTENSIVE THERAPY

Hypertension (high blood pressure) affects 60 million American men; 26 percent of men between the ages of eighteen and seventy-five have significant hypertension. Untreated hypertension represents a major risk factor for the development of stroke, heart attack, and heart disease.

Drugs that lower blood pressure work to overcome the overzealous internal systems responsible for the problem. That would be fine if these medications restricted their activity to lowering blood pressure. Unfortunately, chemicals in many effective blood-pressure-lowering medications create a dissonance in the neurologic and hormonal environment crucial for normal male sexual function.

Although we do not know exactly what causes blood pressure to rise, we have been able to study men with normal and high blood pressure and have learned the following.

- The amount of blood pumped out of the heart (cardiac output) is increased early on in the development of hypertension. Medications that decrease cardiac output, like the beta-blocker propranolol (Inderal), lower blood pressure.
- Blood released from the heart flows through the arterial circulation to deliver oxygen to all parts of the body. The arterial channels of hypertensive men are narrowed (constricted), creating a greater resistance so that blood pressure must increase to blast its way through. Drugs that reverse arterial constriction (vasodilators), like hydralazine (Apresoline), decrease vascular resistance and allow blood pressure to fall. Other drugs, like clonidine (Catapres) and guanethidine (Ismelin), lower blood pressure by dampening the neurologic signals that make arteries constrict.
- Two powerful internally secreted chemicals, norepinephrine and angiotensin II, can, under the appropriate circumstances, cause a man's arteries to constrict and his blood pressure to increase. Drugs that nullify or at least blunt the impact of blood pressure stimulation by norepinephrine (prazosin [Minipres]) and angiotensin II (captopril [Capoten]) can lower blood pressure.
- Excessive salt (sodium overload) has long been suspected of playing a pivotal role in the development of hypertension. Desalting the

body with a diuretic medication (fluid pill) like hydrochlorothiazide is an effective treatment to control salt overload and help normalize blood pressure.

Today, physicians have at their disposal a wide variety of drugs capable of lowering blood pressure. Many have sexual side effects. Avoiding treatment because of fear of sexual side effects is not the answer. Untreated hypertensive men are especially vulnerable to similar sexual problems. It is only recently that the significance of this observation has been fully appreciated.

STUDIES OF SEXUAL FUNCTION OF
HYPERTENSIVE MEN BEFORE AND AFTER TREATMENT

The regularity with which antihypertensive medications affect sexual ability has prompted doctors to wonder how this comes about. Is it the fall in blood pressure, the type of medication used, or some other factor unique to men with high blood pressure that is responsible for their loss of sexual function?

Although antihypertensive medications have been available for almost fifty years, it was not until the early 1980s that several research groups decided to examine the *sexual performance of untreated hypertensive men*. They uncovered some unexpected information.

Men known to have high blood pressure and scheduled to be enrolled in one treatment program or another were, for the first time, asked to complete questionnaires that addressed health-related issues regarding lifestyle, stresses, smoking and drinking habits, and prior illness. The survey also asked about any recent changes in sexual desire, difficulty obtaining or sustaining an erection, and problems ejaculating. Similar questionnaires were administered to men with normal blood pressure.

It turned out that 17 percent of *untreated* hypertensive men reported difficulty achieving or sustaining an erection, compared with only 7 percent of men with normal blood pressure. *Even before they receive any blood-pressure-lowering medication*, hypertensive men describe erectile difficulties, ejaculatory problems, and depressed libido about twice as often as other men of the same age. Thus, the framework for sexual function of hypertensive men is precarious even before treatment.

What happens to the sexual function of hypertensive men when they take blood-pressure-lowering medication? The answer seems to depend on what type of medication is used and whether one or more than one antihypertensive medication is prescribed.

Physicians at the Veterans Administration have devised the Sexual Symptoms Distress Index (SSDI), which differs from other questionnaires because it does not rely solely on yes-or-no responses. Hypertensive men were

---

asked to indicate how upset they were about a specific symptom relative to their sexual function. During the previous month, had they experienced any decreased interest in sex, problems in acquiring or maintaining an erection, or difficulty with ejaculation? Possible responses varied from "not at all" to "extremely"; scores ranged from 0 to 16. A higher number indicates greater distress.

About 40 percent of untreated hypertensive men described some dissatisfaction with sex, whereas 60 percent of men who had received some antihypertensive therapy gave a positive response to these same questions.

Subsequent findings were equally enlightening. In one study, men were treated first with a single antihypertensive medication—captopril (Capoten), methyldopa (Aldomet), or propranolol (Inderal). When blood pressure was not satisfactorily controlled with any of these medications alone, a second drug, the diuretic hydrochlorothiazide (HydroDIURIL), was added. To gauge sexual distress, the SSDI was administered before, during, and after therapies.

Patients receiving captopril, methyldopa, or propranolol alone had no further deterioration in sexual function. Those who were initially potent remained potent. Even those with already marginal SSDI scores were unchanged over the first treatment period (lasting twenty-four weeks). However, men taking methyldopa or propranolol experienced a significant deterioration of sexual function when the diuretic was added. (The diuretic had no effect on men taking captopril.) This was not entirely unexpected.

Physicians already knew that methyldopa or propranolol, when administered in high doses, could impair male sexual function. Captopril does not appear to be burdened with any similar intrinsic properties. For that reason, hypertensive men treated with captopril or any other similar medication like enalapril (Vasotec) seem to tolerate the addition of a diuretic without suffering any further sexual dysfunction.

DIURETIC MEDICATIONS

There are three types of diuretic medications useful in the treatment of hypertension: hydrochlorothiazide and other thiazides, furosemide (Lasix), and spironolactone (Aldactone). To date, furosemide has demonstrated no sexual side effects. However, there is a definite increase in impotence among men treated with thiazides.

Spironolactone has well-documented antiandrogen (anti-male hormone) properties. Men treated with spironolactone are incapable of appreciating the full impact of their own testosterone. This may explain why decreased libido is the single most common sexual side effect reported by them. Despite its side effects, spironolactone has not been stricken from the pharmacologic registry. This medication distinguishes itself from other diuretics by its ability to allow the body to flush out excess sodium while capturing potassium. All the other diuretic medications create a potassium deficiency, a condition that can cause irregular heart rhythms, constipation, muscle cramps, and—as if this were not enough—impotence.

METHYLDOPA

Methyldopa (Aldomet) is generally accepted as an effective antihypertensive medication, but it interferes with the function of the naturally occurring body chemical dopamine, which is important for normal nerve function and hormone release.

The body converts the drug methyldopa to a look-alike chemical called methyldopamine, which then shoulders aside the body's own dopamine. Methyldopamine is referred to as a false neurotransmitter and, like a false prophet, confuses the body by providing scrambled and inaccurate information. The result is that systems crucial for erection do not function properly. Methyldopamine tricks the body into releasing excessive amounts of the sexually inhibiting hormone prolactin. (See Chapter 12.) In addition, methyldopamine creates sufficient biochemical bewilderment in nerve endings to interfere with the way nerves that regulate erections communicate with one another. This then provides a favorable environment for the development of neurogenic impotence.

The most common sexual side effects of methyldopa are decreased libido and impotence; these side effects are not universal, however. The frequency of methyldopa-induced sexual dysfunction varies from study to study, with reports ranging from as low as 3 percent to as high as 37 percent. In most studies, sexual side effects can be anticipated to occur in about 20 to 25 percent of methyldopa-treated hypertensive men.

BETA-BLOCKERS

A group of medications referred to as beta-adrenergic blockers have enjoyed widespread popularity in treating high blood pressure and many heart problems. Among these medications, the beta-blocker propranolol (Inderal) has been available for the longest period, and most of our current knowledge has been derived from the experiences of hypertensive men treated with this drug.

Impotence induced by propranolol appears to be dose related. Sexual potency has been preserved in most men taking doses of up to 160 milligrams a day. When the dose is increased to 320 milligrams a day, impotence and reduced libido occur. Men with hypertension are advanced to this higher dose only if more conventional doses have not adequately controlled their blood pressure. It is not known whether it is the severity of high blood pressure alone or in combination with the increased dose of propranolol that is responsible for the sexual problems.

Metoprolol (Lopressor) is the only other beta-blocker currently acknowledged to cause sexual side effects by impairing erectile and ejaculatory function. As with propranolol, the sexual side effects of metoprolol seem dose related, with decreased libido and impotence more likely to occur at doses greater than 50 mg daily.

ALPHA-BLOCKERS

Guanethidine (Ismelin), guanadrel (Hylorel), prazosin (Minipres), and terazosin (Hytrin) disrupt the body's ability to release or respond to norepinephrine. This results in a significant fall in blood pressure, an effect that may be long-lasting. The drugs also paralyze the ability of the bladder sphincter to close, preventing semen from being ejaculated from the penis. When taken for a long time, guanethidine may also interfere with the neurologic impulses required for erection, eventually leading to neurogenic impotence. Almost 100 percent of men treated with guanethidine have retrograde ejaculations and experience impotence. The drug is now used only for men whose high blood pressure is resistant to all other antihypertensives.

Prazosin (Minipres), tetrazosin (Hytrin), and doxazosin (Cardura) have also been implicated as causes of impotence and retrograde ejaculation, but less frequently. However, since Labetalol (Normodyne, Trandate) has both beta- and alpha-blocking properties, it too can cause retrograde ejaculation.

RESERPINE

Reserpine is an ancient Hindu medicine originally used to treat insomnia, hyperactivity, and insanity. It was this latter property that initially attracted Western pharmacologists. Reserpine (Serpasil) was one of the first major tranquilizers introduced for the treatment of severely disturbed psychotic individuals. As psychiatrists gained familiarity with this medication, they rapidly became aware that their reserpine-treated patients had very low blood pressure and often fainted. In 1955, the pharmaceutical industry elected to capitalize on this side effect; it abandoned reserpine as an antipsychotic medication and reintroduced it as an antihypertensive drug.

A plethora of blood-pressure-lowering medicines are available today, but in the late 1950s, no other antihypertensive medications existed. Thus, reserpine enjoyed widespread popularity. However, it produced a number of significant and troublesome side effects, including depression, impotence, decreased libido, and an inability to ejaculate.

Reserpine interferes with the normal biochemical interactions of the neurotransmitters in the brain, which allow brain cells to communicate with one another. Reserpine-treated patients, like methyldopa-treated patients, commonly have increased levels of prolactin, a sexually inhibiting hormone. Reserpine also has a stultifying effect on the nerves that regulate erections and ejaculations. It can also lower libido. Reserpine is used rarely, only when other antihypertensive medications fail to control blood pressure.

CLONIDINE

Normally, neurologic impulses arising from the medulla (a portion of the brain stem) maintain blood pressure in an acceptable range. When this system overreacts, blood vessels throughout the body narrow and the force needed to propel circulating blood through these constricted arteries must increase. Clonidine (Catapres) lowers blood pressure by blunting the overactive neural signals originating in the medulla.

Clonidine is capable of exerting similar dampening effects on neurologic impulses elsewhere in the body, particularly those responsible for erection and ejaculation. The sexual side effects of Clonidine appear to be both patient and dose specific. Some patients experience sexual dysfunction at any dose. Others note some sexual function impairment only at doses greater than 0.6 mg per day.

CALCIUM CHANNEL INHIBITORS

Verapamil (Calan, Isoptin), nifedipine (Procardia), and diltiazem (Cardizem) belong to a class of recently developed medications called calcium channel inhibitors. These drugs may lower blood pressure by dilating or widening blood vessels. Isolated cases of impotence induced by calcium channel blockers have been reported, but no consistent pattern of sexual side effects has been reported with the calcium channel inhibitors listed above or the newer generation of antihypertensive medications in this category.

ANGIOTENSIN-CONVERTING ENZYME INHIBITORS

One group of antihypertensive medications known as angiotensin-converting enzyme (ACE) inhibitors—captopril (Capoten) and enalapril (Vasotec)—have not caused sexual side effects to date. However, lisinopril (Zestril), a long-acting ACE inhibitor, decreases libido and causes impotence in 1 percent of treated men. The general consensus is that among all blood-pressure-lowering medications, the ACE inhibitors are least likely to interfere with sexual function.

The blood-pressure-lowering effect of these ACE inhibitors is complex. They prevent the transformation of one internal chemical, angiotensin I, to another, angiotensin II. Angiotensin I has no effect on blood pressure, but angiotensin II is the most powerful blood-pressure-elevating chemical known.

SELECTION OF AN ANTIHYPERTENSIVE MEDICATION

What compels physicians to prescribe an antihypertensive medication with sexual side effects when they could just as easily prescribe a medication that does not have any adverse effects on male sexual function? Why are all these antihypertensive medications with sexual side effects still cluttering up pharmacists' shelves? Shouldn't they be relocated to some drugstore purgatory where they can atone for all the grief they have caused?

It is impossible to speak for all physicians, but it is likely that the following considerations enter into the ultimate decision regarding selection of a blood-pressure-lowering medicine.

Harnessing hypertension and bringing blood pressure into the normal range is the primary goal of any antihypertensive therapy. Often this can be accomplished by prescribing a single medication without any sexual side effects. However, hypertension is not always so readily managed. Nothing is gained by prescribing a medication that allows a temporary preservation of sexual function at the expense of unrestrained and uncontrolled hypertension. The risks of eventual stroke or heart attack are too great. It is in those instances, when hypertension cannot be adequately controlled by the more sexually benign medications, that a decision to add medications with potential sexual side effects must be considered. The choice is not easy. Often a satisfactory compromise can be reached so that moderating the doses of medication allows blood pressure to be controlled and sexual function retained.

Abrupt discontinuation of some of the antihypertensive medications can have dire consequences, such as striking rebound elevations in blood pressure. Patients are at risk for headache, heart symptoms, stroke (rarely), and recurrence of sexual problems.

Martin, whose father and grandfather had died of complications of hypertension, was not surprised when he learned that his blood pressure was elevated. He eagerly accepted the doctor's recommendations for an antihypertensive medication, spironolactone (Aldactone). He had no problems for three or four months, during which time he and his wife enjoyed a constant level of sexual activity. Then gradually, almost imperceptibly, he started to lose interest in sex. He no longer made sexual advances to his wife and indeed rebuffed most of her advances to him. She became agitated and suspected he was having an affair, which he vigorously denied. On reflection, they realized that the onset of his sexual apathy emerged shortly after he started to take spironolactone. He discontinued his medication, and in two or three weeks, sexual desire returned. But now Martin had a new sexual problem. He could no longer acquire an erection. Blood pressure was once again elevated, requiring treatment. An alternate antihypertensive drug less likely to cause sexual side effects was substituted. As blood pressure normalized, erections and sexual intercourse resumed.

FINASTERIDE (PROSCAR)

The hormone dihydrotestosterone, a normal by-product of testosterone metabolism, causes prostate enlargement. Lowering DHT levels, therefore, should be useful in reining in a major hormonal stimulus to continued prostate growth. Finasteride (Proscar) inhibits the conversion of testosterone to dihydrotestosterone, causing an 80 percent fall in blood DHT levels and a decrease in prostate size, and for this reason has been useful as a treatment for men with a condition called benign prostatic hyperplasia (BPH). (See Chapter 23.) Finasteride does not diminish total testosterone output, so it was unexpected when, in the initial trials of this medication, a small number (about 4.3 percent) of finasteride-treated men said they became impotent, whereas only 1.8 percent of treated men reported similar sexual problems while taking placebo. The results were surprising not because 4.3 percent of men old enough to experience BPH complained of impotence but because so few of the comparably aged placebo treated men insisted that their sexual function was entirely normal! Considering data amassed during multiple studies described in Chapter 5, it seems highly unlikely that the placebo-treated men in this study were entirely forthright about their sexual prowess. Subsequent studies with Rigi-Scan recordings before, during, and after treatment showed identical erectile function in finasteride and placebo-treated men.

PSYCHIATRIC MEDICATIONS

Most medications useful in the treatment of anxiety, depression, mania, psychotic states, and other psychiatric disorders have sexual side effects. Sexual function, however, is rarely entirely normal in psychiatric patients. Like untreated hypertensive males, men plagued by anxiety, depression, and other psychiatric disorders commonly have impaired sexual function.

Psychiatric, or psychoactive, drugs interact with the network of chemicals called neurotransmitters that are present in the brain and elsewhere in the nervous system. Neurotransmitters allow nerve cells to interact with one another. Many experts postulate that psychiatric illness reflects an ill-defined breakdown in the normal chemical communication among brain cells. This disruption favors a pattern of random, chaotic neurochemical signals that may cause depression, paranoia, psychosis, mania, or other forms of psychiatric dysfunction. Psychoactive medications are thought to be effective by virtue of their ability to redress this internal chemical turmoil and help realign neurochemical impulses so that normal communications can resume.

Psychiatric medications also interrupt the neurochemistry required for the smooth progression of the normal male sexual response cycle. Like antihypertensive medications, some psychiatric medications have a negative effect on libido and/or impair the capability to have erections. But the most consistently reported sexual side effect is delayed ejaculation or a complete inability to ejaculate.

ANTIDEPRESSANT MEDICATIONS

Decreased libido and impotence are common in men suffering from depression. Sexual function usually returns to normal when the depression lifts with treatment. Antidepressant medications fall into three general classes of drugs: tricyclic antidepressants (Imipramine, Desipramine, Amitriptyline, Nortriptyline), monoamine oxidase (MAO) inhibitors (Phenelzine, Isocarboxacid, Tranylcypromine), and atypical antidepressants (trazodone). Sexual side effects are common with all these drugs. Even the newest antidepressants, those characterized as selective serotonin reuptake inhibitors (SSRIs) such as fluoxetine (Prozac), paroxetine (Paxil), and sertraline (Zoloft) have been reported to inhibit sexual desire and potency.

The scenario sounds ominously familiar, something like an instant replay of the hypertension-antihypertensive therapy conundrum. There are indeed similarities, but there are also notable differences.

- Although it is true that compromised sexual function is one of the hallmarks of depression, it is equally apparent that for the sexually dysfunctional man, resurrection of sexual prowess occurs only when his depression is alleviated. Impotent hypertensive men often experience, but cannot depend on, a similar improvement in sexual function when their blood pressure is normalized.
- The trend in tracking sexual function of hypertensive men before, during, and after therapy has not yet established a strong foothold in psychiatric literature. As a result, most of our information regarding the sexual side effects of psychiatric drugs has been derived from either anecdotal individual case reports or sidebars to scientific papers

describing both the effectiveness and adverse effects of new antidepressant medications.

- The scale of studies exploring antidepressant-induced sexual side effects is not comparable. The experiences of thousands of hypertensive men now provide the foundation for our knowledge of the sexual side effects of antihypertensive medications. The largest single report of psychoactive drug-induced impairment in sexual function is based on interviews of fifty-seven men who were already receiving the antipsychotic medication thioridazine (Mellaril) at the time of the interview. Impaired ejaculation was reported by twenty-eight of the men (49 percent).

- Paradoxically, the most common sexual side effect of psychoactive drugs has proven to be a boon to some men with other specific sexual dysfunctions. We know that antidepressant and antipsychotic medications commonly cause delayed or retarded ejaculation. This side effect is a godsend for men suffering from premature ejaculation. Unfortunately, none of the sexual side effects of antihypertensive medications can be similarly adapted to improve the lot of other sexually dysfunctional men.

- Priapism is one sexual side effect attributed to psychiatric medications not shared by the antihypertensives. This painful persistent erection has been recognized with increasing frequency in men who take antidepressant medications. Several tricyclic and MAO inhibitor antidepressants have been reported to cause priapism on rare occasions. Trazodone (Desyrel), an atypical antidepressant, has also been implicated as causing priapism.

SELECTIVE SEROTONIN REUPTAKE
INHIBITORS (SSRI) AND SEX

An entirely new class of antidepressant drugs—the selective serotonin reuptake inhibitors designated as SSRI—has proven to be extraordinarily effective in alleviating symptoms of depression in both men and women. SSRI antidepressants include fluoxetine (Prozac), sertraline (Zoloft), and paroxetine (Paxil), among others. Drugs in this category were at first thought to have relatively few sexual side effects because only 1.9 percent of those originally treated with fluoxetine described sexual side effects. However, now that SSRIs are increasingly viewed as the antidepressants of choice, prescribing doctors and their depressed patients have gained additional experience with these medications. It is now apparent that SSRIs are not sexually innocuous medications. In one study, 54 of 160 (34 percent) patients noticed new sexual problems during fluoxetine treatment. Diminished libido, inability to acquire an erection, and delayed or absent orgasm were among the side effects reported.

TREATING SSRI-INDUCED SEXUAL DYSFUNCTION

Several different treatment options have been devised to correct SSRI-induced sexual dysfunction. Adjusting SSRI dose, juggling the schedule of SSRI administration, adding yohimbine (see Chapter 21), or substituting another antidepressant, bupropion (Wellbutrin), have all been reported to provide relief from SSRI-induced sexual dysfunction.

On occasion, increasing amounts of SSRI are required to alleviate depression, and when that happens, the onset of sexual side effects coincides with escalating SSRI doses. Decreasing SSRI dose alone may suffice to restore sexual function without sacrificing any of the mood-elevating benefits brought about with antidepressant therapy.

Dr. Alan Rothschild of Maclean Hospital, Belmont, Massachusetts, has achieved the same effect by giving his patients a "drug holiday." He instructed thirty patients who experienced sexual side effects while taking either fluoxetine, sertraline, or paroxetine every day to stop taking medication on Friday and Saturday (the drug holiday) and resume their normal dose at 12:00 noon on Sunday. Significant improvement in sexual function was noted by patients who took a weekend holiday from sertraline and paroxetine, but not from fluoxetine. Depression did not worsen during the brief drug holiday, leading the author to conclude that one way to restore sexual function in sexually impaired sertraline- or paroxetine-treated patients was to ease up on the SSRI burden for a brief period of time. Exactly why the same technique was ineffective in fluoxetine-treated patients is not clear.

Another antidepressant medication, bupropion (Wellbutrin), alone or in combination with fluoxetine, has been used to treat men with SSRI-induced sexual dysfunction. Bupropion is an antidepressant medication different in structure and function from SSRI antidepressants and has been touted as being free of sexual side effects, a claim that has been supported to some degree by clinical experience.

Drs. Lawrence Labbate and Mark Pollack described this phenomenon by reporting their experience with a depressed fifty-year-old man who had less depression two months after starting fluoxetine, but after six months of continued treatment noted diminished libido, erectile impotence, and problems achieving orgasm. Fluoxetine therapy was continued and small doses of another antidepressant, bupropion, were added. Libido, normal erections, and satisfactory orgasms returned within ten days of instituting bupropion therapy. When fluoxetine was discontinued, depression returned, and when bupoprion was stopped, sexual function deteriorated, indicating that for this patient a combination of fluoxetine and bupropion was essential to control depression without disrupting sexual function.

Building on this experience, psychiatrists at several medical centers pooled their experience to see what would happen when patients experiencing sexual dysfunction on fluoxetine stopped that medication and instead used bupropion as their only antidepressant. Patients first discontinued fluoxetine and were on no antidepressant medication for two weeks. It was during this interval, off SSRI medication, that sexual function started to improve. Thereafter, bupropion therapy was instituted, and patients' estimates of their orgasms, libido, and overall sexual function were evaluated in 25 of 39 patients (64 percent) who started and completed the eight-week trial. Orgasm, libido, and sexual satisfaction were said to be significantly improved in the majority of patients who completed the trial. Some failed to complete because when they stopped fluoxetine and went on bupropion, depression returned. Others were excluded from analysis for a variety of reasons. The improvement in sexual function after discontinuing fluoxetine and starting bupropion, while gratifying, must be interpreted cautiously, because the design of the study does not resolve the question: Did SSRI-induced sexual dysfunction improve because fluoxetine was stopped or because bupropion was started? Only a placebo-controlled study will provide the answer. In the absence of such a study, depressed men who develop sexual side effects during SSRI treatment should alert their doctors to the nature of their problem, and working together, they should be able to find a way to control depression without disrupting sexual function.

ANTIPSYCHOTIC MEDICATIONS

Schizophrenia and other major emotional disorders can be treated by three groups of medications referred to as antipsychotic drugs: phenothiazines, thioxanthenes, and butyrophenones. Medications from each group have been incriminated as causes of sexual dysfunction, but exact knowledge of the patient's normal sexual function prior to initiation of the drug is often lacking. Thus, the best evidence comes from the occasional patient who reports problems with sexual function when he starts treatment with a different antipsychotic medication. Inhibition of ejaculation is a common sexual side effect associated with thioridazine (Mellaril) and other phenothiazine medications as well. In a few patients, thioridazine also inhibited libido and erections.

The grandfather of all phenothiazine medications, chlorpromazine (Thorazine), is also known to cause inhibited ejaculation. Chlorpromazine has been evaluated in a carefully controlled study that found it does not interfere with erections or libido.

Medications, Chemicals, and Sexual Potency

Fluphenazine (Prolixin) has been saddled with the designation of a libido-inhibiting medication as a result of a report that described the effectiveness of fluphenazine in inhibiting the desire of men convicted of sexual crimes. A large dose of fluphenazine given by injection did produce some reduction in their libido.

Nevertheless, inhibited ejaculation remains the single most common side effect of the mainstream antipsychotic medications.

MEDICATIONS THAT ALTER
SEXUAL FUNCTION BY INCREASING PROLACTIN
OR DECREASING TESTOSTERONE PRODUCTION

Many of the drugs (neuroleptics) used to treat schizophrenia disrupt the body's natural tendency to keep serum prolactin levels in check. As a consequence, serum prolactin levels rise during treatment with these and other medications that interfere with the normal dopamine-induced suppression of pituitary prolactin secretion. (See Chapter 12.)

Metoclopramide (Reglan), a medication commonly given to control nausea and vomiting, also causes higher-than-normal serum prolactin levels. Whenever men or women have elevated serum prolactin levels, sexual and reproductive function suffers, causing men to become impotent and women to stop menstruating normally. The frequency with which these side effects occur in schizophrenic men and women with medication-induced increases in serum prolactin levels is illustrated in Table 16.2.

MEDICATION AND TESTOSTERONE

Other medications such as the antifungal medication ketoconazole (Nizoral), the anticancer drug suramin, and many of the medications used to control advanced prostate cancer cause impotence by abruptly lowering serum testosterone levels. Ketoconazole and suramin work to limit the testicle's ability to make testosterone, whereas leuprolide (Lupron), buserelin (Superfact), and nafarelin (Synarel) shut down the pituitary gland's natural pulsatile secretion of LH. Without this natural stimulus, the testicle's Leydig cells simply cease testosterone production. Other medications such as flutamide (Eulexin), commonly used in conjunction with gonadotropin agonists, is an antiandrogen and understandably further cripples a man's libido and sexual function. Usually, before men with prostate cancer embark on what is referred to as androgen ablative therapy to control the spread of their prostate cancer, they are advised that inhibiting testosterone production or action will cause them to become impotent and have diminished libido. Those who wish to retain erectile function can be offered the option of penile injection therapy or vacuum-assisted erection devices to allow them to have sexual intercourse.

LITHIUM

Lithium, usually in the form of lithium carbonate (Lithobid, Eskalith), is used to treat patients with mania. Mania is a condition of hyperactivity and disordered thinking that may occur spontaneously, as an independent illness, but it more often occurs in conjunction with depression. People affected with the dual illnesses of depression and mania are said to have a "bipolar disorder." Antidepressant therapy is appropriate when they are in the depressed phase of their illness, but when the manic phase supervenes, treatment with lithium is warranted.

Some patients in a manic phase complain that lithium induces sexual side effects, but the data supporting this conclusion are shaky at best. When patients are manic, they have an exaggerated sense of their own sexual prowess. Therefore, it is impossible to obtain accurate baseline information regarding the sexual function of actively manic patients unless their partners can provide corroborating evidence. As the mania and hyperactivity come under control, the patient's thinking becomes more properly attuned to reality.

It is difficult to know whether the impotence reported by some patients in the course of lithium therapy is actually caused by the medication. In the most widely quoted study, two of ten lithium-treated patients developed impotence. Potency returned in both, one who stopped and another who continued lithium treatment. For this reason, it remains unclear whether lithium alone has any negative effect on male sexual function.

MINOR TRANQUILIZERS

Billions of minor tranquilizers are taken every day to relieve anxiety, relax muscle tension, and help people fall asleep. Included are chlordiazepoxide (Librium), diazepam (Valium), lorazepam (Ativan), alprazolam (Xanax), and clorazepate (Tranxene). It is unclear whether these medications have any effect on male sexual function.

ANTIULCER MEDICATIONS

Physicians often prescribe cimetidine (Tagamet) for gastritis and ulcers because it inhibits acid production by the stomach. Cimetidine also inhibits testosterone production, and Tagamet-treated men often complain of impotence. When cimetidine therapy is stopped, the stimulus for testosterone secretion resumes and potency is restored.

Medications, Chemicals, and Sexual Potency

Ranitidine (Zantac) and famotidine (Pepcid) are similar to cimetidine. Both drugs are equally effective in decreasing production of stomach acid, but neither appears to cause sexual side effects.

DIET MEDICATION

Sexual side effects have been reported to occur with a wide range of new medications with bewildering frequency and inconsistency. Thus, the appetite-reducing diet medication fenfluramine (Pondimin) has been reported to cause both *loss of and inappropriately increased libido* in women and impotence in men. The fenfluramine-induced *increase in female libido has been reported only in bulemic women,* that is, women who resort to overeating and self-induced vomiting to control their weight. Fenfluramine controls the urge to overeat, but when given in doses high enough (120 mg per day) to achieve this effect, it seems to also enhance libido to the point that women become sexually obsessed and frantic, preferring to die from bulimia than suffer the sexual consequences of the drug. In contrast, the dominant sexual side effect of overweight men taking fenfluramine is impotence.

It is likely that the differences in sexual side effects is not so much related to gender as it is to the individual's underlying condition, for fenfluramine acts as an aphrodisiac only in women with bulimia.

CHOLESTEROL-LOWERING MEDICATIONS

Clofibrate (Atromid-S) lowers serum cholesterol levels. Unfortunately, the same properties that allow these medications to limit cholesterol production also interfere with the testicle's ability to manufacture testosterone. As expected, men treated with clofibrate often complain of diminished libido and impotence. Recently, a few isolated case reports have implicated gemfibrozil (Lopid) as a cause of impotence, but this has not been confirmed in any larger placebo-controlled studies.

None of the other cholesterol-lowering drugs appears to interfere with sexual function.

WHY DO MEDICATIONS CAUSE IMPOTENCE?

Our current knowledge of the neurologic, vascular, and hormonal interplay necessary for normal male sexual function, though imperfect, is still sufficiently advanced to allow us to understand how prescription drugs and other ingested chemicals can disrupt all or part of the sexual response cycle and cause impotence and infertility.

The physical systems necessary for potency and fertility are remarkably resilient but not infinitely elastic. Some prescription drugs used to treat high blood pressure and emotional disorders have sexual side effects; others do not. Nevertheless, control of blood pressure and emotional disorder is of paramount importance to health. If physicians can achieve this goal without compromising sexual function, they will do so. But this is not always possible. Occasionally, once inroads in the control of blood pressure or emotional disorders have been achieved by a medication with sexual side effects, a physician can adjust the dosage to sustain the therapeutic benefit; doses of the sexually noxious drug are gradually discontinued, and a second drug without sexual side effects is introduced. This tricky business requires close collaboration between doctor and patient.

In addition to the pills supplied by physicians to treat medical conditions, prostate surgery performed to alleviate major, sometimes life-threatening, illnesses can, as an unintended effect, create impotence. In situations where a physician, either by prescribing a medication or by performing surgery, causes an unanticipated side effect, the resultant problem is said to be "iatrogenic" (from *iatros*, Greek for "physician.")

However, physicians are not the sole purveyors of impotence-causing chemicals.

SELF-ADMINISTERED SUBSTANCES THAT AFFECT POTENCY

Cigarettes

Heavy cigarette smoking damages the large arteries supplying blood to all areas of the pelvis and limits the amount of blood available for erections. In addition, and perhaps more important, cigarette smoking damages the tiny blood vessels in the penis that must enlarge to accept the substantial onrush of blood expected during the course of normal erection.

Autopsy studies of heavy smokers show that the small arterioles in the penis are universally narrowed and scarred, no longer retaining the elasticity needed to expand. In contrast, the small penile blood vessels of nonsmokers are normal. This is true for both young and old men alike.

It is no longer necessary to rely solely on anatomic specimens to demonstrate the negative impact of cigarettes on male sexual function. The same information can be obtained by examining the smoking habits of men enrolled in impotence clinics. In two separate surveys, cigarette smoking among impotent men was two times higher than in the potent men. Over 58 percent of impotent men turn out to be active smokers, and 81 percent will admit to heavy cigarette use in the past.

The rate of blood flow into the penis can be measured and calculated as a penile brachial index (PBI) (see Chapter 10). Impotent men who are heavy smokers have a clearly subnormal PBI, indicating that blood flow is inadequate for normal erections.

It is believed that when men stop smoking, penile blood vessels can reconstitute themselves to allow for normal blood flow and restoration of erectile capability. As with any other type of cigarette-induced vascular disease, the critical factor allowing recovery seems to be the number of cigarettes smoked and the duration of the smoking habit.

It is not yet clear how much cigarette smoking a man can tolerate without compromising his sexual function. In dogs, the inhaled smoke from only two cigarettes impairs canine erectile function. In the human, casual smoking may not have a deleterious effect. However, irreparable damage to the penile blood vessels and impaired erectile capability appear to be inevitable for men who smoke packs or fractions of packs a day for several decades.

Alcohol

The negative effect of alcohol consumption on sexual function has been known for many years. Shakespeare was well aware of the initially disinhibiting but ultimately intrusive role of alcohol. In *Macbeth*, the porter says, "It [drink] provokes the desire, but it takes away the performance."

It is possible that moderate alcohol consumption provides some tranquilizing benefit to alleviate sexual anxieties. However, the adverse effects of excessive alcohol consumption on sexual performance have been well documented and commonly experienced. Many currently fully potent men can recall an isolated episode of alcohol-induced impotence. This is primarily due to the soporific effect of alcohol. Inebriated or only slightly tipsy men planning to have sex find that there is a point when the sedative effects of alcohol overcome its disinhibiting effects. In such cases, libido is squelched in favor of a good night's sleep.

Several critical functions necessary for normal male sexual activity are temporarily or irreparably impaired by excessive alcohol consumption. Alcohol inhibits the ability of the testicle to produce testosterone, the major hormone responsible for sex drive or libido. Alcoholic men with low serum testosterone levels have little or no interest in sex.

Alcohol-induced liver damage causes a shift in testosterone metabolism so that this vital male hormone is shunted away from the path that leads to the creation of the even more potent male hormone dihydrotestosterone and into a direction that favors the increased production of a female hormone, the estrogen estradiol.

Inappropriate high serum estrogen levels cause alcoholic men to have enlarged breasts (gynecomastia) and a characteristic flushing of the face and palms.

The reproductive function of the testicle is also impaired by heavy drinking. Infertility is a common result.

Alcohol damages the nerves that allow erection and ejaculation to occur. Many alcoholics are unable to produce semen by masturbation because they can no longer ejaculate forward. The nerve damage caused by alcohol results in retrograde ejaculation.

Many of these changes are reversible with abstinence. Recovery of potency and fertility is most likely in those men whose drinking has not damaged the liver or the nerves that allow erections or ejaculation to take place.

A precise itemization of the total amount of alcohol a man must consume to qualify as a heavy drinker or an alcoholic is not readily available. Most men would like to believe that an alcoholic is someone who drinks more than they do. This is an unfortunate delusion. However, it is still not known exactly how much a man can drink with impunity or at what point his cumulative alcohol consumption is sufficient to usher him across his own sexual and reproductive Rubicon.

Marijuana

Tetrahydrocannabinol (THC), the active ingredient in marijuana, is thought to have a positive effect on male sexual function by increasing sensate focus. However, substantial evidence has now accumulated to indicate that chronic THC use has an adverse effect on both male sexual function and fertility. An enlargement of the male breast (gynecomastia) and a progressive decrease in serum testosterone levels have been noted in chronic marijuana users. In animals, THC use has a negative effect on sexual interest and performance and has a curiously devastating impact on the fertility of male offspring.

Mice exposed to THC in doses equivalent to three marijuana cigarettes daily have high miscarriage rates, and their offspring have a fourfold increase in chromosomal abnormalities. A trend of progressive decrease in fertility extends through the first and second generation of male mice whose parents have been exposed to marijuana. Translation of this mouse research into human terms should be available shortly as the first and second generations of male children born to parents of the Woodstock generation reach reproductive age.

Opiate Drugs

Morphine, heroin, and methadone fall into a class of drugs known as opiates. They have a profound negative effect on the hormonal regulation of male sexual function. All serve to depress the normal pattern of secretion of the hypothalamic hormones that trigger the release of LH and ultimately testosterone. Low testosterone production, decreased libido, and impotence are all common among chronic heroin, morphine, and methadone addicts.

Cocaine

Cocaine enjoys a reputation as an aphrodisiac. However, substantial evidence is accumulating to indicate that chronic cocaine use, alone or in combination with alcohol, ultimately causes sexual dysfunction. Cocaine alone stimulates secretion of the sexually inhibiting hormone prolactin. Cocaine also causes spasms in arteries; blood flow to the penis cannot be sustained if arterial spasms persist. Studies in detoxification centers have demonstrated that partner sex, masturbation, and orgasm frequency decline with chronic cocaine use. Sexual function can return to normal after cocaine detoxification and abstinence. A drug-free interval of nine months to one year is required for restoration of libido and potency.

TABLE 16.1   Sexual Side Effects of Common Prescription Medications

Generic Name	Brand Name	Sexual Side Effect
Antihypertensive Medications		
Diuretics		
Spironolactone	Aldactone	Decreased libido, breast swelling, impotence
Thiazides	Diuril, HydroDIURIL, Naturetin, Naqua, many others	Impotence
Furosemide	Lasix	None
Centrally Acting Methyldopa	Aldomet	Decreased libido, impotence
Clonidine	Catapres	Impotence
Reserpine	Serpasil, Raudixin, Ser-Ap-Es	Decreased libido, impotence, depression
Alpha Adrenergic Blockers		
Prazosin	Minipres	"Dry" (retrograde) ejaculation
Terazosin	Hytrin	"Dry" (retrograde) ejaculation
Beta-Adrenergic Blockers		
Propranolol	Inderal	Impotence, decreased libido
Metropolol	Lopressor	Impotence, decreased libido
Combined Alpha- and Beta-Andrenergic Blockers		
Labetolol	Normodyne, Trandate	Inhibited Ejaculation

(continues)

TABLE 16.1 *(continued)*

Generic Name	Brand Name	Sexual Side Effect
Nonandrenergic Vasodilators		
Hydralazine	Apresoline	None
Sympathetic Nerve Blockers		
Guanethidine	Ismelin	Impotence, "dry" (retrograde) ejaculation
Angiotensin-Converting Enzyme (ACE) Inhibitors		
Captopril	Capoten	None
Enalapril	Vasotec	None
Lisinopril	Zestril	Impotence in a small percentage (1 percent) of cases
Psychiatric Medications		
Antidepressants		
Tricyclics		
Amitriptyline	Elavil	Inhibited ejaculation, impotence
Amoxapine	Ascendin	Decreased libido, impotence
Desipramine	Norpramin	Inhibited ejaculation
Doxepin	Sinequan	Inhibited ejaculation, impotence
Imipramine	Tofranil	Inhibited ejaculation, impotence
Maprotriline	Ludiomil	Inhibited ejaculation

Nortriptyline	Aventyl, Pamelor	Inhibited ejaculation
Protriptyline	Vivactil	Inhibited ejaculation, impotence
Atypical		
Trazodone	Desyrel	Priapism
Monoamine Oxidase (MAO) Inhibitors		
Isocarboxazid	Marplan	Inhibited ejaculation
Phenelzine	Nardil	Inhibited ejaculation, decreased libido
Tranylcypromine	Parnate	Inhibited ejaculation
Sertonin Reuptake Inhibitors		
Fluoxetine	Prozac	Anorgasmia (8 percent), sexual dysfunction 1.9%, impotence 1.7%
Sertraline	Zoloft	Male sexual dysfunction 15.5%
Paroxetine	Paxil	Ejaculatory disorders12.9%, other male genital disorders 10.0%
Perphenazine	Trilafon	Inhibited ejaculation
Trifluoperazine	Stelazine	Inhibited ejaculation
Thioxanthene Group		
Chlorprothixene	Taractan	Inhibited ejaculation
Thiothixene	Navane	Inhibited ejaculation, impotence

(continues)

TABLE 16.1 *(continued)*

Generic Name	Brand Name	Sexual Side Effect
Other Antidepressant Medications		
Venlafaxine	Effexor	Abnormal ejaculation/orgasm 12%, impotence 6%,
Bupropion	Wellbutrin	Impotence 3.4 %
Butyrophenone		
Haloperidol	Haldol	Inhibited ejaculation
Antipsychotic Medications		
Phenothiazine Group		
Thioridazine	Mellaril	Inhibited ejaculation, priapism, decreased libido
Chlorpromazine	Thorazine	Inhibited ejaculation
Mesoridazine	Serentil	Inhibited ejaculation, decreased libido
Fluphenazine	Prolixin	Inhibited ejaculation, decreased libido
Anitmania Medication		
Lithium carbonate	Eskalith, Lithobid	Possible impotence
Antiulcer Medications		
Cimetidine	Tagamet	Decreased libido, impotence
Ranitidine	Zantac	None
Famotidine	Pepcid	None

Cholesterol Lowering Medications

Clofibrate	Atromid-S	Impotence
Cholestyramine	Questran	None
Colestipol	Colestid	None
Gemfibrozil	Lopid	None
Probucol	Lorelco	None
Lovastatin	Mevacor	None

Diet Medications

Mazindol	Sanorex	Impotence, painful erections
Phenteremine	Fastin, Adipex, Others	Impotence, decreased libido
Fenfluramine	Pondimin	Decreased libido, impotence, increased libido in women with bulimia
Dexfenfluramine	Redux	??

TABLE 16.2 Reported frequency of sexual dysfunction in schizophrenic men and women who had medication induced increases in serum prolactin levels

Symptoms reported by 26 Men	Percent
Cannot have an erection	38%
Cannot maintain an erection	42%
Decreased orgasm	58%
Symptoms reported by 27 Women	
Decreased orgasm	22%
Irregular Menses	78%
Painful orgasm	7%

17

Psychologic Factors Affecting Potency and Ejaculation

The recognition of the physical—vascular, neurologic, and hormonal—determinants of normal male sexual function has for the moment taken center stage and relegated to the background the important role of psychologic or emotional factors that can conspire to disrupt a man's sex life. It wasn't always this way. Subtle variations in a man's psychology, his emotional life, or the way he related to his sexual partner were once considered to be the only explanations for impotence. Today, with a broader understanding of both the physical and emotional underpinnings of a healthy sex life, we can now build on the pioneering work of the psychologists, psychiatrists, and sex therapists who were the first to venture into the area of the sexuality of men and women. In this chapter, you will learn how a man's psyche can interfere with his sex life, be able to recognize the signs of an emotional conflict, and read about ways to cope with or find help for the depression, anxiety, or panic that still so commonly interfere with sex.

Our current understanding of the male sexual response cycle is based in large part on the contributions of psychiatrists, psychologists, and behavioral scientists. Until recently, only they had the opportunity to delve into issues relevant to male sexual function. Others did not challenge the mental-health profession's exclusive dominion over sexual matters. Sex was discussed in psychiatry and psychology textbooks only.

As a result, medical textbooks published before 1980 were not inclined to devote much attention to the subject of impotence because at that time it was commonly believed that 90 percent or more of impotence was psychologic in origin. This limited perspective has been reconsidered. Current medical textbooks discuss impotence extensively and thoroughly. Today, physicians recognize that in addition to psychologic problems, physical or organic (vascular, neurologic, or hormonal) abnormalities can disrupt the male sexual response cycle.

Whereas men with organic types of impotence have physical conditions that require correction, men with so-called psychogenic impotence are physically capable of sex but are blocked by some emotional discord. Psychogenic impotence is a generic diagnosis encompassing a constellation of problems, including performance anxiety, lack of sensate focus, recent or deeply rooted emotional conflicts, and depression. Anxiety and other emotional factors may impede sexual satisfaction by causing premature or delayed ejaculation. Effective treatment is available once a correct diagnosis is made.

SYMPTOMS AND DIAGNOSIS

Psychologic factors must be considered instrumental in a man's impotence if he:

- Has normal erections in the morning, evening, during masturbation, with an alternate sexual partner, after viewing erotic films, or any other time but is incapable of acquiring an erection when he attempts to make love with his primary partner.
- Has experienced a *sudden* loss of potency in the absence of direct injury to the spine or penis.
- Is embroiled in a fractious relationship with his partner.
- Feels under undue stress.
- Finds sexual intercourse an anxiety-provoking experience.
- Describes symptoms or shows signs compatible with a diagnosis of depression.

It is not always obvious when emotional problems are causing sexual difficulties. Being impotent is in itself a depressing and anxiety-provoking experience. All impotent men, when first evaluated, appear anxious and, if not overtly depressed, despondent about their loss of sexual function. This is true even for those men whose impotence is caused by neurologic, vascular, or hormonal abnormalities. In their case, any psychologic problems are a *reaction to* and not a *cause of* their impotence.

Sometimes psychogenic impotence is the diagnosis by default. After normal nocturnal penile tumescence, penile blood flow, and hormone tests have exonerated neurologic, vascular, or hormonal systems, psychogenic impotence emerges as the only remaining fallback diagnosis. On other occasions, the recognition of organic or psychologic causes of impotence may be solely a reflection of the type of doctor who evaluates the man; the mindset of the examining physician exerts a powerful influence on the ultimate diagnosis. Urologists, internists, and endocrinologists are more likely to look for and find organic rather than psychologic causes of impotence. Psychiatrists are more attuned to recognition of subtle psychologic problems.

EVALUATION AND TREATMENT

A detailed medical history is the first step in understanding the nature of the psychologic conflict responsible for the current sexual problem.

Batteries of pencil-and-paper tests, in the form of self- or therapist-administered questionnaires, are also available to help establish a psychologic profile of men with sexual problems. The Multiaxial Descriptive System for Sexual Dysfunction Manual (MADSSDM) provides a format for the precise classification of sexual problems. Questions are designed to illuminate specific details of a man's current and prior sexual activity, desires, fetishes, and concerns. More elaborate probes have been devised to assess his level of sexual knowledge and misconceptions. Still others explore the nature of the man's sexual fantasies and experiences and ask him to describe his level of satisfaction with his current and prior sexual partners.

Like many similar probes, the Florida Sexual Health Questionnaire (FSHQ) developed by Dr. Michael Geisser consists of a series of questions designed to assess a man's current and past sexual function. This panel consists of twenty questions, some more important than others, and has been useful in segregating men who have psychologic from those whose impotence is caused by physical problems. The very first question is: How often do you think about sexual intercourse? The possible answers are:

1. Never
2. Rarely (every 2–3 months)
3. Occasionally (once a month)
4. Fairly often (every 2–3 weeks)
5. Usually (once or twice a week)
6. Always (almost every day)

Men who check off "1" are either depressed or suffering from a significant decline in testosterone production, for only depression or a major disruption in testosterone output marginalizes a man's sexual interest so severely.

Other questions are similar in format and are arranged so that the man has the opportunity to check off the frequency of his spontaneous nighttime or morning erections, whether or not he has problems with premature ejaculation, and how often he has problems in acquiring or maintaining an erection, with a slightly different range of possible responses:

1. Always
2. Usually (75 percent of the time)
3. Fairly often (50 percent of the time)
4. Occasionally (25 percent of the time)

5. Rarely (10 percent of the time)
6. Never

A complete questionnaire appears in the Appendix at the end of this chapter.

Healthy men tend to rack up high scores, whereas men with physical problems cannot bring their scores above 70. Men with psychogenic impotence also score high on the FSHQ.

When an impotent man's FSHQ score exceeds 72, psychogenic impotence is likely. This is a particularly useful cutoff score, because sometimes it is not possible to determine whether psychologic or physical problems have the upper hand. For example, the sexual dysfunction of diabetic men is often, but not invariably, caused by physical problems. Diabetics are not immune to psychologic pressure, and when their FSHQ scores are greater than 72, it is likely that the negative influence of underlying emotional issues requires attention. In that case, counseling or psychotherapy may be the best way to help that diabetic man retrieve his lost sexual function.

These questionnaires are valuable research tools but do not by themselves confirm a diagnosis of psychogenic impotence. Information provided by these questionnaires can only establish the baseline level of sexual dysfunction. During and after therapy, the questionnaires can be readministered to determine whether medication, psychotherapy, or sex therapy was effective.

A wide variety of services is now offered impotent men with psychologic problems. Psychiatrists, psychologists, sex therapists, and specially trained counselors can all provide help; discussion between therapist and patient (or "talk therapy") is the primary form of treatment for psychologic problems. Sex therapists can furnish the patient with additional sexual information and education. The patient may need medications, either mild tranquilizers or more powerful antidepressants. In such cases, the services of a psychiatrist are necessary.

At the outset, it must be determined whether the sexual problem is primary or secondary.

PRIMARY IMPOTENCE

Men with primary impotence have never experienced normal psychosexual maturation, nor have they ever successfully masturbated or engaged in a satisfactory sexual relationship. For many years, primary impotence was believed to be a relatively rare problem. In his *Sexual Behavior in the Human Male*, Dr. Alfred Kinsey reported that less than 0.4 percent of men under the age of twenty-five had primary impotence. It is possible that this figure underestimated the prevalence of this disorder.

A recent reawakening of interest in the subject of male sexual problems and the availability of treatment has unearthed a cache of men with primary impotence. In one recent study of 573 consecutive men seen at an impotence clinic in a German military hospital, 67 (11.7 percent) had primary erectile dysfunction. All 67 men gave a history of a total absence of fully sustained erections since early childhood or puberty. Surprisingly, physical abnormalities were detected in 57 (85 percent) of them. Only 15 percent had pure primary psychogenic impotence. However, even those with organic causes of their impotence also had significant psychologic difficulties, possibly as a secondary reaction to their lifelong inability to function sexually. The results of the German study have not yet been confirmed elsewhere. In most physicians' experience, psychologic problems dominate in men with primary impotence.

Effective treatment of men with primary impotence is extraordinarily difficult and often fails. Men with primary impotence who have vascular or neurologic problems must first have the physical defect corrected. Vascular surgery is possible in some cases to reestablish blood flow to the genitalia. Disrupted neurologic connections are less amenable to correction. Circuitous methods to bypass the nerve damage either by inserting a penile prosthesis or by using intrapenile injections to stimulate erections can be considered. Either technique allows the man to experience erections.

Treatment of physical problems is a start, but it does not provide a fully satisfactory or comprehensive treatment. Psychotherapy is necessary to help the man arrive at some understanding of the physical and emotional factors that have contributed to his long-term inability to function sexually. With insight gained from therapy, he should be able to enjoy some sexual satisfaction.

Ralph was thirty-seven years old when he was seen in consultation, ostensibly for evaluation of infertility. The reason for the barren marriage surfaced when Ralph indicated that he and his wife had never had sexual intercourse. Further probing revealed an almost unfathomable depth of sexual naïveté.

Ralph had grown up in a strictly religious household and was made to feel ashamed of the erections he had as an adolescent. He did not know what masturbation meant. His teenage years at an all-male military school provided no enlightenment, as he was shy and reclusive. When asked if he knew how men and women had babies, he responded, "I just get on top and then do it."

Studies indicated that Ralph was able to have erections and had a normal complement of hormones. An enormous chunk of life, critical for normal psychosexual development, was either not developed or repressed. Ralph was referred to a group of psychologists to see if they could resurrect fragments of his lost adolescence, a daunting task even for the most confident therapist.

This condition, primary impotence, though startling and dramatic, is the exception and not the rule.

SECONDARY IMPOTENCE

The majority of sexually dysfunctional men have secondary impotence, which means that they did engage in sexual activity at one time and were able to acquire and sustain an erection satisfactory for masturbation or intercourse. Then something happened to stifle their natural sexual urges, inhibit erectile capabilities, or meddle with the ejaculatory process.

Details of the vascular anatomy, neurologic connections, and patterns of hormone secretion required for normal male sexual function have already been spelled out. With specific testing, we can recognize abnormalities in blood flow to the penis, neurologic impulses, and hormone disorders. The psychologic prerequisites are somewhat more difficult to define. Dr. Steven Levine, a psychiatrist at Case Western Reserve University in Cleveland, has identified the psychologic underpinnings for a satisfactory sexual life as "a willingness to make love, capacity to relax, and the ability to concentrate on sensation."

Yet how can we determine whether somebody's "willingness to make love" is impaired? How do we gauge his "capacity to relax," or a man's "ability to concentrate on sensation?" These emotional factors cannot be measured with any precision. All we can do is provide some sense of their impact on sexual function by way of illustration, using performance anxiety as one prototype of psychogenic impotence.

PERFORMANCE ANXIETY

Performance anxiety is one of the most common sexual problems. A man, fully potent for most of his life, suddenly experiences a sexual failure. He is surprised to find that while having sex he can neither achieve nor sustain an erection satisfactory to complete the sexual act.

Men respond to this problem in different ways. Some assume that the failure was a temporary nuisance that will resolve itself spontaneously. They do not dwell on one isolated incident and indeed have no difficulty having an erection the next time they attempt sexual intercourse.

Other men become preoccupied with their ability to achieve an erection. The sexual act shifts from a sensual, erotic experience to a worrisome encounter. The man becomes obsessed with the transition of his penis from a limp to an erect state. Each time he attempts intercourse, he wonders whether he will be able to have an erection, and if so, for how long. These concerns are difficult to extinguish. The man becomes so consumed with them that all other components of the sexual act lose importance. He is, in a sense, staring at his penis like a spectator waiting to see if the erection will occur and praying that once it does occur, it will not fade.

The term *spectatoring* has been coined to describe this phenomenon. The focus on the penis consumes the man to the exclusion of all other sexual thoughts. The "willingness to make love" has been replaced by an "anxiety over the ability to make love." The cycle is vicious. The more he concentrates on his penis to see if it will become erect, the more he is destined to fail. A series of failures begets more anxiety, which in turn guarantees further failure.

What commonly follows is a cascade of events that makes things worse. First he withdraws, avoiding routine intimate and even conventional physical contact, such as hugging and kissing. His anxiety about his inability to perform becomes intense. Soon he ceases all sensual contact and feels broken and diminished by his impotence.

One pragmatic treatment approach accepts a man's sexual dysfunction and impotence as a fact and does not inquire into the source of the problem. Treatments are designed to help him restore his willingness to make love, his capacity to relax, and his ability to concentrate on sensation. These are the sensate focus exercises popularized by Masters and Johnson.

SENSATE FOCUS EXERCISES

Twenty-plus years after their landmark book *Human Sexual Inadequacy*, William Masters and Virginia Johnson's treatment programs are still used. Some have quibbled with certain aspects of their program, but the fundamental principles remain sound.

Lack of sensate focus was considered by Masters and Johnson to be the most common, potentially remediable, sexual problem experienced by men. Men can often be distracted during sex by unrelated, troublesome thoughts. These nettlesome concerns inhibit a man's ability to concentrate on sensation. As a result, a man experiencing lack of sensate focus does not achieve an erection during foreplay. Even if an erection sufficient for penetration does occur, it cannot be maintained while his mind is preoccupied.

The original Masters and Johnson technique was developed for couples who were willing to devote two weeks to an intensive daily sexual-therapy program. Male and female co-therapists were a critical component of the treatment. Today, similar programs continue the dual-therapist approach; other equally successful programs are directed by a single therapist and usually extend over several weeks to months. Common to all programs is a set of ground rules:

1. Couples must agree to establish a moratorium on sexual intercourse during the treatment period. They are not permitted even to attempt intercourse until directed to do so by the therapist.
2. They must have no extramarital affairs during the course of therapy.

3. The use of alcohol, mood-altering drugs, or nonprescription medications must stop.
4. Both partners must agree to set apart a specific time of the day to do individual homework assignments.
5. The couple must start with a clean slate, setting aside any disagreements or grievances.
6. They must be explicit in telling each other what does and does not stimulate them.

Although it is true that Masters and Johnson are properly credited with popularizing sensate focus programs today, similar exercises were first proposed more than two hundred years ago. In 1788, the English surgeon Dr. John Hunter first prescribed "six amatory experiences without coital connexion." Even in the eighteenth century, physicians recognized the need to reestablish a sense of erotic arousal with "amatory exercises" in a setting that temporarily prohibited sexual intercourse "without coital connexion."

Today, the same principles have been resurrected. The original sensate focus exercises have been modified and adapted primarily to accommodate the busy schedule of working men and women. The goal is unchanged. The sensate focus exercises seek to reawaken sexual desire and allow couples to become comfortable and relaxed during the sexual experience.

The treatment begins with a reexamination and discussion of female and male sensual anatomy. Men and women are encouraged to identify those forms of stimulation that excite and those that diminish their sexual desire. Discovering maneuvers that turn on and turn off sexual interest is most important at this early phase. This information is especially useful for couples who are no longer aroused by the pattern of lovemaking that they once found exciting.

It is also critical that the man be absolved of any anxiety he may harbor about achieving erections. The physiology of erections and their *involuntary* regulation by neurologic, vascular, and hormonal influences are stressed. At this time, the man is encouraged to dispel all notions that he should be able to have an "erection on demand." Rather, he is encouraged to concentrate on the sensations that arouse him and communicate them to the woman. She, in turn, must help him appreciate what excites her.

The actual sequence of sensate focus maneuvers is programmed as different levels of exercises performed over several days or weeks. As noted, during this time, attempts at intercourse are forbidden. The goal of the exercises is to reawaken sexual desire and allow couples to become comfortable and relaxed during sex.

The sensate focus exercises are as follows:

Step 1. Lie together naked, hold each other, breathe together, but do not touch sexually sensitive areas.

Step 2. Explore all parts of the body manually or orally but exclude the breasts and genitals. The partners are encouraged to take turns so that both can find ways to relax and arouse each other.

Step 3. Breast caressing. Manual or oral stimulation of the breast is allowed at this time.

Step 4. The woman is encouraged to caress the man's penis and scrotum. The goal is not to achieve erection or orgasm but to create an atmosphere for a pleasurable experience.

Step 5. Manual caressing of the genitals to bring both partners to orgasm. During this phase, concern is raised about premature ejaculation. The woman is instructed in the "squeeze" or "start-stop" exercises to delay the moment of ejaculation.

Step 6. Intercourse is allowed, but the goal is simply vaginal penetration. Only a minimum amount of thrusting is permitted. To make matters easier for the man, he is advised to lie on his back with the woman on top.

Step 7. An extension of Step 6. Intercourse with prolonged thrusting to orgasm. Again the woman is on top.

Step 8. Allows intercourse with the man on top.

Therapists usually instruct patients to proceed very slowly through the sensate focus sequence and encourage repetition of each step for several nights before moving on to the next. If problems surface, the couple is encouraged to backtrack until they find a comfortable pace of progression. The therapist will want to explore the specific details of areas of conflict or anxiety. It may be necessary to shift the entire sequence into low gear and spread the sensate focus exercises over several weeks to months. Once performance anxiety has established a foothold, it can be tenacious. Cooperation, patience, and understanding are necessities.

Men experiencing performance anxiety and couples whose previously vibrant sex life is now more appropriately described as humdrum generally respond well to the sensate focus exercises. Couples whose sex life is impeded by interpersonal conflict and anger respond poorly or not at all. Depressed men, men with organic impotence, and men who have little or no interest in restoring potency do not respond.

VIAGRA FOR MEN WITH PSYCHOGENIC IMPOTENCE

The man who has lost confidence in his ability to engage in sexual intercourse because of his preoccupation with his ability to acquire and then sustain an erection and has lapsed into the ritual of "spectatoring" whenever he attempts to make love is an ideal candidate for Viagra. His concerns regarding the durability of his erection can be put to rest if he is willing to wait for the Viagra to take effect. Then, with the caressing and genital stimulation of normal foreplay, his penis will become erect and will remain so until he has completed intercourse and ejaculated. If, however, he is impatient or brings to the bedroom the anxieties of past sexual failures, he will continue to have problems. In that case, coupling a dose of Viagra with the sensate focus exercises described should allow him to regain his lost self-assurance and enjoy sex once again.

EXERCISES TO DELAY EJACULATION

Psychologists and sex therapists cite an 80 to 85 percent success rate in helping men overcome their tendency to ejaculate before maximal sexual excitement has been achieved. Two maneuvers—the squeeze technique and the start-stop technique—help men acquire a sense of confidence and control about timing of ejaculation. Both exercises utilize partner-initiated masturbation to stimulate arousal and are often performed in conjunction with a sensate focus program.

The squeeze technique encourages penile stroking and genital caressing up to the point of orgasm. When the man senses that he is about to ejaculate, he signals his partner, who lightly circles the fingers of her free hand around the glans, the bulbous tip of the penis. When the man senses he has achieved some control of his impulse to ejaculate, stimulation resumes until he reaches a sense of containment of semen.

The start-stop technique also begins with partner-initiated penile stroking to activate an erection. When the man is near ejaculation, he instructs his partner to stop. After a few moments (or minutes), he gives the signal to start, and the process is repeated. As the exercises progress, the interval between the start and stop signals lengthens until finally the man acquires the ability to determine the moment of ejaculation.

The couple may repeat the squeeze or start-stop exercises as often as they like during a session; ultimately, the man will ejaculate. Gradually, as the man becomes used to experiencing prolonged pleasure from sexual stimulation, he will gain confidence and control over the timing of his ejaculation.

INSIGHT THERAPY

Impotent men with more deeply rooted emotional problems do not benefit from sensate focus therapy. They must come to terms with the seeds of their discontent through short-term or in-depth therapy. Insight therapy involves an exploration of the factors responsible for original and current erectile failure. The man is obliged to reexamine all aspects of his sexual life.

Andrew's sexual problems began after his forced retirement. He was unable to make love to his wife the night he received the news. His retirement plan provided a comfortable income but no solace. In his preretirement days, he went to bed confident that he would be at work the following morning. Sexual intercourse was never a problem. Now he went to bed worrying not only about the next day but about the rest of his life. His morning and nighttime erections were as firm as ever, but he could not muster an erection when he attempted to have sex. He felt like a failure.

The sense of worthlessness engendered by his obligatory retirement was overwhelming, and Andrew plunged himself into a frenzy of activity to reaffirm his value as a man. Unfortunately, the intensity of his activity consumed all of his intellectual and sexual energy, leaving no room for his wife. A realignment of priorities was in order. Andrew was encouraged to restructure his daily activity and carve out a specific time of day to focus some of his considerable energy on his sexual feelings for his wife.

Crises have a way of galvanizing a relationship between caring couples, and Andrew was able to reaffirm his love for his wife and rechannel his energies appropriately so that his erectile function and their sexual happiness became "better than they had ever been before retirement."

All the circumstances surrounding Andrew's sexual problems were of recent onset and readily recalled so that his therapist had little difficulty piecing together the psychodynamics of his impotence and formulating a treatment plan. This is not always the case.

On occasion, the psychologic root cause of impotence is buried deep within a man's subconscious and is revealed through the more elaborate psychiatric probing available only with psychoanalysis.

In 1985, Robert was forty-four, single, and impotent. Married briefly, then divorced, he was something of an enigma. He was healthy, worked full-time, and had no difficulty meeting and dating women. Morning erections were normal and he could masturbate, but he was unable to have an erection during sex. When a relationship became serious, Robert became emotionally aroused but could not translate this sense of sexual excitement into an erection. Eventually, he became embarrassed and stopped dating altogether.

No clues regarding the origin of his sexual problems were forthcoming from the standard psychiatric interviews. Eventually, the psychiatrist suggested psychoanalysis to see if the process of free association would divulge the source of his repressed anxiety about sex.

Psychoanalytic sessions are, by nature, rambling and not immediately productive. However, after several sessions, as Robert was recalling events of his childhood, he blurted out, "Don't pull your pants down. Don't let them see you with your pants down. If you have to pee, make sure no one is looking."

Here was the clue the psychiatrist needed. As a child of four, Robert and his family were trapped in Poland during World War II. His father's greatest fear was that because he, Robert, and his brothers had been circumcised, the Nazis would immediately recognize them as Jews. It was for that reason that his father admonished Robert and his brothers never to expose their penises.

Information imprinted in the subconscious of a terrified little boy is difficult to extricate. It was this fear inculcated in Robert as a youngster that prevented him from undressing as a prelude to having a satisfactory sexual relationship with any woman. Only by recognizing and confronting his subconscious fears about exposing his penis was Robert able to feel comfortable and successful in a sexual relationship.

DEPRESSION

Depression is different from sadness. We all get periodically despondent, unhappy, and disheartened over life's disappointments. After a period of brooding and feeling sorry for ourselves, we usually resume normal function.

Depression, however, disables a person. People who are depressed frequently feel worthless, helpless, and guilt ridden. They cannot mobilize the energy, enthusiasm, and concentration needed for most activities, including sex. Impotence, predictably, reinforces the depression.

Depressed people have abnormal sleeping patterns. On the one hand, many depressed people develop insomnia; either they are unable to drop off to sleep or they tend to wake in the middle of the night and cannot fall asleep again. On the other hand, a significant number of depressed people sleep far too long and too much, yet still feel fatigued. They never feel refreshed after a good night's sleep. Depressed individuals may be plagued by a variety of other physical symptoms, including headaches, persistent dry mouth, stomach aches, excessive belching, passing wind, occasional palpitations, frequent constipation, and inexplicable weight loss. Symptoms such as these should not be ignored, for they may be harbingers of serious physical problems. However, when medical investigation fails to disclose any physical cause, a diagnosis of depression must be considered.

Health professionals rely on information from patient interviews to establish the diagnosis of depression and then turn to standardized formats like the Hamilton Depression Scale (HAM-D) to gauge the severity of depressive symptoms. The HAM-D explores and grades different aspects of depression, including mood, sleeping problems, feelings of guilt, suicidal thoughts, and sexual dysfunction, and then assigns a numerical score to reflect the intensity of each symptom. The greater the depression, the higher the score. As treatment alleviates depression, HAM-D scores return to normal.

The severity of the depression determines the therapeutic approach. Some depressed men may be incapacitated or suicidal. They may well require hospitalization. Less-severely impaired men who are troubled primarily by their depression-induced impotence and inability to function at work and in relationships can be treated as outpatients. Generally, treatment involves a combined approach utilizing psychotherapy and antidepressant medication.

Wide ranges of drugs capable of stabilizing mood and relieving depression are available. The combination of antidepressant medications and psychotherapy is usually effective, and sexual potency frequently returns as treatment lifts the depression.

However, antidepressant medication can create another sexual problem. About 25 to 50 percent of men treated with antidepressants experience some difficulty in ejaculating. This is sometimes overcome by switching to another medication.

APPENDIX

The Florida Sexual Health Questionnaire

A. How frequently do you think about sexual intercourse?

1. Never
2. Rarely (every 2–3 months, on average)
3. Occasionally (once a month, on average)
4. Fairly often (every 2–3 weeks)
5. Usually (weekly or biweekly)
6. Always (every day)

B. Ejaculation with sexual intercourse occurs:

1. Never
2. Rarely (10% of the time)
3. Occasionally (25% of the time)
4. Fairly often (50% of the time)
5. Usually (75% of the time)
6. Always

C. Ejaculation with masturbation occurs:

1. Never
2. Rarely (10% of the time)
3. Occasionally (25% of the time)
4. Fairly often (50% of the time)
5. Usually (75% of the time)
6. Always

D. The ejaculate volume during intercourse or masturbation is usually:

1. Nonexistent
2. One drop
3. Between 2 and 5 drops
4. 1/4 teaspoon
5. 1/2 teaspoon
6. Greater than 1/2 teaspoon

E. The semen ejaculate during intercourse or masturbation is usually:

1. Clear and watery
2. Clear mucous
3. Very thick clear mucous
4. White mucous
5. Thick white mucous
6. Yellow- or green-tinged thick mucous

F. Sexual intercourse with partner occurs:

1. Never
2. Every two months
3. Monthly
4. Every two weeks
5. Weekly
6. Twice weekly or more often

G. Vaginal penetration with intercourse occurs:

1. Never
2. Rarely (10% of the time)
3. Occasionally (25% of the time)
4. Fairly often (50% of the time)
5. Usually (75% of the time)
6. Always

H. Nightly or early morning penile erections occur:

1. Never
2. Every two months
3. Monthly
4. Every two weeks

5. Weekly
6. Twice weekly or more often

I. Masturbation without sexual intercourse occurs:

1. Never
2. Every two months
3. Monthly
4. Every two weeks
5. Weekly
6. Twice weekly or more often

J. Premature ejaculation before vaginal penetration occurs:

1. Always
2. Usually (75% of the time)
3. Fairly often (50% of the time)
4. Occasionally (25% of the time)
5. Rarely (10% of the time)
6. Never

K. Difficulty in obtaining an erection for sexual intercourse occurs:

1. Always
2. Usually (75% of the time)
3. Fairly often (50% of the time)
4. Occasionally (25% of the time)
5. Rarely (10% of the time)
6. Never

L. Difficulty in maintaining an erection for sexual intercourse occurs:

1. Always
2. Usually (75% of the time)
3. Fairly often (50% of the time)
4. Occasionally (25% of the time)
5. Rarely (10% of the time)
6. Never

M. Is male infertility a problem (past or present)?

1. Long-standing problem

2. Intermittent problem in the past
3. Current problem for the past five years
4. Current problem for the past two years
5. Current problem for the past year
6. Never a problem

N. In regards to your physical development during adolescence (growth of facial hair):

1. No facial hair
2. Minimal facial hair (above lip, chin only) shaving required less than every two weeks
3. Moderate facial hair (lip, chin, sideburns) shaving required less than every two weeks
4. Normal facial hair, shaving weekly or less
5. Normal facial hair, shaving 2–4 times per week
6. Normal facial hair, shaving daily or twice a day

O. In regards to your physical development during adolescence (growth of pubic hair, penis, and testes):

1. No notable growth
2. Initial growth normal, but not completed (sparse pubic hair, small penis and testes)
3. Normal development, but delayed until after age 17
4. Normal development but recent (last 5–10 years) decrease in penis or testes size
5. Normal development and no change in penis or testes size
6. Normal development and recent (last 12 months) increase in penis or testes size

P. Please rate the firmness and rigidity of penile erections prior to intercourse or masturbation:

1. Never firm or rigid
2. Rarely (10% of the time)
3. Occasionally (25% of the time)
4. Fairly often (50% of the time)
5. Usually (75% of the time)
6. Always firm or rigid

Q. When was the last time you and your partner had intercourse?

1. One or more years ago
2. Six months ago

3. Two months ago
4. One month ago
5. Two weeks ago
6. Within the last week

R. How frequently would you like to have sexual intercourse?

1. Not at all
2. Once a month
3. Once every two weeks
4. Once a week
5. Twice a week
6. More than twice a week

S. Overall, how satisfactory is your sexual relationship to you?

1. Extremely unsatisfactory
2. Moderately unsatisfactory
3. Slightly unsatisfactory
4. Slightly satisfactory
5. Moderately satisfactory
6. Extremely satisfactory

T. Overall, how satisfactory do you think your sexual relationship is to your partner?

1. Extremely unsatisfactory
2. Moderately unsatisfactory
3. Slightly unsatisfactory
4. Slightly satisfactory
5. Moderately satisfactory
6. Extremely satisfactory

18

Penile Implants

For years, men suffering from impotence or erectile dysfunction would turn to urologists, surgeons specializing in what were considered to be men's problems, including urinary difficulties brought on by a large prostate gland, prostate and testicular cancer, and impotence. Focusing on ways to alleviate the mechanical problems of acquiring and maintaining an erection, urologists devised ingenious methods to allow impotent men to enjoy sex once again. They developed silicone penile prostheses and vacuum devices and were at the forefront in the implementation of penile injection therapy. All these modes of treatment are discussed in the next three chapters. Chapter 18 provides information on penile implants. Penile injection therapy is reviewed in Chapter 19, and vacuum devices are the subject of Chapter 20.

Surgical implantation of penile prosthetic devices has been and is still an accepted means of restoring erectile capability in impotent men. In 1989, U.S. surgeons implanted an estimated 27,500 penile prostheses. That number has declined only somewhat since the advent of penile injection and MUSE therapy. The fate of penile prosthesis surgery after Viagra remains to be determined. However, since about 30 to 35 percent of impotent men who try Viagra do not respond well enough to resume sexual intercourse, there will always be a sizable number of impotent men who will want to have penile prosthesis surgery or some other erection assistance to help them enjoy sex again.

Dr. William Scott of the Johns Hopkins Medical School and Dr. Michael Small, professor of urology at the University of Miami Medical School, and his associate Dr. H. M. Carrion are recognized as the patron saints of modern penile prosthesis implant surgery. Dr. Scott fashioned a silicone inflatable penile prosthesis (IPP), which he first implanted in early 1973. Drs. Small and Carrion developed their unit shortly thereafter. The Scott and Small-Carrion devices are the prototype for most of today's penile prostheses.

The original Scott prosthesis, a multicomponent device, had a fluid reservoir implanted in the lower abdomen. A tube from this reservoir was connected to a bulb in the scrotum. The penis remained in a normal flaccid state until intercourse was desired. Then an erection was created by pumping the scrotal bulb to transfer the fluid from the reservoir to the penile implant. (See Figure 18.1.)

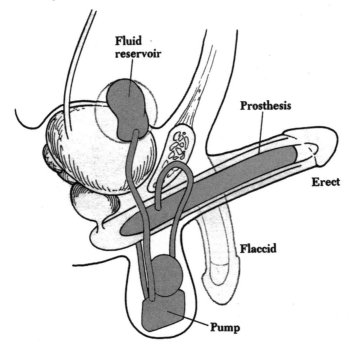

FIGURE 18.1   Multicomponent inflatable penile prosthesis.

The Small-Carrion prosthesis did not rely on hydraulics to convert the penis from a flaccid to an erect state. Once inserted in the penile corporal bodies, the device provided a perpetual erection. Although highly desirable during moments of sexual intimacy, this proved to be something of a burden at other times. The first recipients of Small-Carrion penile implants found it necessary to gird themselves in tight-fitting underwear or wear baggy pants to camouflage their protruding penis. Concealment was the watchword for these men.

Since its inception, penile implant surgery has become so popular that in less than fifteen years, the procedure has generated its own legacy of legends, mythology, and misconceptions. Since penile prosthetic implants are still an integral component of the current spectrum of therapeutic options offered to impotent men, it is important for the potential penile-implant recipient to ask the following questions:

- What aspects of sexual function are improved or unchanged following prosthesis implantation?

- What types of prostheses are currently available?
- How are prostheses implanted?
- Are there any complications of prosthesis surgery?
- Am I an appropriate candidate for prosthesis surgery?
- What factors determine patient-partner satisfaction or dissatisfaction following surgery?
- Is the silicone used in penile implants in men as hazardous as the silicone used in breast implants in women?

Penile prostheses serve only one function: They provide the penile shaft with sufficient rigidity to allow for vaginal penetration. They do not increase penis size, nor do they enhance any other aspect of the male sexual response cycle. One of the common misconceptions about penile prosthetic surgery is that men who receive prostheses will be endowed with a penis of prodigious length and girth. This is not the case. Prostheses cannot lengthen the penis since the rods are inserted in the corpora cavernosae of the nonerect penis; they must be confined to this limited anatomic space.

In this way, the erectile capability created by a penile prosthesis differs from spontaneous erections. The naturally occurring spontaneous erection causes a discernible increase in penile length and girth. The discrepancy between a man's recollection of the size of his prior erections and the erection afforded by the penile prosthesis may cause some disappointment. The prosthetic erection provides only the rigidity needed for penetration, nothing more.

Men with penile prostheses do not experience enhanced arousal, nor do they have any sense of amplified ejaculation or orgasm. Indeed, most recipients indicate that those aspects of sex may be somewhat less satisfactory than before. This disappointment, however, is usually overshadowed by the sheer relief of once again being able to have erections.

TYPES OF PENILE PROSTHESES

The Small-Carrion and Scott penile prostheses are still used but are not the only options. There are a number of different devices on the market today. Four discrete categories of prostheses—semirigid, malleable, inflatable, and hinged—are currently available. All the units listed below have been judged safe and effective by an expert group of urologic surgeons recruited by the American Medical Association to participate in the recent Diagnostic and Therapeutic Technology Assessment panel.

- The original *Small-Carrion* prosthesis consists simply of two rigid rods.

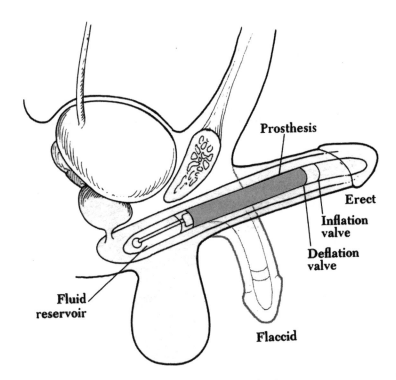

FIGURE 18.2   Self-contained inflatable penile prosthesis.

- Penile prostheses with abdominal fluid reservoirs include the *Scott-AMS 700* and a similar device manufactured by the Mentor Corporation.
- The *Jonas* prosthesis is a semimalleable device that depends on a network of internal silver wires to allow for some degree of flexibility.
- The *OmniPhase* and *DuraPhase* prostheses have internal cables that allow the device to bend to a flaccid state when not in use. These units are activated by adjusting the cable to produce penile rigidity. Other malleable devices like the *AMS 600* and *Mentor* have similar designs.
- The *Finney* prosthesis is hinged and converts from flaccid to rigid state merely by locking the hinge in place.
- Newer inflatable prostheses like the *Hydroflex* and *FlexiFlate* have internal fluid systems and are designated as self-contained penile prostheses (SCPP). The SCPP transforms the penis from a flaccid to an erect state by manipulation of a valve implanted in the tip of the penis. (See Figure 18.2.)

TABLE 18.1   Types of Penile Prostheses

Type	Name	Advantages	Disadvantages
Rigid	Small-Carrion	Permanent erection	Permanent erection, difficult to conceal, slips out of vagina
Malleable	Jonas Mentor AMS 600	Easy to insert, Minimal patient education, relatively inexpensive, adequate rigidity	Penis permanently firm, penile pain, can irritate or rupture the urethra, numbness of glans, failure due to fracture of internal wires
Inflatable: extrapenile reservoir	Scott AMS 700 Mentor	Attempts to mimic normal erections, adequate rigidity	Frequent mechanical failure requiring reoperation, surgery complex, manual dexterity required
Inflatable: intrapenile fluid reservoir	Hydroflex Flexiflate	Readily concealed, adequate rigidity	Requires manual dexterity to operate
Hinged/ Segmented	Omniphase Duraphase Finney	Surgery not complex, little manual dexterity required, flaccid at rest, adequate rigidity	Does not increase penile length or width

Individual urologic surgeons may at one time or another favor one prosthesis over another. However, no single device has yet emerged as the dominant unit of choice. Each device has its own intrinsic advantages and disadvantages. (See Table 18.1.) The rigid, malleable, hinged, and controlled expansion cylinder devices do not increase penis length or girth. These devices come in a variety of lengths; the urologist chooses from an inventory of prosthetic units a rod customized for each individual patient. The Scott and the comparable Mentor multicomponent inflatable penile prostheses (IPPs) both allow some increase in penile girth and rigidity without changing penis length.

Most urologists take pains to discuss this issue in detail. It is important for potential recipients to understand this preoperatively lest they harbor any illusions of acquiring significant augmentation of penile anatomy and sexual prowess. Such fantasies can never be fulfilled by any of the currently available prosthetic devices.

HOW PROSTHESES ARE IMPLANTED

Normal erections occur as increased blood flows into and is trapped in the two corpora cavernosae and the corpus spongiosum. Penile prosthetic devices, whatever kind, all attempt to duplicate this process by outfitting the penis with silicone surrogates for the two corpora cavernosae. (The corpus spongiosum is not replaced during implant surgery.) Prior to implantation, the tissue in the penile cavernosa must be stretched to accommodate the rods.

Patients receiving either the Scott or Mentor inflatable prosthesis require one additional surgical procedure. The bulb for activation or transfer of fluid from a reservoir to the prosthetic shaft is surgically implanted in the scrotum.

Most prostheses are inserted by making a surgical incision either in the lower abdomen or at the junction of the penis and the scrotum and then advancing the rod forward toward the tip of the penis. Some of the newer self-contained penile prostheses, on the other hand, may be inserted by making an incision around the tip of the penis and pushing the prosthetic rods backward toward the bony joint at the end of the torso. The patient usually requires general anesthesia and stays in the hospital three to five days. Some surgeons give patients a spinal block (or spinal epidural anesthesia) and send them home on the same day, but this practice is not widespread. Inflammation, a reaction to the insertion of a foreign body in the penis, causes some postoperative pain, which is controlled by medication. The pain subsides as the inflammation wanes. Following surgery, the patient must allow four to six weeks for healing. During this interval, the silicone rods become firmly embedded and anchored in the penile shaft. Then the prosthesis is ready for use.

SUCCESS RATE

Recipients of penile prostheses are generally pleased with the results. All acquire a rigidity of the penile shaft adequate for penetration. Initial reports from urologic surgeons were glowing, with success rates reported at 90 to 95 percent. Long-term follow-up has tempered this enthusiasm to some degree. Today, patient and partner satisfaction is closer to 60 to 75 percent.

COMPLICATIONS OF PENILE PROSTHESIS SURGERY

A surprisingly large number of men will require repeat surgery. The most common complications are mechanical failure of the prosthesis, postoperative infection, and penile pain.

Mechanical complications occur most often in multicomponent inflatable prostheses and reflect malfunction in the workings of the rods, cylinders, or hydraulic system or kinks in the tubing. The prosthesis must be

TABLE 18.2   Results of Penile Prosthesis Surgery

Type	Reop %	Complications %
Inflatable IPP	41	6.8
Small-Carrion	11	10
Jonas	10	7
Self-Contained	18	10

removed and replaced with either a new, identical unit or an alternative type of prosthesis; the choice is up to the urologist and patient.

Postoperative wound infection is less common today than in the past. Now implant recipients receive antibiotic treatment during and immediately after surgery.

Postoperative pain does occur in some patients. It is usually localized in the tip of the penis (the glans); however, discomfort in the penile shaft, scrotum, base of the penis, or abdomen is not uncommon. In one series of 179 penile prosthesis implants performed at the Mayo Clinic, 61 patients reported complications with the prostheses' mechanisms. Another 42 patients experienced pain, most commonly at the tip of the penis but occasionally in the penile shaft, scrotum, base of the penis, or abdomen. Of these men, 32 rated their pain moderate or severe.

Pain can herald a more serious problem. It may imply that the position of the prosthesis compromises the function of other vital structures. Pressure on the urethra will cause pain and is a warning of some underlying problem. Paraplegic patients, however, do not perceive pain. As many as one-third of impotent paraplegic men with penile prostheses experience damage to their urethra within six months after surgery.

Research indicates that complications as well as the need for reoperation seem to depend on the type of device implanted, the duration of the follow-up, and the group of patients studied. For example, patients implanted with the older, rigid Small-Carrion prosthesis rarely require reoperation. The reoperation rate is much higher with inflatable penile prostheses (IPP). (See Table 18.2). The malleable and self-contained penile prostheses (SCPP) are the least prone to mechanical breakdown. However, even when these devices were relatively new and most urologists had little more than two to three years of experience with them, reoperation rates were 14 to 22 percent.

LONG-TERM COMPLICATIONS OF PENILE PROSTHESIS SURGERY

All penile prosthetic devices are made of silicone. Now, silicone has proven to be remarkably versatile, and this same material, in liquid form, has been used by plastic surgeons for breast implants, to *reconstruct* the breast after breast cancer surgery and also to *augment* the appearance of the breast in other women. When used for purposes of breast reconstruction or augmentation, liquid silicone must be encased in a plastic bag. The silicone-containing plastic bag is then inserted under the skin to reshape the breast. On rare occasions, silicone has leaked out of the bag and drifted into other parts of the body. Women who have had silicone breast implants have subsequently developed serious medical problems such as immunologic diseases and second cancers that they have attributed to the silicone used in breast implants. For the silicone to be responsible for such problems, it must first leak out of its bag and then enter the body's veins, arteries, or lymph nodes and activate abnormal immunologic responses in the body's lymphatic system. Such leakages do occur, and it is possible that this is what has caused the serious systemic disease in women who feel they have been injured by silicone breast implants. Although confined to a relatively few women, this is nonetheless a serious problem. Today, the FDA has approved silicone for use in women undergoing breast reconstruction surgery but discourages its use in women who desire augmentation breast surgery.

It is reasonable to inquire: Is the silicone used in penile implants in men as hazardous as the silicone used in breast implants in women? For silicone to wreak havoc in the man as it does in some women, the penile prosthesis silicone must shed some particles. These individual *silicone particles* must migrate, invade, and set off an inflammatory response, first in the fibrous capsule surrounding the prosthesis, then moving on and insinuating themselves into local lymphatic tissue (lymph nodes) to trigger immunologic reactions. Surprisingly, this problem has not been as extensively evaluated in men as it has been in women. Only 25 penile prosthesis recipients have been evaluated to date.

1. Seventeen of 25 (72 percent) had silicone particles in the fibrous capsule surrounding the penile implant.
2. None of these silicone particles had provoked inflammation.
3. In 11 of 17 cases, encasements called granulomas had formed around the silicone to prevent further spread.
4. Three groin lymph nodes and one lymph node near the aorta had silicone granulomas.
5. Autoimmune disease did not develop in any of these men.

While it is reassuring to learn that no man in this small series developed any immunologic disease or adverse systemic reaction to silicone penile prosthesis implantation, the discovery that particles from the prosthesis can migrate to the capsule and to locations as remote as a lymph node near the aorta was unexpected. The implications of this observation are that physi-

TABLE 18.3 Three most common causes for reoperation in 555 men who first had penile prostheses installed starting in 1975 and 137 men who had penile prostheses installed between 1985 and 1989.

1975—Cause of reoperation for 555 men	*Percent of men requiring reoperation*
Mechanical	56.7 %
Fluid loss	7.7 %
Infection	11.5 %
1985–1989—Cause of reoperation for 137 men	*Percent of men requiring reoperation*
Infection	35.7 %
Mechanical	34.7 %
Patient Dissatisfaction	13.8 %

SOURCE: From RW Lewis, *Long Term Results of Penile Prosthesis Surgery.* Urologic Clinics of North America, 1985; 22: 847–856.

cians caring for penile prosthesis recipients must recognize that silicone particles can separate from the penile prosthesis. Most will remain harmlessly encased in local granulomas, but a few are capable of drifting beyond the confines of the penile shaft and into local or remote lymph nodes. Adverse immunologic reactions, when they occur, begin in lymph nodes, but immunologic disease has not to date been noted in men who have had penile implants.

UPDATE ON PENILE PROSTHESIS SURGERY

With continued experience, physicians have learned much more about who is and is not a good candidate for penile prosthesis surgery. For example, impotence is common in diabetic men who can usually resume sexual intercourse after a penile prosthesis is implanted. However, diabetics are prone to develop infections, particularly when their diabetes is not well controlled. One test commonly performed to assess the adequacy of diabetic control is a test called a glycohemoglobin, which should be no higher than 6.9 percent. Diabetic men strive for but do not consistently achieve this goal. If they are far off the ideal mark and have a glycohemoglobin over 11.5 percent, the chance of infection is so high that some urologists will refuse to install a penile prosthesis. Only when diabetic control is more satisfactory, as judged by a closer-to-normal glycohemoglobin, will surgery be contemplated.

In the early days of penile prosthesis surgery, problems inherent in prosthesis design resulted in mechanical failures, and this structural breakdown was the primary reason some men who had penile prosthesis surgery had to have the defective implant removed and a new one installed in a second operation. With technical advances in prosthesis design, mechanical failures now occur less frequently and infection is now the major reason for repeat penile prosthesis surgery. The three most common problems requiring a second operation in men who have had penile prostheses implanted starting in 1975 and 1985 are listed in Table 18.3.

The data in the tables are as reported by Dr. Ronald Lewis from the experience of the Department of Urology at Mayo Clinic. Men who are having their first penile implant should anticipate a reoperation rate of 10–15 percent between five and ten years after the original surgery, whereas those who have already had one penile prosthesis revision should be advised that fully 25 percent of them can anticipate a need for reoperation in less than five years. The majority of men who have penile prostheses implanted do not require any more surgery, making patient and partner satisfaction the primary determinants of the success of the surgery.

SATISFACTION FOLLOWING PENILE PROSTHESIS SURGERY

Although surgical success rates for some devices now approach 90 to 95 percent, patient satisfaction does not parallel this impressive figure. A major problem is disappointment with postoperative penile length and width. Some men never attempt intercourse after the prosthesis is implanted; others have intercourse for only a brief time and then abandon sexual activities. Additional areas of disaffection with prostheses have surfaced in response to specific questions.

The majority of urologists are men, and in the beginning, the male perspective distinctly colored the reported results of prosthesis surgery. Female health-care professionals saw things differently. They approached the issue of satisfaction after implantation by interviewing both partners. Some couples were not having intercourse at all. Of those who were having intercourse, 25 percent reported restriction in positions because of the decreased penis size. Fifteen percent of the men experienced diminution of orgasmic intensity. Still, 79 percent of men said that they would, if given the opportunity, undergo the operation again. Only 59 percent of their partners had no hesitation.

Some urologists claim that satisfaction depends on the type of prosthesis, with IPP recipients being generally more satisfied than those who receive other prostheses. Because they are easily concealed and readily activated, one would have anticipated that the multicomponent IPP would have emerged by now as the dominant, if not the only, penile prosthetic device implanted.

This has not turned out to be the case, for two reasons. Significant problems with the internal hydraulics of IPPs remain, and mechanical failures are common. Perhaps more troublesome is the fact that a certain amount of manual dexterity is required to inflate the IPP.

Originally, in an effort to mimic the genital caressing that is a natural component of sexual foreplay, the man's sexual partner was encouraged to play an active role in pumping the scrotal bulb so that fluid could be transferred from the abdominal reservoir to the prosthesis, a maneuver intended to mimic a stimulated erection. This has not been as warmly embraced as expected.

Sexual partners are often unwilling to participate in the pumping procedure. Some are simply not deft at manipulating the scrotal bulb. As a result, inadequate amounts of fluid are transferred from the reservoir to the prosthesis shaft, and a suboptimal erection ensues. In such cases, failure of the device has been ascribed not to mechanical problems of the unit itself but to the inadequate level of participation of sexual partners. Those who have been unwilling to become involved as vigorous squeezers of the scrotal bulb have been decried as "timid pumpers." Other factors may also have a significant impact on postoperative sexual satisfaction. Any of the following put the couple's satisfaction at risk:

- Extreme obesity
- Psychogenic impotence
- Impotence not the only sexual problem
- Sexual dysfunction in woman
- Severe marital conflict
- Unreasonable expectations
- Partner opposed to surgery
- Woman pressuring man to have surgery
- Couple ceased all sexual touching

Obese patients are often displeased following penile prosthesis surgery because the length of the unit protruding beneath their lower abdominal fat pad is limited. Most prostheses are approximately eight inches in length. If there is an extensive overhanging fat pad, then perhaps only an additional four inches of rigid penile tissue will protrude for purposes of sexual intercourse. If the patient's partner is also obese, it will be very difficult for the couple to find a position in which penile-vaginal penetration and adequate vaginal containment is possible. For obese couples, postoperative sexual gratification may be limited.

Inappropriate expectations are high on the list of reasons for postoperative patient-partner dissatisfaction. The prosthesis provides only the penile rigidity necessary to achieve vaginal penetration. Patients who anticipate that the equipment will allow them to recapture the real, or imagined, sexual prowess of their youth are likely to be displeased.

Patients whose impotence is attributed to psychogenic factors do not derive as much long-term benefit from prosthetic surgery as those whose impotence is caused by either neurogenic or vasculogenic factors.

On occasion, impotent men have sexual problems other than erectile dysfunction. Lack of spontaneous arousal, limited libido, and ejaculatory disorders are not corrected by penile prosthesis implantation.

The level of preoperative patient-partner interaction is a critical determinant in evaluating postoperative satisfaction. If, for example, the female partner has her own sexual dysfunction, such as pain during intercourse, then she may be fearful of experiencing vaginal penetration again. A man may choose to have a penile prosthetic implant without notifying his partner. Such a decision is commonly interpreted as a rejection of the partner. In addition, some women are fearful that their previously impotent partners, now outfitted with penile prostheses, will seek other lovers. Limited studies exploring this question have indicated that penile prosthesis recipients are no more susceptible to seduction than other comparably aged potent men, nor do they routinely seek out new sexual opportunities more often than their potent peers.

On the other hand, some female partners of impotent men, frustrated after long periods of sexual abstinence, may pressure the men into surgery. Any discordance in patient-partner desires for penile prosthesis surgery is considered a major risk factor for postoperative dissatisfaction.

Couples who have distanced themselves sexually from each other and have ceased hugging, touching, and all sensual and erotic contact may not be able to retrieve all aspects of normal sexual function merely by placing a prosthetic rod in the penis. Clearly, satisfaction is maximal only when both partners are involved in all discussions and decisions from the beginning.

CANDIDATES FOR PENILE PROSTHESIS SURGERY

Prostheses have been implanted in men with virtually every known type of impotence, but some men are more appropriate candidates for surgery than others. Urologic surgeons prefer to implant devices in men whose impotence is a result of a physical cause, either neurogenic or vasculogenic. Included in the category of neurogenic impotence are men with diabetes mellitus, spinal-cord injuries, and multiple sclerosis, along with paraplegics and men whose pelvic nerves have been damaged or severed during prostate or lower abdominal surgery. Vasculogenic impotence applies to men with either decreased penile arterial inflow or increased venous outflow; vascular surgery is the preferred form of treatment for these men. But they are not always willing to go through the somewhat more complex surgical procedures and may elect prosthetic implantation instead.

As noted, patients with Peyronie's disease have no difficulty achieving an erection. The problem is that the erection bends, so the penis deviates, often creating a J-shaped erection unsuitable for intercourse. Peyronie's disease occurs when fibrous bands grow in the outer lining of the penis and tug at the penile shaft. The bands can be removed surgically, but this is only a temporary solution because these strictures tend to recur at the same or different locations in the penis. Implanting a prosthesis is often the only way to circumvent the problem.

Men with endocrine disorders, whose potency can be restored with appropriate hormonal therapy, and men with overt psychologic problems, who require psychotherapy, psychiatric medications, or both, are the only groups to whom physicians do not routinely offer penile prosthetic implants.

THE FUTURE OF PENILE PROSTHESIS SURGERY

The initial brouhaha attending the introduction and early years of penile prosthesis surgery has subsided. It is now possible to reflect and cast a sober eye on the role of penile prostheses in the treatment of impotent men. It is clear now that surgical skills alone are not enough to solve the problem of impotence.

The penile prosthesis industry is highly lucrative and competitive. The five penile-prosthesis manufacturers collectively accounted for $60 million in worldwide sales up to 1998.

It is too early to know whether the availability of Viagra will dampen enthusiasm for penile prosthesis implantation. Still, the most optimistic estimates indicate that Viagra is effective in restoring erectile function in about 65 percent of impotent men. Among those 35 percent of impotent men who have a suboptimal response to Viagra are men who have become impotent as a result of:

- Radical prostatectomy
- Neurogenic impotence
- Diabetes mellitus

Thus, the remaining 35 percent of men with erectile dysfunction who do not respond satisfactorily to Viagra are precisely those men who have, in the past, been considered to be ideal candidates for penile prosthesis surgery. However, these are the same men who may also respond to penile injection therapy or intra-urethral alprostadil (medicated urethral suppository, or MUSE) therapy. With so many treatment options now available to correct erectile dysfunction, significant adjustments in strategy will be needed to decide exactly what treatments are best for the 30 percent of men who do not benefit from Viagra.

COST OF PENILE PROSTHESIS SURGERY

Penile prosthetic surgery is expensive. The cost of the prosthesis, hospitalization, and urologic surgeon's fees can be as high as $10,000 to $12,000. This figure is applicable to those men who have their surgery and three to five days of postoperative care in the hospital. Most medical insurance plans cover the cost of surgery only for patients with documented organic impotence. With improved anesthetic skills and pressure to cut down on the high cost of hospitalization, some urologists have been experimenting with same-day ambulatory outpatient surgery. It is too early to determine whether this novel approach will safely replace the more traditional three-to-five-day hospitalization.

19

Penile Injection

Puncturing one's penis with a needle is not for the squeamish. Piercing the penis with a needle and then injecting a chemical to enhance one's sexual potency sounds more like a bizarre, sadomasochistic nightmare from the annals of Krafft-Ebing's *Psychopathia Sexualis* than a doctor-recommended treatment of impotence. Nevertheless, many men, with guidance from their physicians, practice self-injection of the penis to achieve an erection. Three types of medications—phentolamine (an alpha-blocker), papaverine (a smooth-muscle relaxant), and alprostadil (a prostaglandin)—may be loaded into syringes and injected directly into the penile erectile chambers to provoke an erection.

Phentolamine, papaverine, and alprostadil are all effective in stimulating erections because they overcome neurologic signals that normally keep the penis in a limp or flaccid state and help encourage the release of intrapenile chemicals like nitric oxide and cyclic GMP to increase blood flow into the corpora cavernosae. Neurologic control of erections is vested in the sympathetic nervous system.

To understand how the sympathetic nervous system works, it is useful to create a simple scary example. Imagine that you are alone at night walking down a dark street. There is no sound. Then, as you are absorbed with your thoughts, someone comes up behind you and says, "Boo!"

Your sympathetic nervous system immediately swings into action to cause, among other reactions, an increase in pulse rate and blood pressure. The change in pulse and blood pressure is caused by internally produced adrenalinelike compounds with unique properties designated "alpha" or "beta." Beta forces cause you to have palpitations and an increase in pulse rate, while alpha influences raise your blood pressure.

What does this have to do with erections? The penis is richly endowed with extensions of the sympathetic nervous system, specifically nerves of the alpha type. Alpha signals either facilitate or inhibit normal erections.

When the alpha forces dominate, the penis remains at rest. An injection of a medication that blocks the erection-inhibiting alpha nerves makes it possible for a full and unrestrained flow of blood to be directed into the

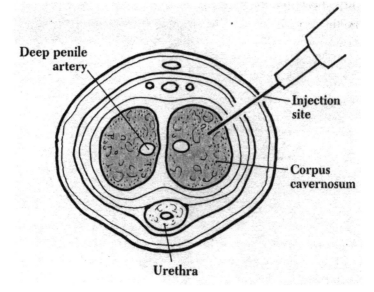

Deep penile
artery

Injection
site

Corpus
cavernosum

Urethra

FIGURE 19.1   Penile injection directly into corpora cavernosae.

erectile bodies of the penis. Medications like phentolamine, an alpha-blocker, and prostaglandin El, a muscle relaxant with probable alpha-blocking activity, cause erections by blocking the nerve signals that maintain the penis in a limp state.

It is somewhat more difficult to understand exactly how papaverine works. There are no papaverine receptors in the penis. Papaverine, unlike alpha-adrenergic compounds or prostaglandins, is not made by the body. However, papaverine has one characteristic that is useful in inducing an erection; it is a *smooth*-muscle relaxant.

The body has two types of muscles, striated and smooth. Striated muscles are literally striped in appearance and are, for the most part, under voluntary control. The muscles of the arms, legs, and face are striated muscles. Smooth muscles are not under volitional control. For example, the muscles in the intestines are smooth muscles. The muscles lining the penile blood vessels that must dilate for an erection to occur are also smooth muscles. It is presumed that papaverine induces an erection by causing these intrapenile smooth muscles to relax, thereby allowing or encouraging increased blood flow into the penis.

To be fully effective, alprostadil (Caverject) or other similar medications must be injected directly into one of the penile erectile bodies, the corpora cavernosae. (The medication will naturally migrate over to the other side of the penis so that symmetrical erection is acquired.)

A cross section of the penis illustrates the corpora cavernosae surrounded by the thick outer fibrous sheath (tunica albuginea). (See Figure 19.1.) The

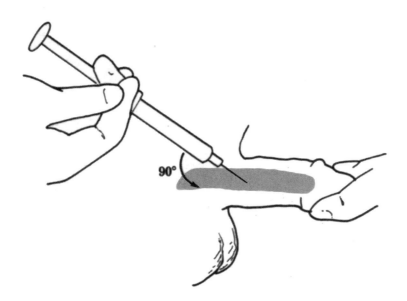

FIGURE 19.2   Proper technique for penile injection.

needle is inserted at a ninety-degree angle to the penile shaft and must penetrate the tunica albuginea to make contact with the corpus cavernosum. Men are taught to advance the needle into the penis and wait for a slight "give" in the resistance. When they sense this change in tension, they know that they have punctured the tunica albuginea. The medicine is then injected. (See Figure 19.2.)

An erection occurs within twenty to thirty minutes. No sexual stimulation is needed. Thus, penile erections differ from Viagra, which is first effective one hour after the pill has been swallowed. Most urologists recommend that injection be performed no more than twice a week. If desired and tolerated, Viagra can be used daily. The side effect profile of the two treatments designed to enhance a man's erectile capability does differ with penile pain and priapism being prominent adverse effects experienced by men using intrapenile injection and dizziness and occasionally blue-tinted vision occurring in men who take Viagra. (See Table 19.1.)

CANDIDATES FOR INTRAPENILE INJECTIONS

Sixty-five to 75 percent of impotent men can have an erection induced by the intrapenile injection of combined papaverine and phentolamine. Preliminary reports from Japan suggest that 86 percent acquire erections with prostaglandin E1 (Caverject) alone. The men most likely to respond to injections are those with neurogenic impotence. Injection can induce erections in men with vasculogenic impotence, but only if the dose of

TABLE 19.1   Comparison of Intrapenlie Injection and Viagra

Treatment	Intrapenile Injection	Viagra
Administered How?	Direct penile injection	Pill–oral medication
Time from administration to erection	15–30 minutes	One Hour
Sexual Stimulation required?	No	Yes
Side Effect	Penile pain	Dizziness, Blue tinted vision
Priapism	Common	Uncommon

NOTE: Prostaglandin El (marketed as alprostadil [Prostin VR Pediatric]) as well as Papaverine, phentolamine, and syringes with very small needles are available in most pharmacies.

medication is significantly greater than that needed for other men. Intrapenile injections are not an effective long-term treatment for men with vasculogenic impotence because the injections will eventually fail to stimulate erections even if a large amount of drug is used. In addition, for reasons that remain unclear, about one-third of men with psychogenic impotence do not respond adequately to intrapenile injections.

In the age of Viagra, intrapenile injections are a fallback option for the 35 percent of men who fail to respond to or cannot tolerate the side effects associated with Viagra. Others who are in a hurry to have sex and do not want to wait the full hour before the Viagra effect kicks in will be happier with a program of intrapenile injections.

PATIENT AND PARTNER SATISFACTION

More than half of the patients enrolled in one penile injection program reported that they were either "very satisfied" or "satisfied" with the program; one-third considered the treatment "not acceptable." Men seem more pleased than women with penile injection programs. They describe an increase in erectile function, intercourse frequency, and improved self-image.

Some women note that they are turned off by the artificiality of the procedure. On the other hand, some get into the spirit of things; one said, "When I'm in the mood I simply leave a syringe on the pillow and he gets the message."

Seven years after the first intrapenile papaverine injections were given, doctors had enough experience to recognize that this form of treatment is not a panacea. Specific problems reported include lack of a sustained erectile response over time, high patient drop-out rate, and complications.

Different doses of drugs have been administered. Doses effective in inducing the first erection are not consistently effective in maintaining satisfactory erections with each successive injection. A need to increase the dose after a while or switch from one medication to another seems to be standard. Even men who have a fully satisfactory response do not always stay with this form of treatment; about one-third drop out early on, and up to 70 percent lose interest in or do not continue this therapy indefinitely.

COMPLICATIONS

Three different complications have been attributed to intrapenile pharmacotherapy: penile nodules and scarring (sclerosis), abnormalities of liver function, and prolonged erection (or priapism).

Penile Nodules

Men who continue to inject papaverine-phentolamine develop nodules along the shaft and scarring in the body of the penis. To date, nodules have not developed with prostaglandin El (caverject) injections, but problems may surface as physicians and patients gain more experience with the drug.

Abnormal Liver Function Tests

It was originally believed that papaverine or papaverine-phentolamine injected directly into the penis would remain there and not enter the bloodstream. This has proved not to be the case. Some of the mixture enters the general circulation and causes damage to the liver. Up to 40 percent of men who continue long-term treatment can expect to develop at least one abnormality of liver function—mild inflammation. Liver-function tests return to normal when treatment stops. Prostaglandin El, however, is fully metabolized in the penis and does not circulate.

Priapism

From the very beginning it was apparent that some men who injected papaverine were susceptible to prolonged erections lasting for six to twelve hours. The prospect of a twelve-hour erection may, at first, tantalize some men with fantasies of nonstop, daylong fornication. However, men who have chemically induced prolonged erections know that this is not possible. Prolonged erections are often extremely painful and hence neither sexually exciting nor erotic.

Prolonged erections were most commonly observed in men with neurogenic impotence. This is truly unfortunate. There is no way of restoring the nerve connections to the penis that have been severed as a result of spinal trauma, diabetes mellitus, or pelvic surgery. However, the anatomy and blood supply to the penis remain intact. Intrapenile papaverine injections seemed an ideal solution for these men. Men with neurogenic impotence do achieve a most dramatic and prompt restoration of erectile function after the first papaverine injection. The problem is that they are too responsive, which makes them so susceptible to priapism.

Mindful of this, physicians have been adjusting the treatment schedules to lower the dose of papaverine and phentolamine. Papaverine doses initially calibrated at 80 mg are now down to 25 mg or less. Still, problems with priapism persist.

Priapism is a medical emergency and requires immediate intervention. An erection that persists beyond six hours deprives the penis of adequate oxygen. Reversal of priapism usually requires the infusion of additional chemicals to counteract the effect of papaverine or phentolamine. Often, this treatment alone allows blood to drain from the penis.

Surgery is required for those men whose priapism remains even after medical treatment. On occasion, Draconian surgical maneuvers have been necessary to decompress the swollen penis and reverse the erection. Some patients have had major distortions in penile anatomy, and many have been left permanently impotent.

Those men unfortunate enough to have experienced these severe reactions have sought redress. Their attorneys have initiated litigation against the physicians who recommended participation in the penile autoinjection program in the first place and the Eli Lilly Corporation, the pharmaceutical company that manufactures and distributes injectable papaverine.

Upset that papaverine had caused serious patient disability and corporate liability, Lilly rewrote its package information form to express displeasure at the use of its medication for purposes of inducing a penile erection. The current package insert provided with each vial of papaverine now states the following under the "contraindications" section:

> Papaverine hydrochloride is not indicated for the treatment of impotence by intracorporeal injection. The intracorporeal injection of papaverine hydrochloride has been reported to have resulted in persistent priapism, requiring medical and surgical intervention.

This disclaimer shifted the onus of continued use of papaverine for intrapenile injection away from the manufacturer and squarely on the shoulders of prescribing urologists and their patients. This action did not, however, sound a death knell for all intrapenile injection programs.

All three medicines work, but no single drug or combination of drugs has yet emerged as the treatment of choice. In comparison studies of intrapenile injections of papaverine alone, papaverine-phentolamine combination, and prostaglandin El given to the same impotent men, the papaverine-phentolamine combination and prostaglandin El were clearly superior and roughly comparable. Differences between the two surfaced when the number and types of complications were examined.

Whereas none of the men who received prostaglandin El experienced prolonged erections, 7 to 10 percent of those taking the papaverine-phentolamine combination did. This finding should have allowed prostaglandin El to emerge as the drug of choice. Unfortunately, 19 percent of men injected with prostaglandin El experienced pain in the penis.

There is one overriding problem plaguing enthusiasts of intrapenile injection for the diagnosis and/or treatment of impotence. Only one of the drugs, prostaglandin E1 (Caverject), has been approved for this use by the FDA. As just mentioned, the manufacturers of papaverine include a specific warning *against* its use for purposes of inducing an erection. Prostaglandin El, originally approved for the treatment of a rare form of congenital heart disease in newborn infants, is now also approved for intrapenile injection treatment of impotence. Marketed as Caverject and available in preloaded syringes, it can be obtained in local pharmacies with a doctor's prescription.

The lack of government and pharmaceutical approval for the other agents used for intrapenile injection has disappointed but not deterred urologists. According to published reports, as of December 1989, more than 4,000 men in the United States, Europe, and Japan have participated in intrapenile injection programs and have received a total number of injections in excess of 60,000. Urologists who have been at the forefront of research are convinced that this treatment is both safe and effective.

In 1996, approximately ten years after penile injection therapy was introduced and enthusiastically endorsed, doctors started asking a series of critical questions:

1. Is it necessary to inject a specific chemical or medication into the penis to produce an erection?
2. How much or how little medication is required to guarantee sufficient penile swelling and rigidity to allow for satisfactory sexual intercourse?
3. Will men and their partners, previously accustomed to a pattern of mutual sexual excitation during spontaneous lovemaking, adjust to a ritual of preemptive, exclusively male sexual arousal in future sexual encounters?
4. What are the short-term and long-term side effects of a program of penile self-injection?

To answer these questions the collective experience of physicians at fifty-one separate medical centers was pooled to provide an extraordinarily detailed and comprehensive analysis of the effectiveness and acceptance of penile self-injection as a treatment for male sexual dysfunction. Men who were impotent because of inadequate blood flow to the corpora cavernosae (vasculogenic impotence), those who had impaired nervous system signals to the genital area (neurogenic impotence), and others who had emotional factors disrupting their sexual function (psychogenic impotence) and multiple causes (mixed impotence) participated.

Is it necessary to inject a specific chemical or medication into the penis to produce an erection?

Men received intrapenile injections of either a placebo or different doses of alprostadil (Caverject). The first intrapenile injections were given in the clinic, and the quality of the penile swelling (tumescence) and stiffness (rigidity) that ensued were observed and graded by the technician administering the injection. In addition, Rigi-Scan assessments of penile tumescence and rigidity provided more precise quantitative data on the strength and vigor of the erectile response. No man had an erection following a placebo injection, confirming the need for a specific medication to activate the erectile process.

How much or how little medication is required to guarantee sufficient penile swelling and rigidity to allow for satisfactory sexual intercourse?

Five percent of men had erections induced by the very small doses of alprostadil, whereas in others, larger doses, tailored to each man's need, were required to produce vigorous and sustained erections (defined as 70 percent rigidity lasting for more than ten minutes). As soon as each man's optimum dose was established in the clinic, he received further instruction in the technique of penile self-injection, was provided with free medication and syringes, and was encouraged to use penile self-injection to rekindle his sexual life at home. This was the critical phase of the study, because the activation of an erection under scientific observation in a clinic does not address the issue of how useful and acceptable penile injection will be to impotent men and their partners.

EFFICACY AND ACCEPTANCE OF PENILE INJECTION

Will men and their partners, previously accustomed to a pattern of mutual sexual excitation during spontaneous lovemaking, adjust to a ritual of preemptive, exclusively male sexual arousal in future sexual encounters?

Six hundred and eighty three men and their sexual partners entered a six-month study designed to evaluate the short- and long-term benefits, as well as the potential side effects, of a program of at-home intrapenile injection therapy to restore erectile capacity for sexual intercourse. During this time period, 13,762 intrapenile injections preceded sexual intercourse. According to the men and their sexual partners, the sexual intercourse that ensued was deemed fully satisfactory by 87 percent of men and 86 percent of their sexual partners.

However, despite the high success rate, not every man who started penile self-injection at home continued treatment. Only 471 of the original 683 (69 percent) of men completed the six-month study. The 31 percent of men who could not complete the study stopped treatment because of "penile pain, lack of efficacy, dislike of self-injection, violation of the protocol, difficulty in scheduling visits, problems with partners, no need for the drug, difficulty with injection technique, intercurrent illness, lack of sex drive and death unrelated to the drug."

SIDE EFFECTS OF PENILE INJECTION

What are the short-term and long-term side effects of a program of penile self-injection?

Pain in the penis proved to be the dominant side effect occurring in 50 percent of all men who participated in this study. Other side effects included occasional black-and-blue marks on the penis, prolonged erection (lasting four to six hours), priapism (defined as an erection lasting more than six hours), edema of the penis, and other penile disorders, including numbness, swelling, irritation, sensitivity, redness, itching, yeast infection, and a few instances of penile deformities, including scarring leading to the development of Peyronie's disease, curvature, or deviation of the shaft of the penis.

What appears to be Caverject's formidable side-effect profile is tempered to some degree by the adverse effects seen when other single- or multiple-drug regimens are used for penile self-injection. Liver damage, a rare but worrisome side effect of papaverine therapy, is not a problem with alprostadil. Priapism does occur with alprostadil (Caverject) but apparently less frequently than with papaverine.

Still, many physicians, responsive to their patient's complaints regarding the penile pain that accompanies intrapenile alprostadil injections, have resorted to fashioning pharmacological cocktails with graded amounts of papaverine, phentolamine, and alprostadil (Tri-Mix) in an effort to minimize side effects while maximizing erectile response and enhancing patient acceptance of intrapenile injection therapy.

MEDICO-LEGAL IMPLICATIONS OF INTRAPENILE INJECTION AND THE FUROR SURROUNDING THE LATORRE AMENDMENT

The vast majority of men who continue to use intrapenile injection therapy to enhance their sexual lives would no doubt be surprised to learn that their enthusiasm is not shared by all men embarking on this form of treatment. The high dropout rate alluded to above indicates that about one-third of men who start treatment decide not to stay with therapy even when the medication and syringes are supplied to them free of charge. There is yet another group of men who have experienced significant adverse effects so troublesome that they have felt compelled to seek redress for their grievances within the legal system. Lawsuits claiming permanent injury to the penis resulting from prolonged erections, inadequately or improperly treated priapism, or severe liver damage have been sobering for urologists and the pharmaceutical companies that supply the chemicals that men inject into their penises to achieve an erection. In addition, to everyone's surprise, Eli Lilly, the primary manufacturer of papaverine, no longer content with relying on the wording in its package insert discouraging men from using intrapenile papaverine for purposes of achieving an erection, discontinued manufacture of papaverine altogether. Other pharmaceutical houses, based for the most part in Mexico, jumped in to fill the void left by Lilly's abrupt departure so that those eager to use papaverine had a constant supply of this chemical for intrapenile injection therapy.

But this was not the only legal hurdle for those advocating this treatment for their impotent patients. There was the matter of Dr. Latorre and his patent.

Although the English physiologist G. S. Brindley has been properly credited with introducing the principle of intrapenile injection therapy to modern medicine, he was not the first physician to experiment with the idea of injecting a chemical into the penis for purposes of achieving an erection. That distinction belongs to an Italian physician named Latorre, who self-injected numerous medications all without success. Undaunted by his failures, he *patented the process of penile injection*. This patent, ignored for years, was discovered generations later and peddled around the community of physicians interested in providing a remedy for sexually dysfunctional men. Eventually, an enterprising group known as Men's Health Resources acquired the rights to the Latorre patent and demanded compensation of up to $1,000 per year from each and every urologist prescribing any form of intrapenile injection therapy. (Alprostadil, however, is somehow exempt from the Latorre amendment). Urologists bridled at what they perceived to be corporate extortion for what is now a standard treatment of impotent men and railed against Men's Health Resources both in public and in private.

THE FUTURE OF INTRAPENILE INJECTION THERAPY

Before Viagra, many men relied on penile injection therapy as a quick, effective means of restoring erections, used this treatment as a path to sexual fulfillment, and continue to employ this treatment on a regular basis. Indeed, before Viagra, when 656 men with erectile dysfunction were offered a full range of treatment options including penile injection therapy, penile prostheses, vacuum-assisted erection devices, or vascular surgery, 514 (78 percent) chose penile injection, followed by 10 percent who opted for penile prostheses, 3.8 percent who selected sex therapy, and 3.2 percent who indicated a preference for vacuum erection devices. A smaller percentage, 1.4 percent, were deemed suitable candidates for vascular surgery, and 2.1 percent rejected all treatment options.

In this particular study, only 48 (9.3 percent) men who started were dissatisfied with penile injection therapy. This low dropout rate stands in sharp contrast to the experience of others. Another large survey of 708 men found that the dropout rate in the first year after starting penile injection therapy was 41 percent, and of those who discontinued, reasons cited were "discontent with self-injection concept (38 percent), cost (31 percent), and unnaturalness of therapy (26 percent)." For those who continued with penile injection therapy, the dropout rate over the ensuing years was 31 percent at two years and another 28 percent at three years. It was the perception of those performing this survey that greater and more sustained acceptance of intrapenile injection therapy could be achieved if cost were minimized and programs of patient and partner education and support were emphasized.

To my knowledge, similar surveys have not been performed since the introduction of Viagra. Our experience has been that when men who have responded well to intrapenile injection are given the opportunity to try Viagra, they will stay with this medication. This has been so even when they consistently experience a Viagra-related side effect such as blue-tinted vision. However, for the 35 percent of men who do not benefit from Viagra, a return to intrapenile injection with Caverject may be one means of resurrecting their sex life. The other option is to rely on one of the other alprostadil delivery systems.

OTHER ALPROSTADIL DELIVERY SYSTEMS

Knowing that alprostadil works and recognizing that many men balk at plunging a needle into their penis has prompted new developments. There is now a more user-friendly means of delivering alprostadil to a man's penis to absorb alprostadil from the inside.

The urethra is the hollow tube in the middle of the penis through which men urinate. The erectile bodies, the corpora cavernosae, flank the urethra. If an alprostadil pellet is inserted into a man's urethra, enough will diffuse out into the corpora cavernosae to create an erection. This is the principle behind the MUSE (medicated uretheral suppository) system. A man inserts the MUSE device into the opening in his urethra, presses a button, and the alprostadil pellet remains. (The plastic device is then removed from the urethra.) Alprostadil from the pellet is released and diffuses into the penile erectile bodies to stimulate the blood flow needed to create an erection. (Figure 19.3.)

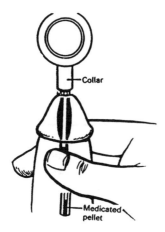

FIGURE 19.3 The MUSE device for instilling alprostadil into the urethra. Following urination, a man inserts the stem smoothly into his urethra and presses a button to release alprostadil, which spreads into the penis to activate an erection. (Modified from Padma-Nathan H., Hellstrom W.J.G., Kaiser F.C., et al. "Treatment of men with erectile dysfunction with transurethral alprostadil." *N. Engl. J. Med.* 1997; 336: 1–7)

Initial studies have compared the erectile response achieved when the MUSE system was used to place either a placebo or an alprostadil-treated pellet within the urethra. Originally, roughly equal numbers of men were tested in the clinic to determine the dose of alprostadil pellet needed to produce an erection. Using a 1–5 erection rating system, where a rating of 4 or 5 is satisfactory for intercourse, 48.8 percent of men receiving the highest dose of alprostadil (1,000 mcg) acquired a four-fifths erection that began within seven minutes after insertion of the alprostadil pellet, was at maximum dimension within twenty-three minutes, and lasted seventy-nine minutes before returning to the nonerect state.

Thereafter, the men and their heterosexual partners were instructed to try out the new system at home. They were provided with a supply of MUSE devices and alprostadil or placebo pellets and evaluated over a three-month period. As was true with the early reports of intrapenile injection programs, the initial reports of efficacy and satisfaction with the MUSE system were glowing, with a high degree of patient and partner satisfaction. Reports of 64.9 percent of men having sexual intercourse following intraurethral alprostadil were impressive. Surprisingly, sexual intercourse was reported by 18.6 percent of previously impotent men who received intraurethral placebos. The number of placebo responders in this group is remarkable, considering the total lack of erectile response when men receive intrapenile placebo injections (see above).

The MUSE system for treating impotence was FDA approved in 1997, one year after Caverject and one year before Viagra. When first introduced, MUSE was a novel treatment option for impotent men and had somewhat greater compliance than penile injection therapy. Today, both Caverject and MUSE are recommended primarily for those men who do not respond to or cannot tolerate Viagra. In such men, penile injection with either Caverject, papaverine-phentolamine, or MUSE can be effective when used properly and can be just what they need to enjoy sexual intercourse again.

20

Vacuum Devices

Impotence has plagued mankind for thousands of years. The distress caused by this symptom has provided the stimulus for the development of a series of innovative and ingenious treatments designed to allow men to recapture sexual vigor. Some therapies have evolved as spin-offs of sound scientific research. A few trace their origins to traditional folk remedies; many "guaranteed cures" turn out to be hoaxes. Today, the impotent man is offered an extraordinary range of therapeutic options, quite literally running the gamut from A (aphrodisiacs) to Z (zinc). Bringing up the end of the therapeutic alphabet are vacuum devices, vitamin E, yohimbine, and zinc. This chapter will describe the use of vacuum devices. (For more on vitamin E, yohimbine, and zinc see Chapter 21.)

THE VACUUM CONSTRICTOR DEVICE (VCD)

Any system encouraging blood to flow into and be captured in the penis should produce an erection. This is the principle behind the vacuum constrictor device (VCD) now offered as a noninvasive means of restoring erections for some impotent men.

Devices resembling the VCD have been shuttling in and out of favor for more than seventy years. The original concept has been traced to the inventor Otto Lederer, who in 1917 was granted a patent for a unit that would allow "persons considered completely impotent to perform sexual intercourse in a normal manner." It is not known whether the Lederer device was ever produced. A newer product, undoubtedly a variation on the original theme, was developed by a man to help him deal with his own impotence. It is marketed under the name ErecAid and sells for about $400. The Encore vacuum erection device is about half that cost. All work using the same principle.

There are several components to the ErecAid device. (See Figure 20.1.) A cylinder designed to fit over the limp penis is connected to a hand-operated vacuum pump. Suction from the pump creates a negative pressure within the cylinder, and this encourages an increased flow of arterial blood into

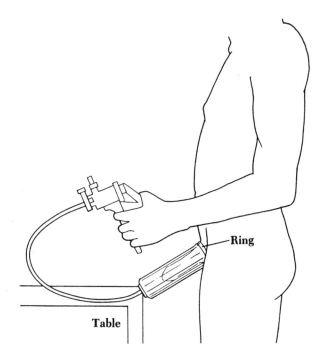

FIGURE 20.1   Use of the Erec-Aid vacuum device to create an erection.

the penis. Venous outflow is prevented by tight bands that fit over the base of the penis. A petroleum jelly-like substance lubricates the system and seals the base of the cylinder. When a user achieves an adequate erection (and with the rubber bands inhibiting venous outflow still attached), he removes the cylinder. The vacuum-induced erection is maintained for up to thirty minutes.

Some dexterity and skill are required to operate the VCD. The user must place the unit on some nearby surface while the limp penis is stuffed into the vacuum chamber. With the penis and the chamber perched at an angle, his hands are free to pump air out of the chamber and affix the restraining bands to the base of the penis. (See Figure 20.2.) Often, significant pressure must be applied. Three to seven minutes in the vacuum chamber are required to achieve erections of optimum rigidity. An alternate VCD, the Encore VTU-1, is shown in figure 20.2.

LIMITATIONS OF THE VCD

Not only does vacuum-induced pressure in the VCD cause most men to experience penile discomfort, but the erection achieved by this means is inferior to a spontaneous erection in three significant aspects. First, once the erection has been induced by the vacuum, the rubber bands in place at the

HOW IS THE VTU-1 USED?

1. After attaching the penile tube to the pump and the mounting cone to the end of the penile tube – select the right size constriction ring. Draw it over and down the mounting cone onto the penile tube.

2. Insert the penis into the penile tube making sure to hold the tube firmly against the body to help seal the vacuum.

3. Pump the handle until the desired erection is achieved. The pump features a vacuum cut-off at 12 static inches for your safety.

4. As soon as the desired erection has been achieved, simply twist the removal guide on the penile tube to automatically mount the constriction ring onto and around the base of the penis. The constriction ring will trap blood in the penis to hold the erection.

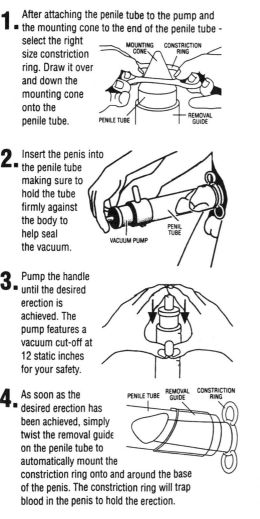

FIGURE 20.2   Sequence of steps for successful use of Encore vacuum device to create an erection.

base of the penis choke off blood flow into the penis. This causes penile skin temperatures to fall to 96°F. One-third of the female partners of men using VCDs found the chilled penis displeasing during intercourse.

Second, another drawback is that as the penis becomes engorged and congested by the VCD-induced suction and inhibition of venous outflow, penile circumference increases more than it would during a normal erection. This gives the penis a sausagelike appearance.

Third, the erection created by the VCD is rigid only from the point at which the rubber bands are affixed. This means that it is not fully upright and rigid like a normal erection but flexible and capable of swiveling or pivoting at its base.

The VCD also does not permit normal ejaculation. Because the rubber bands remain in place throughout the sexual act, semen is trapped in the urethra and can be released only after the bands are removed.

Despite these limitations, the manufacturers of the VCD say that more than 15,000 units have been sold in the United States since 1983.

REPORTS ON PATIENTS' EXPERIENCES

Objective evidence regarding the effectiveness of the device is scanty. There are only a few reports in the medical literature, most by Dr. Perry Nadig, a urologist from San Antonio, of positive VCD experience. One English urologist evaluated the VCD in ten impotent diabetic men who used the unit for three months; they all found it fully satisfactory and were able to have intercourse on the average of six times a month.

Dr. Nadig's experience with the VCD is the most extensive. His first report in the early 1980s described the responses of thirty-five impotent men using the VCD in his clinic. Twenty-seven achieved an erection of sufficient length, girth, and rigidity for intercourse. An additional five experienced some increase in penile length, but rigidity was considered inadequate for intercourse. Twenty-four of them continued to use the device.

By 1989, Dr. Nadig could report on the experiences of 340 impotent men who had used the VCD. Eighty-nine percent achieved erections satisfactory for intercourse. Eighty-one percent purchased a VCD for use at home, and of those who used the unit, most were said to be "satisfied and continued to use the VCD regularly." Dr. Nadig was frank about side effects, including fainting (three cases), infection of the foreskin (one case), and penile pain (most of the men).

Initial interpretation of questionnaires prepared and distributed by the manufacturer of the VCD unit suggests that although 92 percent of men maintain they can achieve a satisfactory VCD-induced erection, only 75 percent continue to use the device. These men limit intercourse to about once every two weeks, perhaps because of side effects or mechanical problems.

Pain and discomfort were common experiences. Black-and-blue marks on the penis occurred in almost all the men. All respondents indicated that they needed a considerable amount of practice time to learn how to use the unit. Once they had acquired the skill to use it, the interval from initiating vacuum suction to the development of an erection ranged from thirty seconds to more than seven minutes and averaged about two and a half minutes.

Only 57 percent of patients rated their orgasm as pleasant; 9 percent described pain; and 12 percent were unable to ejaculate at all.

NEWER VACUUM-ASSISTED ERECTION DEVICES

Technical advances have made it possible to develop an entirely new generation of vacuum devices that are somewhat easier to use and have gained greater acceptance as a way of dealing with erectile dysfunction. All work on the same principle to encourage blood to flow into the erectile chambers of the corpora cavernosae and then use occlusive rings at the base of the penis to prevent blood from flowing out of the penis so that the erection once achieved can be maintained. (Figure 20.2)

A certain amount of mechanical dexterity is required to use all of the vacuum devices effectively, but once men master the technique and become comfortable with using the vacuum and restraining rings, they can create an erection sufficient for vaginal penetration and engage in sexual intercourse. The newer vacuum devices have enjoyed some popularity here and abroad, where reports of efficacy in creating erections have been reported to be as high as 67 percent, and patient and partner satisfaction with vacuum-assisted erections has varied between 25 and 49 percent. Men who have a less than perfect response with intrapenile injection can use vacuum devices to improve the quality and rigidity of their erections.

There are still some who should avoid these devices because vacuum pressure on the penile shaft can create significant problems. Those who are receiving anticoagulant or aspirin treatment are susceptible to extensive intrapenile bleeding when the device is applied. Men who are at risk for the development of priapism, such as those with sickle cell disease and leukemia, are cautioned not to use the unit.

As patient experience grows, it appears that the newer vacuum devices have carved out a niche as a treatment option for men with erectile impotence. They are less expensive, about $200 per unit, easier to use, and, as a result, more acceptable.

We have found VCDs to be most effective in men who:

1. Have had extensive prostate cancer surgery with damage to the neurovascular bundles (see Chapter 24).
2. Have had no response to Viagra.
3. Are unwilling to use or to continue with penile injection or MUSE.

For this group of men, the vacuum devices have proven to be a reliable and useful means of allowing them to have the erections they need for sex.

21

The Lure of Alternative Medicine

Men and women eager to take control of their own health have always looked beyond conventional medicine and embraced nontraditional remedies to provide relief, ease, and comfort. The passage of the 1994 Dietary Supplement and Health Education Act has made it much easier for men and women to obtain herbs, vitamins, dietary supplements, and even male hormones without a doctor's prescription. Some herbal remedies are remarkably effective, whereas others are surprisingly toxic. Today, all of us need to know more about alternative medicine. In this chapter, you will find discussions on:

1. What is alternative medicine
2. Saw palmetto and benign prostatic hyperplasia
3. Adverse effects of herbal medicines
4. PC-SPES and prostate cancer
5. Herbs, minerals, and vitamins to improve a man's sexual function
   A. Ginseng
   B. Vitamin E
   C. Zinc
   D. Yohimbine
6. Over-the-counter male hormones: androstenedione and DHEA
7. Alternative medicine and cancer prevention
8. The cost of alternative medicine

WHAT IS ALTERNATIVE MEDICINE?

For centuries men and women have looked to those in their community who could act as healers. In bygone days, those aspiring to one of the healing professions, shamans, witch doctors, and others acknowledged to possess curative skills passed their knowledge on by word of mouth. Then as understanding of the workings and malfunctions of our bodies increased, there was a demand for a more scientific and structured system. This eventually led to a body of knowledge that formed the curriculum for the modern medical school. Today, young men and women interested in the healing arts must go through rigorous training in a medical school first to become doctors. Then upon graduation, neophyte physicians further increase their skills with additional training as interns and residents. Once they have accomplished all the tasks set before them, they can be licensed as doctors and go about the business of caring for you and me.

Doctors who are conventionally trained are not the only ones eager to step forward to provide succor and treatment for our ailments. Others keen to offer alternative healing techniques now provide an array of alternative options to standard medical practice. The scope of alternative medicine—also called complementary medicine—is broad and includes relaxation methods, chiropractic, massage, spiritual healing, acupuncture, and self-help groups, as well as a host of other innovative strategies intended to improve health and wellbeing. Of particular interest in this book are a growing number of herbs, vitamins, over-the-counter hormones, and dietary and nutritional supplements specifically aimed at helping men and their unique problems.

Men and women with nagging problems for which conventional medicine had few answers have been particularly interested in alternative medical treatments. Individuals with chronic backache, allergies, arthritis, headache, and insomnia often gravitated to alternative medicine when their own doctors failed to provide needed help. A 1993 survey of 1,279 people revealed how often men and women, even those with a regular doctor, were willing to try either an unconventional therapy or visit an alternative medicine provider. (See Table 21.1.)

THE DIETARY SUPPLEMENT AND HEALTH EDUCATION ACT

But the current enthusiasm for alternative treatment options never really blossomed until almost *one year after this report.* It was not a medical breakthrough but an act of Congress that provided the catalyst. Nutritional supplements—sometimes referred to as "nutriceuticals"—owe their widespread popularity to a 1994 law, the Dietary Supplement and Health Education Act. This law, apparently shepherded through Congress by Senator Orrin Hatch of Utah, was passed under intense pressure from a coalition of purveyors of herbs, vitamins, plant extracts, and amino acids and over the objections of the FDA. Supplements enjoy a luxury not accorded to any other health-care product—free entry into the marketplace.

Once a tablet or capsule is designated as a "supplement," it has special privileges and is exempt from conventional regulatory controls. Most medications undergo years of testing to prove that they are both safe and effective before being granted FDA approval for sale to the public. Supplements do not. Indeed, supplements can be sold with little or *no need to prove that they do what they are advertised to do.*

TABLE 21.1   Percentages of Men and Women with Common Complaints Who See a Regular MD, Use an Alternative Treatment, or See a Provider of Unconventional Medicine

Condition	Regular MD	Alternative Rx.	Saw Provider	Type
Back problems	20%	36%	19%	Chiropractic
Allergies	16%	9%	3%	Spiritual healing
Arthritis	16%	18%	7%	Chiropractic, relaxation techniques
Insomnia	14%	20%	4%	Relaxation
Headache	13%	27%	10%	Relaxation, chiropractic
High blood pressure	11%	11%	3%	Relaxation

SOURCE: Adapted from D.M. Eisenberg, R.C. Kessler, C. Foster et al., "Unconventional Medicine in the United States," *N. Engl. J. Med.* 328 (1993): 246–252.

TABLE 21.2   Cost of one year's Daily Supplement Use by One Couple

Supplement	Approximate cost per year ($)
DHEA	$ 240.90
Melatonin	58.40
Beta Carotene	94.90
Vitamin E	124.10
Vitamin C	175.20
Multi Vitamin (Centrum)	262.80
Selenium	58.40
Chromium Picolinate	62.06
Calcium/Magnesium	102.20
Coenzyme Q–10	262.80
St. Johns Wort	394.20
Gingko Biloba	591.32
Siberian Ginseng	164.26
Korean Ginseng	182.50
Garlic	175.20
Bilberry	138.70
Complete Amino Acids	109.50
Phosphatidyl Choline	116.80
EPA & DHA	94.90
DMAE	58.40
Folic Acid (Caplets)	36.50
Total	$ 3,504.02

NOTE: Cost may vary with brand and number of pills per bottle.

A supplement needs only to steer clear of claims that it will either *treat or prevent disease*. Supplement purveyors still have ample latitude to champion their products and can, for example, state that their product "promotes prostate health," "boosts the immune system," "increases energy," or "provides for better peace of mind" as long as the label also stipulates: "*This statement has not been evaluated by the Food and Drug Administration. This product is not intended to diagnose, treat, cure or prevent any disease.*" It is unlikely that anyone reads or pays attention to this disclaimer.

Men and women are drawn to supplements like Pooh to a honey pot, often relying on a heady mixture of herbs, vitamins, hormones, and amino acids to enrich their lives and enhance health. Eager to feel more energetic and stronger, have greater equanimity of mind and a healthier prostate, they accept *without question* the benefits listed on the label.

Individual supplements are also relatively inexpensive, especially when compared to prescription drugs. But devotees are inclined to bundle supplements into a complex daily regimen and that can run into serious money. (An example of one couple's daily supplement schedule and their out-of-pocket cost is illustrated in Table 21.2.)

The supplement industry is *big business*. According to the *Wall Street Journal,* annual supplement sales were projected to *exceed $15 billion* in 1998.

The flood of health-care products, herbs, vitamins, and minerals suddenly reclassified as *nutritional supplements* has started to gain favor among men.

Why?

All men, no matter how sexually competent and physically fit they were yesterday, are always eager to try *anything* that will allow them to be stronger, more virile, and sexually vibrant tomorrow.

If *traditional medical* sources are unwilling or incapable of addressing their concerns, others in the *alternative medicine* arena will step into the breach to offer sexually enhancing and/or strength-promoting herbs, vitamins, and hormones. The erotic marketplace is chock full of rediscovered plant or herbal extracts promising to make any man a better lover, increase his sexual endurance, and even his life expectancy. (Table 21.3)

WHERE DID ALL THESE NEW ALTERNATIVE MEDICINE REMEDIES COME FROM?

Actually, plants and herbs have been used to improve health for centuries. The powerful heart medication digitalis is the product of the foxglove plant *Digitalis purpurea,* the opium poppy made morphine possible, and quinine from the bark of the cinchona tree helps doctors treat malaria. Remarkable advances in health care have been possible with these and other plant-derived medicines.

The new plant-derived therapies differ from their illustrious predecessors in one important respect. Although trendy and in great demand, their *value has yet to be proven.* Still, nutritional supplements are everywhere, on supermarket shelves, in drugstores, throughout specialized nutrition centers, and in multiple Web sites on the Internet.

WHAT IS THE APPEAL OF ALTERNATIVE MEDICINE?

Those of us in traditional medicine claim to but should not be bewildered by the popularity of alternative medicine. As physicians, we rely on double-blind placebo-controlled studies to know with certainty whether a medication really works. Advocates of alternative medicine look elsewhere for confirmation of efficacy. They are more often swayed by their own experiences using one or more herbs and the enthusiastic response of a handful of patients. The major difference between the two disciplines can be summed up in one phrase.

TABLE 21.3   Alternative Medicine Supplements of Interest to Men

Supplement	Alleged to:	Effectiveness	Problem
Saw Palmetto	Ease urine flow in men with BPH	More than placebo similar to Proscar	Does not decrease prostate size
PC-SPES	Lower PSA in men with prostate cancer	? Equal to estrogen therapy	Herbal castration and breast growth
Yohimbine	Impotence treatment	Men with psychogenic or antidepressant induced impotence	Can raise pulse and blood pressure
Ginseng	Sexual stimulant	Anecdotes only	Irritability, problems sleeping
Vitamin E	Aphrodisiac	None proven	Harmless possibly effective as antioxidant
Zinc	Improves male sexual function	Possibly in 3rd world countries where zinc deficiency exists	?
Selenium	? Prevents prostate cancer	Data suggestive but confirmation needed	Side effects unknown

Traditional medicine offers proof, but alternative medicine extends hope.

Alternative medicine provides average citizens with a sense of *empowerment*. Freed from reliance on a traditional physician, they can orchestrate their own health care. Witness the current enthusiasm for *echinacea* to treat the common cold and *gingko biloba* to invigorate memory.

Although herbalists frequently foster a "we-they" schism to distinguish themselves from mainstream medicine, more and more alternative-medicine adventures are being taken seriously. The basic principles of scientific investigation are now used to find out what herbs do and do not work. Today, for example, we know that one herb, saw palmetto, actually helps improve urine flow in some men with enlarged prostates.

SAW PALMETTO AND BENIGN PROSTATIC HYPERPLASIA

Records dating back to the 1700s suggest that Indians in Florida first used extracts of the red berries of the saw palmetto plant to treat male problems like shrunken testicles, impotence, and prostate swelling. Saw palmetto distillates continued to be popular, particularly for the treatment of enlarged prostate glands, throughout the 1800s but faded into obscurity thereafter. The 1990s enthusiasm for botanical treatments reawakened interest in saw palmetto. Doctors wanted to know if this plant product really alleviated the annoying symptoms men experience when their prostate glands enlarge.

So urinary symptoms, rate of urine flow, and prostate size were evaluated before, during, and after treatment with either saw palmetto, placebo, or finasteride (Proscar) in men with benign prostatic hyperplasia (BPH).

Improved urination was reported by 74 percent (242 of 329) of saw palmetto–treated and 51 percent (168 of 330) of placebo-treated men. This confirmed that saw palmetto was not only slightly but significantly better than placebo in relieving many of the pesky urinary urges caused by large prostate glands.

Saw palmetto and finasteride (Proscar) were equally effective in providing symptom relief, but prostate gland size decreased only in men treated with finasteride (Proscar) and not in those men receiving saw palmetto pills.

Differences were also apparent in the side effect profile. Impotence was reported by 4.9 percent of Proscar-treated men and 0.9 percent of saw palmetto–treated men.

Thus, it appears that for some men, saw palmetto provides relief of vexing urinary symptoms and improves urine flow rates as well as finasteride does, but it does not decrease prostate size, though it is less likely to cause impotence. For these reasons, saw palmetto remains a popular alternative medicine option for men with BPH. (See Chapter 23 for more about saw palmetto and the prostate gland.)

Score one for herbal medicine.

ADVERSE EFFECTS OF HERBAL MEDICINES

The saw palmetto experience seems to validate the belief of alternative medicine enthusiasts who preach that "Herbal medicine can offer many of the same therapeutic benefits for treatment of genitourinary disorders as drug therapy *without any of the potentially severe side effects.*"[1]

Unfortunately, this dogma can no longer be accepted at face value. Too many people become ill, sometimes desperately ill, taking herbal products. Toxic and dangerous reactions to supplements include:

- Death in four months after using shark cartilage for childhood brain tumor.
- Worsening of Hodgkin's disease with Matol Biomune OSF Plus, alleged to "create a synergistic effect on the immune system resulting in elevation of natural killer (NK) cell activity."
- Lead poisoning using two tablets daily of "Indian Plants" to treat diabetes mellitus.
- Vomiting and life-threatening chaotic heart rhythms after one week's treatment with dietary supplements (fourteen-herb combination) for "internal cleansing."
- Disorientation within thirty minutes of consuming RenewTrient, a supplement purported to "stimulate the body's own natural production of Growth Hormone, contains butyrolactone." Concerns for safety of this product mounted as similar reports began to filter in. Eventually the FDA was forced to ban the sale of RenewTrient.

We know of these serious side effects only because men and women who became violently ill using these alternative medicines required emergency care in a traditional medical facility.

These sobering case reports of supplement-induced illness continue to appear as scattered case reports in the medical literature. More details of alternative-medicine toxicity are gradually emerging.

Consider the plight of men with prostate cancer who used the herbal remedy known as PC-SPES.

---

[1]Burton Goldberg, ed., *Alternative Medicine: The Definitive Guide* (Puyallup, WA: Future Medicine Publishing, 1993), p. 737.

PC-SPES AND PROSTATE CANCER

PC-SPES, a combination of eight herbs including *chrysanthemum, isatis, Ganoderma lucidum, Panax pseudo-ginseng, Rabdiosa rubescens, saw palmetto, and scutelleria (skullcap),* has been promoted as a natural herbal remedy to stem the tide of advancing prostate cancer. Exactly how, why, and by whom this combination of herbs was first cobbled together is not at all clear, but PC-SPES enjoys great popularity as an underground option for prostate cancer victims who have rejected or failed to respond to conventional prostate cancer therapy.

Most doctors were not aware of PC-SPES until they started learning about this innovative prostate cancer treatment from their patients, who, discouraged by what traditional medicine had to offer, decided to dabble with PC-SPES.

One man's travails proved pivotal. Following surgery, his prostate specific antigen (PSA) was still elevated, a sure sign of persistent prostate cancer. One month later, his PSA level was normal, a stunning and totally unexpected improvement. His baffled doctors asked him what had changed. He told them that he had heard about PC-SPES, decided to try this herbal remedy, and started to feel better almost immediately.

But with continued PC-SPES use, new and troublesome problems cropped up. He no longer had any sex drive, his erections vanished, and his breasts were now bulging and tender. Frightened by this unwelcome turn of events, he returned to his doctors. They discovered that this man was not the only one who had tried PC-SPES. Word of mouth from patient to patient had encouraged others with prostate cancer to try PC-SPES.

Eight men with prostate cancer, all using PC-SPES, agreed to participate in a study to find out what it was about this herbal combination that lowered PSA levels, obliterated men's sex drive, and stimulated painful breast enlargement.

First, doctors wanted to find out if every man who took PC-SPES had a similar response to this herbal combination. They did. Then hormone levels were measured before and after the men stopped PC-SPES.

It turned out that PC-SPES acted just like a female hormone, an *estrogen.* The estrogen effect was responsible for two new problems. First, it stimulated breast growth and, second, shut down each man's testicles, crippling his ability to make hormones. This is what caused his testosterone levels to plummet. As blood testosterone levels declined, so did the natural hormonal stimulus to continued growth of the prostate cancer. This explains why PSA levels fell. PC-SPES had caused an *herbal castration.*

But wasn't that the desired goal?

Yes and no.

Certainly anything that denies prostate cancer cells the hormonal fuel needed for continued cancer growth is desirable, but PC-SPES, though new to the market, is actually *a step backward.* Estrogen therapy, once popular to slow the spread of prostate cancer, was abandoned for three reasons. Side effects like blood clots were common, distressing breast enlargement was inevitable, and survival was not appreciably improved. Other, less toxic, more effective, and safer ways of nullifying testosterone production or testosterone's impact on prostate cancer are readily available today. (See Chapter 24.)

HERBS, MINERALS, AND VITAMINS
TO IMPROVE A MAN'S SEXUAL FUNCTION

Ginseng

Alternative-medicine texts maintain that Panax ginseng has "aphrodisiac qualities for which it has been prized over the centuries," yet little evidence exists to indicate that ginseng is really any better than a placebo. Men complaining of impotence used Korean red ginseng, trazodone, or a placebo. Frequency of sexual intercourse, premature ejaculation, and morning erections were identical with all three treatments. No man had full restoration of sexual potency with ginseng, although ginseng-treated patients reported a "higher level of satisfaction with sexual performance." Man-to-man word-of-mouth endorsements continue to promote ginseng as a sexual stimulant, although evidence of its effectiveness is, for the most part, limited to these anecdotes and testimonials.

Vitamin E

Vitamins ingested in the diet are essential for the normal operation of the metabolic machinery that drives our internal systems. Inadequate vitamin intake leads to symptoms of vitamin deficiency. For example, lack of vitamin C produces scurvy, and diets deficient in vitamin A cause night blindness.

Doctors became fascinated with vitamins because men and women seem to require such minuscule amounts of these substances to remain free of disease. As each new vitamin was discovered, scientists rushed to their laboratories to discover its precise function. To do this, they fed experimental animals diets deficient only in that single vitamin.

The initial studies of vitamin E were carried out in the early 1920s. Male rats fed a vitamin E-deficient diet became sterile. These rats remained potent, however, and could have erections and mount a receptive female rat. But somehow this aspect of the research was overlooked. By convoluted reasoning, the illusion emerged that vitamin E was important not only for rodent sperm production but also somehow enhanced male sexual potency. The public has readily, indeed ardently, embraced this misconception. Manufacturers of vitamin E have done nothing to dispel this notion.

Rats and humans are quite different. Vitamin E, when administered to men suffering from infertility and/or impotence, has not been effective in reversing either condition.

Despite overwhelming evidence, the public seems to want to believe that vitamin E has aphrodisiac qualities. Fortunately, vitamin E is relatively innocuous and can be consumed without any ill effect. Further, vitamin E has desirable antioxidant effects, and in general, antioxidant properties are more likely to be beneficial than harmful

Zinc

The importance of zinc has assumed legendary, almost mythical renown, as a sexual restorative for men. Today, zinc is still commonly used to resurrect flagging sexual function and restore fertility. Much of what we know about zinc comes from studies in rats and mice fed a diet deficient in zinc. Deprived of zinc, these weanling rodents develop testicular and growth failure. Zinc turns out to be an essential trace metal for man, but zinc deficiency states are quite rare.

Zinc deficiency and impotence does occur in men with chronic kidney disease and those with liver failure. In addition, hypertensive men, when treated with the diuretic hydrochlorothiazide, also have lower-than-normal zinc levels.

Would normalizing zinc levels improve sexual function in these zinc-deficient impotent men? The answer is maybe.

Zinc acetate tablets will raise zinc levels in men with chronic renal failure. In one study comparing zinc to placebo, those men treated with zinc reported increased sexual drive, libido, and frequency of sexual intercourse, significantly more so than did men with comparable degrees of zinc deficiency and sexual dysfunction receiving placebo.

Not everyone using zinc has had the same success in restoring sexual function in impotent men with chronic renal failure. Hypertensive hydrochlorothiazide-treated zinc-deficient impotent men fare even less well, with improvements in sexual function occurring rarely and about as often as with either placebo or zinc treatment.

Yohimbine

Man has always been intrigued and tantalized by the fantasy of discovering an aphrodisiac, a substance that would stimulate his or his lover's sexual appetite and desire. Some foods and drugs are believed to have sexuality-enhancing aphrodisiac properties. Those who were privy to the secret ingredients of the sexually stimulating substances were highly valued.

The physician to Louis XIV slipped the monarch a special potion each night before the king received a new lady in his bedchambers. The royal physician's potions were not always effective, causing the king to become displeased, truculent, and vengeful.

At one time, it was believed that the drug yohimbine had aphrodisiac properties. Certainly, yohimbine had the appropriately exotic lineage to satisfy preconceptions of what an aphrodisiac should be. Yohimbine was derived from the bark of a tree that grows only in Africa. It was believed that natives boiled the tree bark in a caldron and then harvested the residue. The yohimbine extract was then administered to men and women who were said to experience a sudden and striking increase in sexual desire.

Intrigued by these descriptions, Western scientists decided to look into the effects of yohimbine in man. Yohimbine, marketed under the name of Afrodex, was tested in 10,000 impotent men. Eighty percent were said to have restoration of potency. That report was published in 1968. Immediately thereafter, Afrodex vanished.

Interest in yohimbine was resurrected in the 1980s. Like other plant-derived products, yohimbine did not undergo extensive testing initially. However, in contrast to other alternative medicines, available as over-the-counter medications, you need a prescription to get yohimbine, which is sold under the name of Yocon or Yohimex. Testing on yohimbine began in earnest only after it was available as a prescription drug. Results have been variable.

In a study of one hundred impotent men, half received yohimbine and the other half placebo. Twenty-one percent of the yohimbine-treated patients had a complete return of sexual function. A surprising 13.8 percent of placebo-treated patients also reported a full return of sexual function. Statistical analysis indicated that yohimbine was not significantly better than placebo in restoring potency.

Was it possible that the dose of yohimbine administered was too low to have produced a positive effect on male sexual function? Apparently not. Larger doses of yohimbine were given in another study involving eighty-two impotent men. With higher doses, 14 percent reported a full return of sexual function. This figure is roughly comparable to the 13.8 percent full response in the placebo-treated patients in the prior study.

Yohimbine is an intriguing drug because it functions as an alpha-adrenergic antagonist. Drugs that block the action of alpha-adrenergic nerves have been successful in inducing erections, but only when injected directly into the penis. (See Chapter 19.)

Does Anyone Benefit from Yohimbine Treatment?   Despite what appeared to be initially disappointing results, yohimbine remains a popular prescription medication for the treatment of impotence. Recent research has established that some men respond better to yohimbine than others. The niche market carved out for yohimbine now includes men with psychogenic, also called nonorganic, impotence, and those originally potent men who became impotent when they started antidepressant medication. Not all men with medication-induced impotence respond as well. Yohimbine is both ineffective and dangerous in hypertensive men who become impotent while taking blood-pressure-lowering pills.

Psychogenic (Nonorganic) Impotence and Yohimbine. Yohimbine has been compared to a placebo in two studies involving 101 men diagnosed with psychogenic impotence. Yohimbine given in a dose of 5.4 mg three times a day allowed 37 percent of men to experience a return of erectile function and resume sexual intercourse within three days to three weeks after the onset of therapy, whereas only 15 percent of placebo-treated men had comparable results. Since the response to yohimbine is relatively prompt, many physicians now feel comfortable offering men with psychogenic impotence a one-month trial of yohimbine to determine whether they will, or will not, notice a return of satisfactory penile erections. Those who respond favorably can continue medication, whereas nonresponders will balk at continued yohimbine treatment because of lack of benefit or side effects. Yohimbine's side effects include anxiety, increased heart rate and blood pressure, dizziness, flushing, nausea, and headache.

In an effort to improve the results achieved with yohimbine alone, yohimbine has been paired with the antidepressant trazodone (Desyrel). In another placebo-controlled study, the yohimbine-trazodone combination was used to treat 63 men with psychogenic impotence. When given together, both medications seemed to be slightly better than either one alone. Patients received placebo or the yohimbine-trazodone combination for eight weeks and then crossed over to receive either placebo or active medication for another eight weeks. Only 55 men completed the trial, and positive results defined as "complete" or "partial" restoration of sexual potency were reported by 32 (56 percent) yohimbine-trazodone- and 10 (18 percent) placebo-treated men. Side effects occurred in 6 (11 percent) the men receiving yohimbine-trazodone and 2 (4 percent) placebo-treated patients. Although the results are tantalizing, it would be premature to encourage the comingling of both medications, for trazodone has a formidable side effect profile of its own. Further studies will be required to determine whether combination therapy is as effective and well tolerated as claimed.

Yohimbine and Medication-Induced Impotence. Sexual side effects are a significant problem for patients receiving antidepressant and antihypertensive medications (Chapter 16), causing so much distress, in fact, that in a desperate attempt to retrieve their lost sexual function, many patients stop taking essential medications, allowing depression to descend and blood pressure to rise.

Physicians are eager not to see the substantial health gains achieved with antidepressant and antihypertensive medications evaporate because of sexual side effects. They have worked hard to reexamine the disruptive influence medications exert on normal sexual function. Psychiatrists found to their dismay that the prevalence of antidepressant-induced sexual problems was greater than anticipated, occurring in about 30 percent of patients treated with the selective serotonin reuptake inhibitor (SSRI) class of antidepressants, which includes fluoxetine (Prozac) and sertraline (Zoloft) among others. For example, in one recent report of 160 patients receiving SSRI antidepressants, 54 (34 percent) complained of either decreased libido, diminished sexual responsiveness, or both.

Eight men who became impotent after starting SSRI antidepressants agreed to take yohimbine in conjunction with their antidepressant medication. Seven men reported "complete" or "partial" return of sexual function, but five experienced side effects of nausea and anxiety, causing two of them to discontinue yohimbine, whereas the remaining five have continued to use the medication with good success for over a year. These reports require validation with a larger cohort of patients in a placebo-controlled study before yohimbine can be recommended for all who experience antidepressant-induced impotence.

The problem is more complex for men with high blood pressure who become impotent while taking antihypertensive medication. Yohimbine provokes increases in blood pressure and cannot be safely prescribed for men with high blood pressure.

In sum, it is fair to say that yohimbine is beneficial in restoring erectile function in about one-third of patients with psychogenic impotence. A brief one-month trial will suffice to segregate those impotent men who will benefit from this medication from those who will not. Yohimbine may also be helpful in reversing the sexual side effects experienced by men taking antidepressant medication, but available data are sketchy and not yet conclusive, whereas yohimbine's blood-pressure-elevating properties makes it unwise to use this medication in impotent men with high blood pressure.

OVER-THE-COUNTER MALE HORMONES: ANDROSTENEDIONE AND DHEA

Testosterone, the most powerful of men's hormones, is readily available as a pill, patch, and injection and will soon be available as a rub-on skin gel, but only by *a doctor's prescription*. Other male hormones like androstenedione and DHEA are available without a prescription. This is yet another legacy of the 1994 Dietary Supplement and Health Education Act. DHEA is reviewed in Chapter 22. What follows is a discussion of androstenedione, the current cult androgen.

Androstenedione

When Mark McGwire, the powerful St. Louis Cardinals slugger, revealed that androstenedione pills were an integral part of his daily training regimen, everyone assumed that it was the androstenedione that allowed him to hit seventy home runs during the 1998 baseball season. Androstenedione, or "Andro," as it is called, became an overnight success. The word was that by taking "Andro" pills, men could build up their own testosterone stores and become better lovers, decrease their flab, and have an increase in the size of their penis. Further, the Andro promoters claimed that the effects of Andro are almost instantaneous, resulting in a 25 percent increase in serum testosterone levels in just sixty minutes. Wow!

Androstenedione "Andro" just will not go away. The storied steroid continues to demand attention as a front-page article, at least in sports pages and on the Internet. Like Beowulf or some Norse saga describing heroic feats of derring-do, Andro has assumed mythic proportions and already spawned its own fables.

Upper-echelon German athletes claim that fifteen minutes after snorting an androstenedione nasal spray, their serum testosterone levels increase by 237 percent! Then there is Lee Stevens of the Texas Rangers, who struggled for nine years in the minors until he finally had his chance to play in baseball's Major League. To everyone's surprise, early in the season this journeyman ballplayer emerged as a hero with a stunning set of statistics—fourteen home runs and forty-eight runs batted in—all made possible, he believed, because of his ritual use of androstenedione. Add this to the seventy-home-run season of baseball's first Andro enthusiast Mark McGwire, and you can readily understand why athletes are attracted to androstenedione.

Others reading of their heroes' testimonials respond as expected and boost sales of androstenedione to gladden the hearts of those who market this product. After all, it is still perfectly legal to buy great quantities of Andro. Athletes and exercise buffs regard Andro as a powerful male hormone, but the U.S. Congress still classifies androstenedione as a harmless dietary supplement.

Supplements, Steroids, and Sports

The byzantine world of supplement regulations—what athletes can and cannot take to improve their performances—varies from sport to sport. Some performance-enhancing hormones like testosterone and erythropoietin (EPO) are banned by all major sports organizations, but other hormones are subject to a selective ban. Androstenedione—banned by the International Olympic Committee—is tolerated by Major League baseball. Why?

Sports organizations use strict criteria to decide what they will and will not condone, primarily based on knowing whether supplement use will artificially enhance a man's performance in a specific sport. Thus, EPO, a hormone known to increase the number of oxygen-carrying red blood cells, benefits athletes like long-distance cyclists, who, if they had more oxygen in their bloodstreams, could pedal faster and longer without getting out of breath. EPO is officially banned by all cycling organizations. Still, each year organizers of major events like the Tour de France announce that one or more of their cycling stars has been disqualified for surreptitiously using EPO.

Does Andro give athletes in other sports a similar competitive edge?

For Andro to be effective it must be proven to have the same effect as testosterone, that is, *act as a muscle-building, strength-enhancing anabolic steroid.* The rules for anabolic steroids follow the same general premise as EPO: prohibiting hormone enhancement to provide one competitor with an unfair advantage over the other. But does Andro really offer athletes an advantage?

Testosterone is banned because when used in massive doses, this anabolic steroid will increase weight, muscle mass, and strength. To decide whether any other hormone will have the same muscle-building effect as testosterone, regulators ask three questions. Is Andro:

1. A "steroid"?
2. Pharmacologically related to testosterone?
3. An *anabolic* steroid? That is, does Andro help build muscle mass and increase strength?

For androstenedione, the answer is yes to questions 1 and 2 but no to question 3.

Of course Andro is a steroid, but so are other naturally occurring hormones. The word "steroid" merely refers to the structure of the hormone. The body makes many different steroid hormones, including cortisone, estrogen, and testosterone.

The production of *all* steroid hormones is the end product of a stepwise construction process, with the building of one steroid as a stepping stone to the next in sequence. Each steroid-producing gland has an internal assembly line of *transforming enzymes* that allows it to change one weak steroid into its more potent successor.

In the steroid chain of command, *androstenedione is the immediate precursor of testosterone.* Those advocating the use of androstenedione reason as follows. If your body has a sudden surge of the steroid that is just one step away from testosterone, it will automatically convert the surplus Andro to testosterone. The reasoning has the same appeal as trickle-down economics, that is,

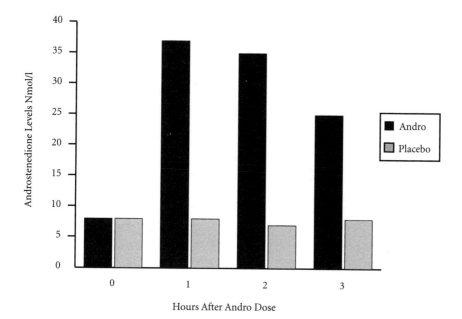

FIGURE 21.1   Serum androstenedione after 300 mg of Andro or placebo. SOURCE: Adapted from D. S. King, R. L. Sharp, M. D. Vukovich, G. A. Brown et al., "Efficacy of Oral Androstenedione on Serum Testosterone and to Resistance Training in Young Men," *JAMA* 281 (1999): 2020–2028.

that the mere availability of more androstenedione will eventually result in more testosterone. This would be a nifty theory were it not for the fact that to turn androstenedione into testosterone, your body needs a specific enzyme and that enzyme resides only within your testicle. Androstenedione pills or nasal sprays are absorbed immediately into your bloodstream and will increase blood androstenedione levels. But all that extra androstenedione cannot insinuate itself into your testicle's steroid production line.

Because of the inability of surplus androstenedione to "cut in line" in the orderly sequence of putting together testosterone, raising blood androstenedione neither interrupts nor augments testosterone output. Men who take a daily dose of 300 mg of androstenedione have a *prompt increase in blood androstenedione level but no increase in serum testosterone level.* (Figures 21.1, 21.2.) Tests of muscle strength before and after androstenedione or placebo show no more improvement in muscle strength in men taking androstenedione than is seen in those treated with a placebo!

All that happens when a man takes extra androstenedione is that his blood androstenedione levels increase. What then does a man do with all that extra androstenedione rattling around in his bloodstream? He disposes of the surplus androstenedione by converting it to a *female hormone called estrone.* (See Figure 21.3.) Too much *estrone* in a man's body can stimulate

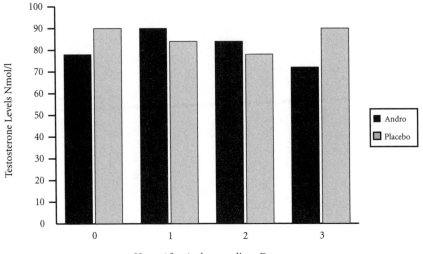

FIGURE 21.2   Serum testosterone before and after androstenedione. SOURCE: Adapted from D. S. King, R. L. Sharp, M. D. Vukovich, G. A. Brown et al., "Efficacy of Oral Androstenedione on Serum Testosterone and to Resistance Training in Young Men," *JAMA* 281 (1999): 2020–2028.

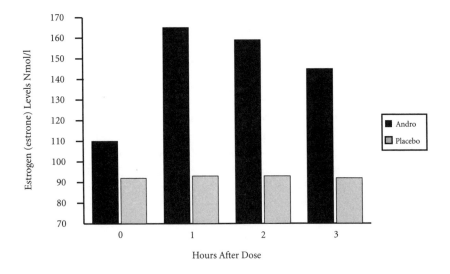

FIGURE 21.3   Estrogen (estrone) levels in men taking androstenedione. SOURCE: Adapted from D. S. King, R. L. Sharp, M. D. Vukovich, G. A. Brown et al., "Efficacy of Oral Androstenedione on Serum Testosterone and to Resistance Training in Young Men," *JAMA* 281 (1999): 2020–2028.

his breasts to enlarge and eventually put a lid on his libido. That is why so many men are leery of signing on for long-term androstenedione therapy.

Mike Simms, another Texas Ranger ballplayer, has tried and been unimpressed with any Andro-induced improvement in his muscle strength or batting average. He is wary of building up extra estrogen in his body and has assiduously avoided Andro. Others eager to believe that they will be the beneficiaries of an Andro "macho miracle" are somehow less concerned about Andro being transmuted to estrone and feminizing their body.

What Will Happen to Androstenedione?

The ready availability and intense publicity surrounding Andro have been a cause of concern for the anabolic steroid experts, who are fearful that the 1994 Dietary Supplement and Health Education Act has inadvertently made it possible for Andro to avoid the clutches and regulatory disciplines of the FDA. They worry that this has provided a back-door opportunity for men to get their hands on an anabolic steroid as an over-the-counter medication.

Doctors have measured hormone levels and muscle strength in men before and after they take Andro. They are convinced that bloodstream androstenedione levels increase dramatically, but the higher blood Andro is not necessarily translated into either an increase in a man's testosterone levels or his muscle strength.

So when Barry McGaffrey, the nation's overseer of illicit drugs, has to decide whether or not to lump Andro with testosterone and other proven and regulated anabolic steroids, he will have to sort out the relative value of information derived from testimonials of baseball players and placebo-controlled medical trials. For the moment, Andro remains readily available and aggressively marketed.

Men who order androstenedione pills hoping that the body will convert the Andro to testosterone are likely to be disappointed.

ALTERNATIVE MEDICINE AND CANCER PREVENTION

Experience with saw palmetto, yohimbine, and even PC-SPES demonstrate that carefully performed studies will help both alternative and traditional medicine practitioners understand which herbs, vitamins, and minerals are truly useful. For example, there is some tantalizing evidence suggesting that selenium supplementation may diminish men's risk of developing *prostate cancer*.

This was discovered by accident. Actually, doctors were trying to determine whether selenium could *prevent skin cancer*. They found over 1,000 men and women who had prior skin cancers and treated half with selenium and half with placebo to see if taking selenium would reduce their risk of future skin cancer. It did not.

But to everyone's surprise, selenium seemed to provide protection against other cancers, in particular, prostate cancer. However, the numbers of men in this study were too small to be statistically significant. Further, knowing how much selenium is enough by reviewing a man's dietary history or his blood selenium levels proved to be unreliable.

Rather, doctors turned to an unusual source—toenail clippings—to gauge a man's internal selenium stores. Using toenail selenium (an index of total body selenium), they found men with low and high selenium stores. Those with the highest toenail selenium levels were least likely to develop prostate cancer. These fascinating studies are intriguing but do not answer one critical question: *Does a man who takes selenium supplements lessen his risk of developing prostate cancer without causing other cancers to crop up?*

Selenium manufacturers are not likely to pony up the cash needed to determine whether selenium does indeed protect against prostate cancer. They can continue to reap profits by selling their product as a protected "nutritional supplement" without incurring the expense of a prolonged clinical trial.

THE COST OF ALTERNATIVE MEDICINE

The Dietary Supplement Health and Education Act has been instrumental in raising public awareness and bringing to the marketplace many innovative health-care products.

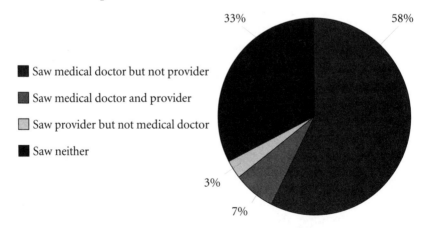

FIGURE 21.4   Percentages of men and women who visited a medical doctor, alternative medicine provider, both, or neither in 1993. SOURCE: Adapted from D. M. Eisenberg, R. C. Kessler, C. Foster et al., "Unconventional Medicine in the United States," *N. Engl. J. Med.* 328 (1993): 246–252.

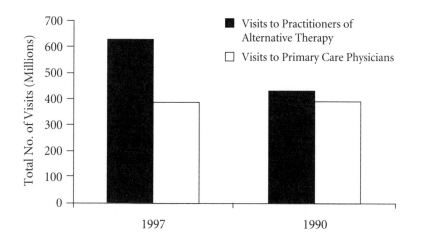

FIGURE 21.5   Total number of visits to alternative medicine and primary care providers in 1990 and 1997. SOURCE: Adapted from D. M. Eisenberg, R. D. Davis, S. Appel et al., "Trends in Alternative Medicine Use in the United States, 1990–1997," *JAMA* 280 (1998): 1569–1575.

The escalating enthusiasm for alternative medicine options can be best illustrated by shifts in care over time. In 1993, for example, 58 percent of Americans visited a traditional medical doctor, 3 percent saw an alternative-medicine doctor, and 7 percent saw both a traditional and alternative-medicine provider. (See Figure 21.4.) Between 1990 and 1997, the number of visits to primary-care physicians remained virtually unchanged, but during the same time, interval visits to practitioners of alternative medicine increased dramatically.

In 1997, visits to practitioners of alternative therapy exceeded the projected number of visits to all primary-care physicians in the United States by 243 million. (See Figure 21.5.)

Of even greater interest are the numbers of men and women who are willing to pay "out-of-pocket" costs for conventional and alternative-medicine services. Men and women drawn to alternative medicine must pay cash for their vitamins, herbal remedies, and visits to alternative-medicine practitioners because most of these services are not covered by health insurance. Figure 21.6 illustrates the Health Care Financing Administration (HCFA) estimate of the money men and women are willing to pay for conventional and alternative-medicine services.

In 1997, out-of-pocket expenses for all physicians' services was $29.3 billion. During the same year, $34.4 billion was spent on alternative-medicine therapies. That figure includes $19.6 billion for alternative-medicine practitioners, $1.7 billion for diet products, $4.7 billion for therapy-specific books, $3.3 billion for high-dose vitamins, and $5.1 billion for herbal prod-

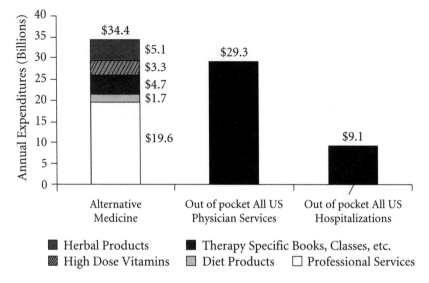

FIGURE 21.6   Health Care Finance Administration estimates of money men and women are willing to pay for alternative medicine (left column) and all outpatient and inpatient medical services in 1997. SOURCE: Adapted from D. M. Eisenberg, R. D. Davis, S. Appel et al., "Trends in Alternative Medicine Use in the United States, 1990–1997," *JAMA* 280 (1998): 1569–1575.

ucts. And the numbers cited have only increased during 1998. From a business standpoint, alternative medicine is a cash cow.

But is it really good medicine or just "feel-good" medicine?

Much of supplements' appeal is due to effective marketing. Comforting words like " natural . . . not a chemical or drug" and "Nature's own remedy" foster an impression of the benign temperament and safety of herbal supplements. Freed from responsibility for premarketing testing, we never learn of a supplement's potential toxicity until men and women become desperately ill and must be rushed to emergency wards.

ALTERNATIVE MEDICINE'S POPULARITY
RANKLES CONVENTIONAL MEDICINE

Prominent medical spokespersons like Drs. Jerome Kassirrer and Marcia Angell, editors of the prestigious *New England Journal of Medicine,* have called for more scrutiny and rigorous scientific studies to determine which of the legion of alternative-medicine supplements are a boon and which a bane to health. Their pleas will fall on deaf ears, for as long as supplement makers can drape themselves in the protection of the law that allows them to sell their products without proof of efficacy, they will continue to do so.

Men and women will continue to buy supplements in record quantities. They do not need the same *proof* of efficacy doctors demand. They want something more important. They want *optimism,* and that is precisely what alternative medicine has to offer.

Consider how men and women have catapulted one alternative medicine, the obscure adrenal hormone DHEA, to prominence in such a short period of time.

22

The Saga of DHEA

The DHEA melodrama, a tale of one drug's rejection, resurrection, and rehabilitation, is quite extraordinary. Spurned by the Food and Drug Administration as being unworthy of approval as a "safe and effective" *drug*, DHEA has risen phoenixlike from the ashes of FDA rejection to become accepted and endorsed by some as a bulwark of alternative medicine. In this chapter, you will find discussion of the following topics:

1. What is DHEA?
2. Who needs DHEA?
3. The DHEA mystery
4. Life, death, DHEA, and the FDA
5. Rancho Bernardo: DHEA gets some respect
6. Restoring youthful DHEA levels in mature men and women
7. DHEA and the Internet

"I'll be honest with you," Margaret began, "I really had serious doubts that these pills would help."

Originally from St. Louis, with "show me" indelibly engraved into her soul, this fifty-four-year-old grade-school teacher had an inbred distrust of all medications. She was not at all pleased when tests from her prior visit suggested that she might benefit from a daily regimen of one pill a day. Just one month earlier, she had sat in my office on the verge of tears as she described her plight. Struggling to compose herself, she first took time to smooth some creases out of her hound's-tooth skirt, liberated a carefully folded floral ascot from the pocket of her camel blazer, paused another moment and began. Margaret spoke softly at first, but as her anguish mounted, her calm, deliberately measured tones receded as the increasing intensity in her voice betrayed her gloom. Wrenching and twisting the ascot, she described her overwhelming sense of exhaustion and fatigue.

"It's sucking me dry." Everything was an effort, from dragging herself out of bed in the morning to going to work. Coping with her fourth-grade class drained her so much that she could only go home, microwave a frozen dinner, pay some bills, attend to a few household chores, crawl into bed, sleep fitfully, then wake in the morning to do it all again. Unmarried, but with many nearby relatives and a cadre of close friends, she no longer had the energy to spend time with either, thereby intensifying her loneliness and despair.

I wondered whether she might be not just blue but severely depressed, so I asked some pointed questions. None of her responses suggested an underlying depression. Then I arranged for some blood tests and, based on the results, recommended that she start taking a medication.

"Well, after the first day nothing happened, but by the second day I started to feel a little bit better and by day three, this enormous burden which had been weighing me down was suddenly and miraculously gone. I started sleeping better, woke each morning eager to start the day, and felt like an entirely new person. And I think the children noticed the difference, because for the first time in I don't know how long, two of the girls and one of the boys told me how nice I looked one day. You can't imagine how good that makes an old teacher feel. And this weekend I have a real date," Margaret blushed. "Those pills have been my salvation," she cooed.

"Yeah, I tried the pills. But they didn't do a thing for me. Used them for two months and nothing," complained Carl, the dapper middle-aged owner of a successful reinsurance firm. He was talking about the same pills that had helped extricate Margaret from her doldrums. However, Carl's problems were not quite the same. Like Margaret, he too felt both his age (he was fifty-nine) and life's everyday travails weighing very heavily on him. Still, he insisted that was not his major problem. He had at one time thought of himself as a sexual dynamo. After all, he was able, until recently, to copulate with his wife at night and the very next day with the young, lithe, and incredibly limber Felicia from fiscal, with whom Carl consulted frequently on pressing fiduciary matters in the privacy of his locked office: "And no calls when Felicia and I are in conference." But even dynamos start to sputter some time, and now Carl was beginning to run down. Although he was sure he could "perform" if he wished to, he simply no longer wanted to. His wife was more understanding than Felicia was. It was on Felicia's recommendation that he stated taking the pills, but nothing changed.

"Damn pills are no damn good!" was how he so eloquently put it.

How come the same pills that proved to be so invaluable for Margaret were so useless for Carl? Was this a gender-specific miracle drug, good for women but not at all helpful for men? Not really. Under the proper circumstances, the very same pill can work wonders in men who really need it.

What pill?

The pill is an over-the-counter *male hormone* called DHEA (dehydroepiandrosterone). Many like Margaret swear by DHEA's miraculous powers. DHEA is purported to be the most popular of all self-prescribed nutritional supplements available in health-food stores and on pharmacy shelves. Continuing impressive sales among those who remain steadfast believers in DHEA's health-enhancing and curative powers attest to the persistent popularity of this little tablet. Others are less impressed. Many have never even heard of DHEA. Where did DHEA come from, and how come only some people know about this "wonder drug?"

The saga of DHEA and its journey from an obscure hormone produced in the human adrenal gland to a life-affirming, life-extending, anti-aging hormone is remarkable.

Lacking FDA approval as a prescription medication, DHEA is now readily available as an inexpensive over-the-counter pill. Touted for its alleged benefits to "help fight disease, improve mood and energy, boost your sex drive and influence longevity," DHEA has undergone an extraordinary transition from the hormone laboratory to the world of alternative medicine, where this hitherto unknown adrenal hormone has been embraced as a welcome adjunct to personal health care. Everyone who has heard about DHEA has a strongly held opinion. People often talk of DHEA in sepulchered tones, as if the wondrous properties of this obscure hormone inspires, nay demands, a reverence often reserved for an item of religious devotion.

Others, particularly those in traditional medicine, have watched dumbfounded as this previously unknown, relatively weak male hormone catapulted from obscurity to prominence within a few short years. After all, most scientific developments leading to new medicines are invariably the products of extensive research conducted in the world's leading research centers or major pharmaceutical firms. DHEA has sidestepped the conventional path and leapfrogged into prominence primarily by ignoring—some would say flaunting—the traditional medical establishment.

The entire field of alternative medicine, chock full of herbs, dietary supplements, and obscure hormones, has quite suddenly emerged as a very appealing option for many men and women seeking nontraditional treatments. Individuals drawn to these nontraditional treatments are often disappointed with the medical profession's inability to provide relief for their fatigue, exhaustion, and episodic moodiness. They therefore look elsewhere for relief. Men and women who opt for alternative treatment seem eager to try anything purporting to alleviate depression or to improve their sense of well-being, sleep, sexual stamina, and muscle mass. (See Table 22.1.) The willingness of the public to embrace these nostrums so avidly is what gives doctors fits, for physicians know very little about the alleged benefits and possible adverse effects of these products.

All of the remedies listed in Table 22.1 have enjoyed varying degrees of popularity, but none seems to have the staying power and appeal of DHEA, a medication that was until recently a shadowy adrenal hormone. You can learn about DHEA from several sources, because the alleged anti-aging

TABLE 22.1   Some Currently Popular NonTraditional Remedies & Alleged Benefits

Substance	Alleged Benefit
DHEA	Anti-Aging, Strength, Libido, Sexual Stamina
Creatine	Strength, Muscle mass
Melatonin	Alleviates insomnia
St. Johns wort	Relieves depression, PMS

properties of DHEA have made this a lively topic in the popular press. Interest in DHEA has spurred on intensive medical research. Prominent medical journals often carry results of placebo-controlled trials in which mature men and women volunteer to take identical-looking pills, some containing DHEA, others containing no active medication (placebos).

Neither the doctors doing the study nor the men and women participating in the study know which pills they are taking, since they all look alike. Because neither the doctor nor the patient knows who is taking DHEA and who is taking a placebo, both are considered "blinded," and this type of study is referred to as a "*double-blinded placebo-controlled*" trial. Sometimes the men and women who used placebo during the first half of the study are then given the opportunity to receive the active medication, in this case DHEA, during the second half of the study, whereas those who took the DHEA initially then take placebo pills for the second half of the trial. Because the same persons take either DHEA or placebo for the first three months and then switch and take the placebo or DHEA for phase 2, the second three-month block, this type of study is referred to as a "*double-blind placebo-controlled crossover study.*" Both double-blind placebo-controlled trials and crossover trials provide reliable results, but they are often published only in medical journals not generally accessible to the average person.

But businessmen eager to *promote the sale of DHEA* often read through these dense scientific tracts and extract snippets of information that cast the most favorable and glowing portrait of DHEA, while selectively ignoring negative commentary, and then prepare a brief, easy to understand synopsis. This abbreviated upbeat version is published in readily accessible paperback books that grace the shelves of local health-food and nutritional-supplement stores.

But that is not the only way to find out about DHEA.

Plug DHEA into any Internet search engine and your computer screen will billow with information and options to extend your search ad infinitum.

What you think about DHEA will depend on where you get your information.

WHAT IS DHEA?

DHEA (the name stands for dehydroepiandrosterone), is a hormone made mainly in the human adrenal glands and released from there into the body's bloodstream. The adrenal glands are two fascinating, vital, and intriguing hormone-secreting organs. Shaped like plump triangles, one each is perched atop the right and left kidney.

Now, the adrenals are unusually busy little hormone factories. The natural tendency is to think of the adrenals as the source of adrenaline—that "pick-me-up" hormone that provides that extra energy and rush we all need to help us cope with everyday stress, danger, or crisis. Adrenaline (also known as epinephrine) is one of the hormones made in the adrenal gland, but it is neither the adrenal's major or most important hormone. That distinction belongs to cortisol (a.k.a. hydrocortisone).

It turns out that the adrenal churns out copious amounts of not one but several important hormones every day. Hormone output within the adrenal gland hormone is discretely compartmentalized. For example, adrenaline is made in the central part of the adrenal gland, an area called the adrenal medulla. We have all had the opportunity to experience the impact of a "turned-on" adrenal medulla at one time or another during our lives. Remember getting ready to ring the doorbell for that important first date, when your heart was pounding like a trip-hammer? That sensation was caused by extra adrenaline squirting out of your adrenal gland and rushing through your bloodstream to tell your heart to shift its rate into overdrive. It is not just the first date that can do this, but anything that creates a conscious sense of excitement, dread, or foreboding, which in turn activate impulses from our nervous system to wring extra adrenaline secretion from our adrenal medulla. Although it is physically nestled within the adrenal gland, the adrenal medulla is actually a collection of nerve cells specially adapted to produce and release hormones. Adrenaline and its parent compound noradrenaline, or norepinephrine, belong to a class of hormones called *catecholamines*. Nerve endings throughout our body and brain are especially equipped to produce and release catecholamines.

DHEA is an entirely different type of adrenal hormone, a *steroid* hormone made in a portion of the adrenal called the adrenal cortex. All steroid hormones share the same funny-looking chicken-wire-type shell. (See Figure 22.1.) Only specialized structures within the body—the ovaries, the testicles, and the adrenal glands—are capable of manufacturing steroid hormones. Estradiol and other estrogens are the ovaries' steroid hormones, whereas testosterone is the dominant steroid hormone produced by the testicles. Both the ovaries and the testicles have the capacity to make DHEA, but most DHEA is made in a special inner zone of the human adrenal cortex, the zona reticularis. Each zone of the adrenal cortex is specially adapted

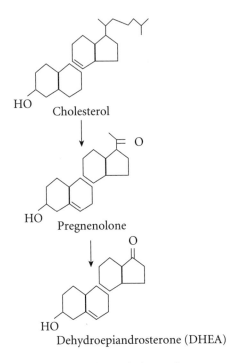

FIGURE 22.1　The creation of DHEA from cholesterol.

to make one major hormone. Thus, cortisol (hydrocortisone) is made in the middle zone, the zona fasiculata, and production of the salt-retaining hormone aldosterone occurs only in the outer zone, the zona glomerulosa, whereas DHEA production is relegated to the innermost zona reticularis. (See Figure 22.2.)

DHEA differs from the other adrenal steroid hormones in several important aspects. Dominant adrenal steroid hormones such as cortisol and aldosterone are considered vital for healthy existence. Until recently, DHEA has not been categorized as a "vital" human hormone. Why?

WHY IS CORTISOL A VITAL HUMAN HORMONE WHEN DHEA IS NOT?

The human adrenal production of cortisol and aldosterone starts during fetal development and continues steadily throughout life. DHEA production, on the other hand, is inconstant. Blood levels of DHEA and its companion steroid hormone DHEA-Sulfate (DHEA-S) levels are unusually high at birth, but only for a fleeting instant. Thereafter, DHEA and DHEA-S levels plummet to low levels and remain in check during most of childhood, but then DHEA bursts on the scene just before the start of puberty, remains vig-

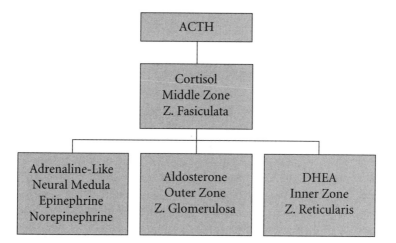

FIGURE 22.2   Sites of production of cortisol, aldosterone, and DHEA within the adrenal cortex.

orous until about age fifty, and abruptly wanes and drops out of the hormonal scene as we age. (See Figure 22.3 on page 302.)

Low DHEA and DHEA-S levels allow all children to grow and develop normally from birth to the preteen years. Indeed, at this time of life, *restraining DHEA production* is critical for normal development. In those rare instances when the adrenals make excessive DHEA during childhood, children suffer. Too much DHEA too early *stunts growth* and may be linked to other serious medical complications such as uncontrollable blood pressure that is either dangerously high or inappropriately low.

However, there is a time when the body of every normal boy and girl is ready for DHEA. For most of us, that time coincides with our tenth or eleventh birthday. Then the human adrenal starts to manufacture DHEA and continues to make copious amounts of it for many subsequent years. Blood levels of this hormone peak just before puberty, remain vigorous during our early adult years, and then about age fifty, just like a flickering candle, start to flame out. From this point on, DHEA levels start to decline, not just in some people, but in everybody, men and women alike.

In this regard, DHEA differs from other adrenal hormones like cortisol, which remain at a constant level throughout life.

However, it is not just the whimsical nature of DHEA and DHEA-S secretion that relegates DHEA to the role of "minor adrenal hormone." A vital human hormone is one that is necessary to maintain well-being and sustain life.

We know that animals that have no adrenal glands and therefore lack adrenal hormones fail to thrive. They become weak, fatigued, lethargic, eat poorly, lose weight, become dehydrated, and eventually die. From this, we

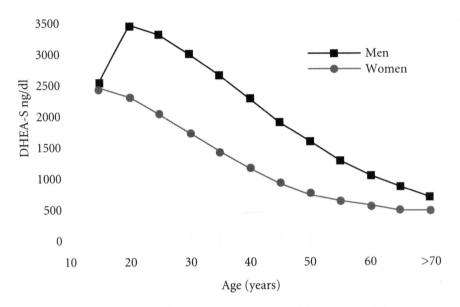

FIGURE 22.3   Variation of DHEA-sulfate levels with age in healthy men and women. ADAPTED FROM: N. Orentreich, J. L. Brind, R. L. Rizer, and J. H. Vogelman, "Age Changes and Sex Differences in Serum Dehydroepiandrosterone Sulfate Concentrations Throughout Adulthood," *J. Clin. Endocrinol. Metab.* 58 (1984): 551–555.

conclude that there is something about the presence of normal adrenals within the body's adrenal glands that is essential for normal health. That something is the proper daily ration of specific adrenal steroid hormones (cortisol in humans and corticosterone in rodents). Health can be restored and death prevented if animals with no adrenals are given back the hormones they need to survive (cortisol in humans and corticosterone in rodents). DHEA will not do the job and for this reason is not a life-saving steroid in either species.

WHY DOESN'T DHEA SAVE LIVES?

There are several reasons DHEA is not a life-saving hormone in animals, but perhaps the most important is that *most animals do not normally produce DHEA at all*. They live out their entire life span and thrive without DHEA. Indeed, DHEA is an alien hormone for most animals. This is an important consideration when interpreting the results of studies purporting to show that DHEA improves immune status and extends lifespan in rats (see below). Normally, only man and some other primates make DHEA.

Furthermore, DHEA is totally ineffective in reversing the weakness, fatigue, low blood pressure, low blood sugar, and weight loss that occurs when the adrenal glands are not present or not working properly. Those symptoms occur when the vital adrenal hormone cortisol is in short supply. Repletion of the body's cortisol promptly alleviates all of the symptoms of adrenal insufficiency and restores good health.

Men and women who have damaged or diseased adrenal glands suffer because they cannot produce sufficient amounts of adrenal hormones to keep them healthy. In medicine, this condition, *adrenal insufficiency,* or *Addison's disease,* is not common but has plagued and weakened some prominent Americans, most notably President John Kennedy. Actually, Kennedy was a congressman when his Addison's disease was diagnosed, and he remained in good health as long as he took his daily adrenal hormone ration. Although his adrenals were malfunctioning and not making adequate amounts of cortisol, aldosterone, and probably DHEA, he did not have to take DHEA supplements. Today's DHEA proponents would probably argue that he would have felt better if he had taken DHEA.

It was only in 1999 that DHEA supplements were recognized as a genuinely valuable *add-on therapy* in others who, like President Kennedy, have the rare medical condition known as adrenal insufficiency. Hydrocortisone, aldosterone, and DHEA, the three most important hormones made by the human adrenal glands of healthy men and women, are lacking in men and women with adrenal insufficiency. One hormone, hydrocortisone, is essential, and a second hormone, an aldosterone surrogate (fludrocortisone [Florinef]), is often prescribed to restore good health in patients with adrenal insufficiency. No one had ever considered replenishing the body's DHEA as part of the mandatory adrenal-hormone supplement regimen for adrenal insufficiency.

But the value of DHEA was never properly tested until 1999, when twenty-four women—with an average age of forty-two and all with documented adrenal insufficiency—agreed to take part in a study. They would first continue their standard adrenal-hormone treatment. Then half received either a single 50-mg DHEA pill or an identical-looking placebo pill every morning for four months. At this time, women who had taken the DHEA pill reported an *increased sense of well-being and improved sexuality.* The placebo-treated women had no improvement. DHEA-treated women also had *more sexual thoughts and fantasies* within one month of starting DHEA. But it was only after four months of continuous DHEA therapy that these women with adrenal insufficiency were able to experience a genuine increase in their overall sexual satisfaction. With this persuasive evidence, doctors are now recommending adding DHEA supplements to care for their patients with adrenal insufficiency.

However, adrenal insufficiency is a very rare disease affecting only a handful of people. The justification for the current widespread use of DHEA in otherwise healthy men and women with normal adrenal function is not as easy to recognize. DHEA may be able to improve the lot of women, and probably men, with adrenal insufficiency, but that does not mean that DHEA can be considered a vital human hormone.

IF DHEA IS NOT A VITAL HORMONE, WHAT IS IT DOING TO OUR BODIES?

The late-childhood surge in DHEA production correlates with the first signs of sexual maturity, the sprouting of hair in the armpit and groin. Because the appearance of these burgeoning adolescent developments occurs in conjunction with the secretion of this adrenal hormone this stage of our development is referred to as the *adrenarche*. In both young men and women, the adrenarche usually precedes full sexual maturation. That requires activation of the gonads, the ovaries in young girls and the testicles in young men, an event referred to as *gonadarche*.

WHAT ELSE DOES DHEA DO?

We know that when DHEA is present in more than normal amounts, hair growth is stimulated. Unfortunately DHEA does not stimulate growth of hair on the scalp, which would be a boon for balding men and women suffering hair loss. Rather DHEA, when present in more than normal amounts stimulates the growth of facial hair, particularly in the beard and mustache area, a major problem for women but often not noticed by men, who are accustomed to having beard hair. For women with persistently elevated DHEA levels, unsightly beard and mustache hair is not the only problem. Sustained elevations in DHEA can disrupt women's normal menstrual cycles, inhibit ovulation, and cause infertility. For these women, return of normal ovulation and enhanced fertility can be achieved with treatments designed to lower blood DHEA levels.

All actions of DHEA, starting with the appearance of armpit (axillary) and pubic (groin) hair when DHEA secretion begins before puberty as well as the unsightly facial hair and disordered menstrual cycles, occur because DHEA acts like a male hormone (androgen).

Each adrenal steroid hormone has its own unique action. For example, cortisol helps modulate blood-sugar (glucose) levels and for that reason is referred to as a glucocorticoid, whereas aldosterone helps regulate sodium and other minerals and is designated as a mineralocorticoid. DHEA acts like a male hormone and for that reason is referred to as an anabolic androgenic steroid. Steroids are classified as anabolic if they help build muscle. Testosterone, as the body's major anabolic steroid, will help build muscle even when present in small amounts. In contrast, DHEA is a weak androgen and can only exert its effects when present in relatively large quantities.

The DHEA Mystery

Other than providing the stimulus for axillary and groin-hair development, what does DHEA do? We do not know for sure, but there are several tantalizing clues suggesting that DHEA may be more important than previously suspected.

The Abundance Theory

After the adrenal gland shifts gears and starts to produce DHEA (adrenarche), it does so with a vengeance. Once DHEA production begins, daily output of this hormone is greater than any other adrenal hormone. Indeed, when the adrenal gland acquires the capacity to make DHEA, it does so in record fashion, churning out ten times more DHEA than cortisol. Surely, it has been reasoned, there must be some physiologic reason that our body is flooded with this adrenal androgen at this time. It is the very fact that so much of this adrenal hormone is suddenly in our circulation that has prompted many well-respected scientists to conclude that DHEA contributes to our well-being when we are young in ways that we still do not fully understand. They argue that DHEA production peaks early and remains in abundance throughout our young adult years, when our faculties are at their sharpest and performance in work and at play is at its peak. Starting about age fifty, many of our physical and mental skills start to decline. It is precisely at this time that DHEA production starts to ebb.

"Aha!" shriek the DHEA advocates with delight. "Declining physical and mental functioning occurring just when DHEA levels are falling? A coincidence? I think not!"

There is no question that the two events—declining strength and stamina and falling DHEA levels—occur at the same age in both men and women. Could our declining strength and increasing frailty be caused by falling DHEA levels? Would we be better off if at age sixty we had the DHEA levels of a twenty-year-old? We are about to learn the answers to these questions.

Life, Death, DHEA, and the FDA

The Food and Drug Administration, which must pass on every new medication to determine if it is safe and effective, has for the most part chosen to ignore DHEA. To achieve approval by the FDA, each new medication must go through a series of rigorous tests designed to see if the drug does what it is intended to do without causing an undue amount of adverse side effects. For example, when a drug company has a new cholesterol-lowering medication, the company has to find thousands of men and women with high cholesterol levels, give all of them the same low-cholesterol diet, and offer half of them the new medication and the other half an inactive but similar-appearing placebo pill. If the new medication lowered cholesterol levels more than the placebo and did so without causing an undue amount of adverse side effects, then it can receive the FDA's seal of approval certifying that it is both a safe and effective cholesterol-lowering medication.

Today, all new medications—whether intended to lower cholesterol, decrease blood pressure, alleviate depression, or improve the lot of men and women with AIDS—must go through this process.

DHEA never did. Lacking any formal pharmaceutical-company interest and willingness to commit the resources to shepherd DHEA through the tedious, time-consuming, and costly testing process required for approval, the FDA had no other option. Instead, lacking any specific information on DHEA, the FDA basically punted and in 1984 cut DHEA loose to be handled like a vitamin, herb, or any other alternative medicine. (See Chapter 21.)

Rancho Bernardo: DHEA Gets Some Respect

That decision to let DHEA fend for itself in the vitamin, nutritional-supplement, alternative-medicine market came just two years before the Rancho Bernardo study was published in the *New England Journal of Medicine.*

It was at a place called Rancho Bernardo that DHEA first made medical news. Here in this California retirement community, Dr. Samuel Yen and his University of San Diego Medical School colleagues set out to study normal aging. To do this, they did two seemingly pedestrian experiments. First, they collected and analyzed blood samples for so-called health risk factors, such as cholesterol, blood count, and hormones, including levels of DHEA and its by-product DHEA sulfate (DHEA-S). They examined men age fifty and older who had chosen to reside in Rancho Bernardo. Then they waited twelve years and returned to Rancho Bernardo to see how everyone was doing.

The first finding of importance was that blood DHEA-S levels fell progressively with age. This was not surprising, for other scientists had noted the natural decline in DHEA-S levels with advancing age. Thus, starting at age fifty, blood DHEA-S levels drift downward, with levels diminishing with each subsequent decade, demonstrating an unequivocal *age-related trend.* No one was spared. With advancing age, DHEA levels declined in all. Those in the youngest age group could be counted on to have the highest serum DHEA levels and with each advancing decade DHEA levels fell progressively. By now that was old news.

What was new and startling about this study was that at any age, some men had *abnormally low DHEA-S* levels. It was this group of men with unusually low DHEA-S levels that caught the investigators' attention, as these people appeared to be singularly vulnerable to premature death, especially from heart disease. Those who were destined to die had the lowest DHEA-S levels. This is illustrated in Table 27.1 in Chapter 27. The predictive association of low DHEA-S level and premature death from heart disease was independent of age and other cardiac risk factors such as cholesterol level.

Does this mean that those with lower DHEA levels are at risk for premature death from cardiovascular disease? Should all men and women have an assessment of their DHEA levels as part of the routine annual physical? Is knowing what your DHEA-S level is as important as knowing your blood pressure, cholesterol profile, and smoking history in determining your risk for heart disease? More important, do people with low DHEA levels improve their chance of survival if they take DHEA pills to raise their DHEA-S level?

Proponents of DHEA think so. Others without a vested interest in DHEA are less sure.

Surveying the Evidence For and Against DHEA as an Important but Not Vital Human Hormone

Experiments with DHEA.   Researchers seeking to find out more about DHEA have slipped DHEA into the drinking water of experimental animals like mice. Some of these mice are genetically destined to develop diabetes mellitus (sugar diabetes). Mice who slurped DHEA did not become diabetic. Other mice, programmed to be obese, transcended their genetic destiny and remained slim merely by consuming DHEA. Like humans, mice tend to gain weight as they age. However, mice treated with DHEA gained less weight than their age-matched placebo-treated littermates.

Likewise, compared to placebo-treated rats, rats treated with DHEA seemed to live longer, have improved immune responses, and be less likely to develop breast cancer. Studies in rabbits show that DHEA rabbits are less likely to develop atherosclerosis. Surely these findings should convince even the most skeptical that DHEA has extraordinary preventive and curative properties.

Perhaps that is true for rodents. But mice, rats, and rabbits do not normally make DHEA. Their remarkable responses to the introduction of an *exotic hormone* prove only that under the proper circumstances, rodents benefit from receiving a hormone that is normally only made in man and other primates.

Human DHEA Studies.   Two lines of evidence support the concept that DHEA may be an important, if not vital, hormone. Patients destined to have or who have already been afflicted with a major medical problem have trouble making as much DHEA as other healthy men and women in the same age group. Earlier, I noted that at any age, men with very low DHEA-S levels were more likely to have, and die from, heart attacks than their age-matched counterparts. In a similar vein, women with low DHEA levels were more likely to have breast cancer as well as a diminution of their immune status, so that they would be less likely to fend off disease. This type of *epidemiologic evidence* is often cited to validate the importance of DHEA in human health.

But does it?

Although tantalizing, as was the case with poor King Tantalus, what you see may not be what you get. In Greek mythology, Tantalus was condemned to spend his life floating in a pool of water, just beneath a tree dangling succulent fruit. The instant he opened his mouth to drink, the pool of water dried up, and when he reached up to pluck the fruit from the overhanging limb, the fruit-bearing branch receded just out of reach. DHEA may be suffering the same fate.

For example, other epidemiologic studies have failed to confirm a relationship between low baseline DHEA-S levels and premature cardiovascular disease. The antidiabetic and immunoprotective properties of DHEA in rodents have not been duplicated in humans.

What Happens to Men and Women Who Take DHEA Pills? Large (high doses) and more moderate amounts (replacement doses) of DHEA have been given to men and women to gauge their responses to supplemental DHEA.

DHEA and Menopause

When six postmenopausal women age 46–61 volunteered to participate in a high-dose DHEA study, they received an initial test dose of 400 mg and then took 1600 mg of DHEA every day for twenty-eight days. Blood DHEA levels rose immediately. Once in the bloodstream, DHEA is rapidly converted to other male and female hormones so that the levels of DHEA-S, testosterone, and a testosterone (T) metabolite called dihydrotestosterone (DHT) also increased. Hormone levels peak at two weeks, then tail off somewhat but remain elevated above baseline for the entire four-week study. The body's metabolic machinery is particularly well equipped to take advantage of this sudden male hormone (androgen) surge as fodder for producing more female hormones. Thus, a modest but unequivocal increase in serum estrogen levels occurs in conjunction with the DHEA-provoked increase in serum androgen levels. Note that blood estradiol values increase promptly and then appear to plateau after two weeks of DHEA therapy. (See Figure 22.4.) This phenomenon, readily demonstrable in postmenopausal women, is

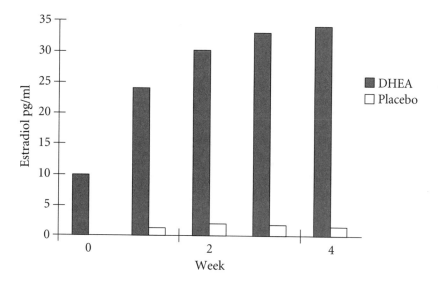

FIGURE 22.4 Serum estradiol levels in menopausal women before and during 4 weeks of DHEA treatment.

gender specific. Young healthy men who take DHEA do not as a rule experience an increase in testosterone or other male hormone levels.

DHEA in Young Men

When twenty-three-year-old men took DHEA in equivalent amounts (1600 mg per day), their serum DHEA-S levels tripled, but serum T and DHT values rose but only modestly. However, even in this healthy group of young men, the consequences of DHEA-provoked increases in serum androgen levels were readily apparent. Body fat declined by 31 percent, yet weight was unchanged, implying that when these young men took DHEA, their muscle mass increased as their percent fat decreased. Total serum cholesterol level also declined, primarily due to a selective decrease in the values of the unfavorable low-density lipoprotein (LDL) cholesterol.

Unfortunately, both this study of young men and the earlier one of menopausal women came under heavy criticism because the amounts of DHEA administered were far in excess of what healthy twenty-year-olds normally produce.

Restoring Youthful DHEA levels in Mature Men and Women

In an effort to quash the criticism levied at the earlier high-dose DHEA studies, Dr. Arlene Morales, working with Dr. Yen, decided to use more moderate "physiologic" amounts of DHEA. She recruited seventeen women and thirteen men who agreed to take either DHEA 50 mg per day or an identical-looking placebo pill for three months and then "switch over" and take the placebo or DHEA for the next three months. Neither the men and women participating in the study nor the doctors conducting the trial were aware of the order in which the DHEA or placebo was given. Hormone levels were checked throughout the study, and participants answered questionnaires about their mood, sense of well-being, and sex drive (libido) at designated intervals throughout the six-month study.

Even with this lower "replacement" DHEA dose, both DHEA and DHEA-S values were higher during the period of DHEA treatment than during control or placebo periods. Increases in the hormones testosterone and dihydrotestosterone were evident once again in women but not in men. However, both men and women reported an "improved sense of well-being" with DHEA but not when taking placebo. Women were slightly better off in this regard, with 82 percent of women and only 62 percent of men experiencing the improvement in well-being. The mechanisms underlying the benefits ascribed to DHEA are not clear. The improved sense of well-being was not due to the impact of sex-hormone-driven improvements in libido, for questionnaires measuring sexual interest and libido showed no changes in sex drive throughout the study.

Feeling better is fine but not enough for some who have greater expectations for DHEA. Particularly troublesome is the lack of documented improvement in sexual function. The cover of one of the more popular DHEA books states unequivocally that DHEA "Boosts Your Sex Drive," yet the pages of that book provide scant evidence in support of this claim. One man named Martin, a DHEA enthusiast, maintains that since starting DHEA, "There's been a remarkable influence on my sexual satisfaction. My libido has improved, and I feel thirty years younger when I'm intimate with some one. Also I noticed that my energy level is better and I'm more relaxed."[1]

Other than this upbeat individual testimonial, no other evidence in support of DHEA's ability to improve sexual function in either men or women is offered. Apparently overlooked is the lack of difference in libido during DHEA and placebo treatment. Despite the lack of supporting evidence, the author of this book concludes, "There is no doubt that DHEA boosts sex drive especially in those who have low DHEA-S levels to start with."[2]

Herein lies both the challenge and the appeal of DHEA. Since everyone over the age of fifty has "low DHEA-S levels to start with," it would not be at

---

[1]Adapted from R. Sahelian, *DHEA: A Practical Guide* (Garden City Park, NY: Avery Publishing, 1996), p. 13.
[2]Ibid., p. 107.

all difficult to recruit men and women over fifty to participate in a project to evaluate the effects of DHEA on sex drive, immune function, aging, and longevity. But to do the study properly, it would be necessary to treat some with DHEA and an equal number with placebo. At the end of three months, six months and one year, the DHEA and placebo group responses could be compared to seek out differences in outcome for DHEA- and placebo-treated patients. If DHEA were indeed helpful in boosting sex drive, fighting disease, and improving mood and energy or in prolonging life, that would be apparent by looking for differences reported by DHEA- and placebo-treated patients at any of these intervals.

If, however, placebo-treated patients fared as well as those who received DHEA, then serious questions would continue to dog DHEA aficionados. Still, only a massive study of this design would provide some degree of closure on the DHEA story.

DHEA AND THE INTERNET

Ignored by the FDA, embraced by some, but by no means all clinical researchers, DHEA has found a happy haven on the Internet. The last time I checked, there were no less than fifty-nine Internet sites offering information on and credit card sales of DHEA as well a plethora of other nonprescription health-care products. Some of these sites offer little more than chat lines with DHEA enthusiasts effusively sharing their positive experiences with this product. Occasionally e-mailers will write in to say that DHEA made them too aggressive or hostile, but more often than not, the news is upbeat and positive. Prowling through the Net provides useful insight into the popularity of this product. Although DHEA has male hormone (androgenic) properties, its sale is not restricted, as is the case with other more powerful androgenic hormones like testosterone. To obtain testosterone, you need a prescription from a doctor with a license to dispense narcotics.

Testosterone does not have any of the addictive characteristics of most narcotics. Nonetheless, its distribution is limited because like narcotics, testosterone and other androgenic hormones have become drugs of abuse. Intended primarily to treat testosterone-deficient men or debilitated cancer patients who have become physically weakened by the muscle-depleting rampage of their malignancy, testosterone and other anabolic androgenic steroids have found favor among athletes and bodybuilders eager to maximize muscle mass as a prelude to improving body shape or athletic performance.

Remember, although DHEA is an androgen, it is a relatively weak androgen and does not fall under the same guidelines used to restrict the sale of more powerful male hormones, and it can be sold without a prescription like a vitamin pill.

A WORD ABOUT LIFE'S LITTLE "PAUSES," WITH ATTENTION TO THE "ADRENOPAUSE"

We grow old, age, and die: Life's depressing but unassailable triad of truisms is under attack. Today, scientists, no longer willing to accept this traditional lore, are seeking to turn the tables on the inevitable. They are probing life-and-death issues as never before to look more critically at exactly what it takes to first weaken a man or woman and then snuff out life. In some cases, hormones can be implicated.

MENOPAUSE AS A PROTOTYPE OF AGING

A woman's ovaries start to fail in her late forties or early fifties and can no longer generate the eggs (ova) or the female hormones (estrogens) of her earlier reproductive years. Deprived of her normal ration of estrogen, a woman is likely to experience some immediately apparent symptoms such as hot flashes, as well as some less obvious consequences of estrogen insufficiency. For example, without adequate estrogens, her bones and heart are not as protected as they once were. Calcium, her skeleton's most important stabilizing and strengthening mineral, takes flight, leaving only a limited supply of calcium to brace her bones. Weakened by a lack of calcium in her bones, she develops osteoporosis, making fractured bones more likely. Estrogens also protect women from heart disease, but when estrogen levels plummet, women become as susceptible as men to cardiac death.

Women can significantly reduce their risk of developing postmenopausal osteoporosis and heart disease by taking estrogen pills to replenish their body's quotient of a natural hormone that was lost when they entered menopause. Recently, evidence has emerged to indicate that estrogens may also provide some protection against developing Alzheimer's disease.

The experience with estrogen hormone replacement therapy (HRT) in menopause has been quite dramatic and extraordinary, impelling other scientists to use the same principles of replenishing our stores of other hormones that naturally decline with age. The pituitary gland's growth hormone, abundant and important in our youth to help the growth of our body *(soma)*, declines to almost undetectable levels as we age, an event that has been referred to as the *somatopause*. Would growth hormone replacement therapy be as beneficial as estrogen replacement therapy? Some think so. Others are concerned about the cost—about $14,000 per year—and the serious side effects.

If estrogen deficiency defines the menopause and age-related decline in pituitary growth hormone is characteristic of the *somatopause*, is it not natural to think of the age-related dwindling in *adrenal* DHEA production as the *adrenopause*? Shouldn't every man and woman over a certain age replenish their stores of DHEA? Would this help them live longer while diminishing their risk of age-related illnesses like heart disease and cancer? The truth is nobody knows, and we are not likely to find out.

Answers regarding advantages and risks of long-term estrogen and growth hormone therapy will be available long before any definitive assessment of or consensus regarding DHEA emerges. It all comes down to basic economics. The pharmaceutical companies that make and distribute estrogens and growth hormone are willing to commit the resources needed to find the answers, for they know that research demonstrating patient benefit will be published in major medical journals and will then translate into more estrogen and growth hormone prescriptions.

DHEA distributors have not as yet felt the same need to prove the value of their product. Rather, they have had the good fortune to rely on the rather substantial word-of-mouth network that has surfaced to tout DHEA and help market this product. Fortunately, DHEA is not costly and has few side effects, most notable the growth of facial hair in women. Thus, risks associated with DHEA's use are mainly cosmetic. Benefits, however, are somewhat more difficult to document.

WHEN IS IT APPROPRIATE TO USE DHEA?

Although all men and women have a natural lowering of DHEA levels with age, some seem to tolerate the lowering of DHEA better than others do. Listlessness, lack of energy, and inability to function effectively in work or personal relationships is characteristic of men and women with low DHEA levels. As an endocrinologist, I see men and women who have many of the symptoms listed above, and when no other cause is apparent, I check their DHEA level. If the level is low, I recommend that they go to their local pharmacy and pick up some DHEA, which is available as an over-the-counter medication. Then I see them again one month later to first see how they are feeling and next check their DHEA level. Patients who benefit from DHEA notice the improvement almost immediately.

CONCLUSIONS

Doctors are, as a rule, not fond of alternative medicine in general and DHEA in particular. Physicians' failure to keep abreast of the developments in alternative medicine stands in stark contrast to their need to remain au courant with the latest advances in traditional medicine. Doctors are for the most part obsessed with keeping up to date with each new scientific discovery to ensure that they do not "fall behind," a chronic concern of conscientious physicians. Why then are they so out of tune and oblivious to progress in "alternative medicine"?

It is primarily because the evidence generated in support of using either DHEA or any of the other alternative-medicine treatments has, so far, not been subjected to the same scrutiny they have come to demand for any other treatment or therapy they recommend. They are unimpressed and rarely recommend DHEA or other alternative medicines.

As a consequence, men and women hear about these nontraditional treatments not from their doctors but from friends, late-night television ads, tabloid magazines, and clerks in health-food stores. Then, impressed with what they hear, they eagerly shell out cash and try the new medication, and if they sense an improved general energy level, sleep better, and have more sexual drive or less depression, they continue to use and often become staunch believers in this new form of alternative medicine. Doctors then find themselves in the embarrassing position of knowing little or nothing about this newfangled treatment and are ill-equipped to pass any judgment on the efficacy or safety of their patients' self-directed remedies.

DHEA continues to enjoy great popularity as an over-the-counter medication. It has no apparent side effects in men, and if one discounts the fact that *high-dose long-term use* of this adrenal hormone causes facial hair to sprout in some women, DHEA has proven to be a remarkably benign medication. Men and women who take DHEA insist that they feel better when taking this medication. Because it is a male hormone (androgen), albeit a weak androgen, DHEA can bolster a man's own sagging androgen output. The body can also convert DHEA into a weak estrogen and in so doing may be of value to menopausal women whose bodies cry out for some sort of estrogen supplementation. Those men and women who want to buff up their own internal male or female hormone levels but do not need, want, or even qualify for traditional testosterone or estrogen therapy often "test drive" DHEA as an inexpensive alternative for a brief period of time. If they feel better and are not troubled by the extra facial and body hair that may result from long-term use of this adrenal androgen, they will likely want to continue using this supplement.

23

The Prostate and Its Problems

A man can add prostate gland enlargement to death and taxes as one of life's inevitabilities. His prostate gland starts bulking up at about age fifty, and once it starts increasing in size, it never stops. By age seventy-five, almost all—90 percent—of men will have big prostate glands due to a condition known as benign prostatic hyperplasia (BPH). If you are dashing off to the men's room more often than usual, have to strain to urinate, or are embarrassed by occasional episodes of incontinence, BPH may be the culprit. Medical treatments (pills, both prescription and herbal) are now available to ease urination and decrease prostate gland size. When pills stop working and you continue to have problems with urination, prostate surgery can provide relief. This chapter focuses on BPH. Chapter 24 deals with prostate cancer. In this chapter, you will find discussions on:

1. Where the prostate gland is and what it does
2. Benign prostatic hyperplasia (BPH)
3. Controlling symptoms caused by BPH
4. Which medication is best to control symptoms of BPH
5. Prostate surgery for BPH
6. The cost of treating BPH

WHERE IS THE PROSTATE GLAND AND WHAT DOES IT DO?

The prostate gland rests in the lower abdomen, nestled between a man's bladder and his rectum. (See Figure 23.1.) Liquid secretions from the prostate gland mix with sperm released from the testicles and contribute to semen. Additional fluid is provided by the seminal vesicles, smaller glands huddled near the prostate. The prostatic and seminal vesicle aqueous secretions provide a convenient and efficient waterway for sperm to be transported out of the testicle and deposited in the vagina at the climax of sexual intercourse.

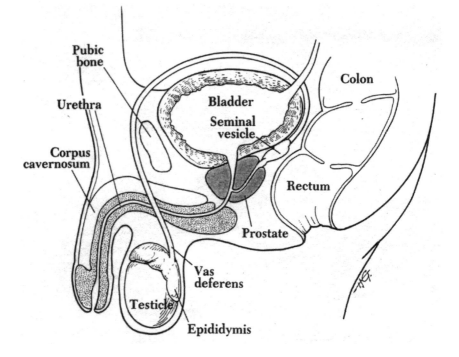

FIGURE 23.1   The anatomy of the normal prostate gland and its relation to the bladder, testicles, and lower bowel.

Most men are unaware of the presence of their prostate until it becomes inflamed, infected, or enlarged. Inflammation of the prostate—prostatitis—often causes rectal pain or pain on urination. Prostatitis is a concern for young sexually active men because it is often, but not invariably, the result of a venereal or sexually transmitted disease. Extremely painful ejaculation is a common symptom. Antibiotics are often the treatment of choice.

BENIGN PROSTATIC HYPERPLASIA (BPH)

Enlargement of the prostate gland, or benign prostatic hyperplasia (BPH), occurs frequently in middle-aged and older men and disrupts normal urine flow. Problems with urination that develop slowly and early on are only annoying. More frequent trips to the men's room during the day and getting up once or twice at night to empty the bladder create a nuisance but do not cause much of a problem at first. Then, as the prostate continues to bulge into the bladder, more symptoms emerge. Irritation at the bladder neck causes local spasm, creating a sense of urgency and a need to bolt to the bathroom to avoid sudden bladder overflow or loss of bladder control. Occasionally, this causes grown men to wet their pants.

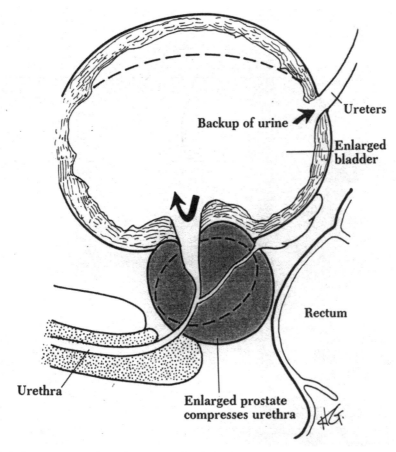

Backup of urine

Ureters

Enlarged bladder

Rectum

Urethra

Enlarged prostate compresses urethra

FIGURE 23.2   An enlarged prostate gland blocks urine flow out of the bladder.

The proximity of the prostate to the lower end of the bladder, specifically the area where the bladder joins the urethra (the tube through which urine flows), is responsible for the vast majority of symptoms of an enlarged prostate. The progressive growth of the prostate creates a bulge, something like a knuckle, at the critical junction between the bladder and the urethra. Urine is, in a sense, dammed up inside the bladder. (See Figure 23.2.)

The enlarging prostate can disrupt a man's ability to urinate either by *obstructing* the flow of urine out of the bladder or by creating an *irritation* at the point where urine leaves the bladder. Symptoms of *obstruction* include:

- an inability to empty the bladder fully
- a *weak urinary stream*
- some *hesitancy in initiating* urine flow

The Prostate and Its Problems   317

- *persistent dribbling*, often characterized by a desire to try to shake the last few drops of urine out of the penis before completing the process of urination
- occasionally, urine trapped within the bladder breaking loose, causing a man to wet his pants, a condition known as *overflow incontinence*

In contrast, *irritative symptoms prey on bladder control,* causing:

- a sense of *urgency* and need to rush to the toilet to urinate promptly
- a tendency to *void in small volumes* frequently

Since both obstructive and irritative symptoms are due to the enlarged prostate, it is important to know exactly what causes prostate growth.

It turns out that there are at least two types of prostate cells. One type, which tends to gather at the area where urine leaves the bladder (the bladder neck), contains a muscle that flexes or relaxes in response to adrenalinelike signals from the nervous system. The remaining prostate cells trap testosterone from the bloodstream and convert it to another hormone called dihydrotestosterone (DHT). As prostate DHT levels increase, these cells enlarge.

If the muscles at the bladder neck can be encouraged to relax or if the DHT stimulus to prostate growth can be blunted, both obstructive and irritative symptoms associated with benign prostatic hyperplasia should diminish. Indeed, that is precisely what happens.

CONTROLLING SYMPTOMS CAUSED BY BPH

Frequent urination and a sense of urgency, a need to rush to the bathroom to avoid urinating in one's underpants, are among the most common symptoms resulting from bladder-neck spasm caused by BPH. Two medications, terazosin (Hytrin) and doxazosin (Cardura), block the nerve signals that cause muscles around the bladder neck to go into spasm. These two medications (which belong to a class of drugs called alpha-blockers) diminish spasm and help muscles in the bladder neck work more efficiently and minimize many of the embarrassing urinary symptoms. Terazosin or doxazosin (Hytrin and Cardura) are therefore commonly prescribed to help control many of the troublesome symptoms of early prostate enlargement, and both allow a man to achieve a renewed sense of control over his urination. With either medication, a man's urine flow and urine volume increase substantially.

Terazosin and doxazosin (Hytrin and Cardura) pills, while effective in minimizing annoying urinary symptoms, are not without risk, for both *al-*

pha-blockers were originally developed as *blood-pressure-lowering* medications. When men take either Hytrin or Cardura, they will have both a relief of bladder-neck spasm and less need to run to the bathroom frequently but will also have a lowering of their blood pressure. Once in the bloodstream, the active ingredient in terazosin or doxazosin relaxes the muscles in a man's bladder neck to minimize symptoms of bladder-neck spasm. This is the desired effect. Terazosin and doxazosin also relax or dilate the arterial muscles that help stabilize a man's blood pressure. This causes an inevitable drop in blood pressure, not a problem for most men, who can tolerate a slight reduction in their blood pressure without having any unpleasant symptoms. However, men with low-normal or frankly low blood pressure can feel dizzy with only a modest lowering of their blood pressure. When a man's blood pressure falls, he may have symptoms of lightheadedness or queasiness or may even faint.

To be effective in controlling urinary symptoms and fending off side effects that might cause an abrupt lowering of blood pressure, doctors tend to prescribe low doses of terazosin or doxazosin at first and then, if the man tolerates and gets used to the medication, cautiously increase the dose to an ideal level that will *diminish urinary symptoms but not blood pressure.*

Men who have high blood pressure and are taking antihypertensive medications should alert their physicians so that appropriate adjustments in the mix of blood-pressure-lowering medications can be made to accommodate the anticipated fall in blood pressure caused by Hytrin or Cardura. Newer alpha-blocker drugs are in development that selectively target the bladder neck and spare the arterioles. These drugs should achieve the same degree of bladder-neck relaxation required to minimize a man's urge to urinate frequently without causing his blood pressure to fall to dangerously low levels.

DECREASING THE SIZE OF A MAN'S PROSTATE GLAND

Since prostate size is responsible for most of the symptoms of BPH, why not whittle down the prostate? Surgical treatment of BPH can decrease prostate size but sexual side effects, including retrograde (or backward) ejaculation and impotence, occur with some regularity. For this reason, men have looked for other treatment options that would decrease prostate size without causing them to become incontinent or experience sexual side effects.

Although both terazosin and doxazosin are effective in controlling many urinary symptoms associated with BPH, neither drug diminishes prostate size. To decrease prostate size, it is necessary to rein in the stimulus responsible for continued prostate growth.

WHY DOES A MAN'S PROSTATE GLAND ENLARGE?

The prostate gland absorbs testosterone from a man's bloodstream. Testosterone, once trapped within the prostate, is converted into another potent male hormone called dihydrotestosterone (DHT). It is DHT within the prostate that stimulates prostate growth. When prostate DHT levels are high, prostate gland size increases.

Some men with a peculiar genetic defect are born lacking the enzyme needed to convert testosterone to DHT. They have low blood DHT levels and small prostate glands and *never develop benign prostatic hyperplasia (BPH)*.

Doctors tried to mimic this quirk of nature, reasoning that if they could safely decrease a man's DHT levels, they should be able to eliminate the major stimulus to his prostate gland growth. That is what led to the development of the medication finasteride (Proscar).

Finasteride (Proscar) inhibits a critical enzyme called 5-alpha reductase. The 5-alpha reductase enzyme is what changes testosterone (T) to dihydrotestosterone (DHT). Shortly after men start taking finasteride (Proscar), their blood DHT levels fall by almost 80 percent. Levels of DHT within the prostate also decline, and with continued finasteride (Proscar) treatment, prostate gland size starts to dwindle. Prostate volume decreases by about 28 percent from pretreatment size. Often this shrinkage in prostate volume is sufficient to alleviate pressure on the bladder and provide relief from many of the obstructive symptoms associated with benign prostatic hyperplasia (BPH).

Men who use finasteride are about half as likely to need emergency prostate surgery to relieve acute urinary obstruction, an agonizingly painful condition that occurs when the prostate gland gets so big that it blocks all flow of urine out of a man's bladder. Many men who use finasteride (Proscar) will avoid prostate surgery, but a handful have to cope with sexual side effects, predominantly erectile dysfunction. (See Table 23.1.)

WHICH MEDICATION IS BEST
TO CONTROL SYMPTOMS OF BPH?

The sexual side effects associated with finasteride use, though occurring in less than 5 percent of men, were sufficiently worrisome to prompt some physicians to reconsider the use of alpha-blockers to treat the symptoms of BPH. The competition between the alpha-blockers terazosin and doxazosin and the 5-alpha reductase inhibitor finasteride to control the lucrative market of medications used to help men counteract the symptoms associated with BPH has heated up quite recently. A large study published in the *New England Journal of Medicine* described the responses of 1,229 men to treat-

TABLE 23.1   Side Effects Reported by Men with BPH Treated for 12 Months with Finasteride or Placebo

Symptom	Reporting Side Effects with Finasteride 5 mg	Reporting Side Effects with Placebo
Decreased Libido	4.7%	1.3%
Ejaculatory disorder	4.4%	1.7%
Impotence	3.4%	1.7%

SOURCE: Modified from Gormley GJ, Stoner E, Bruskewitz RG et.al. The effects of finasteride in men with benign prostatic hyperplasia. N Engl J Med. 1992;327: 1185–91.

ment with placebo, terazosin, finasteride, or a combination of finasteride and terazosin. About 250 men in each group rated their prostate symptoms and urine flow rate before and after one year of treatment with either placebo, terazosin, finasteride, or a combination of both terazosin plus finasteride (Table 23.2). In this study, finasteride was no better than placebo, whereas terazosin alone or in combination with finasteride significantly improved both urinary symptoms and urine flow. However, despite improved urine flow, *prostate size increased during terazosin treatment. Decreased prostate gland size* was apparent only in those *men who were taking finasteride alone or in combination with terazosin.*

Side effects of dizziness and low blood pressure were prominent, occurring in 26 percent of terazosin-treated men. Impotence was reported with roughly equal frequency with placebo and terazosin treatment. However, 7 percent of men treated with combined finasteride and terazosin reported problems with ejaculation, compared to less than 2 percent in the other groups.

WHAT'S A MAN TO DO?

These disparate findings have led some to suggest the following plan of action for men with symptoms of BPH. If a man complains of urinary symptoms, frequent urination, getting up often during the night to void or a sense of urinary urgency, he should have a digital rectal exam to check the size of his prostate. If the prostate is *not enlarged,* then treatment with terazosin alone may be all that is needed to provide relief. However, for men with *enlarged prostates,* treatment with finasteride alone, or in combination with terazosin, seems sensible.

WHAT ABOUT SAW PALMETTO?

A new "natural" herbal remedy, *saw palmetto,* has been promoted as a safe and effective treatment for BPH. Saw palmetto is derived from extracts of a

TABLE 23.2 Placebo, Finasteride, Terazosin and Finasteride + Terazosin (Combined) in Men with BPH

Symptom	% Reporting Side Effects with Placebo	% Reporting Side Effects with Finasteride	% Reporting Side Effects with Terazosin	% Reporting Side Effects with Combined
Dizziness	7 %	8 %	26 %*	21 %*
Weakness	7 %	8 %	14 %	14 %
Impotence	5 %	9 %*	6 %	9 %*
Ejaculatory Problem	1 %	2 %	0.3 %	7 %
Decreased Libido	1 %	5 %	3 %	5 %

* Indicates significantly different from placebo

SOURCE: Modified from Lepor H, Williford WD, Barry MJ et al. "The efficacy of terazosin, finasteride or both in benign prostatic hyperplasia." *N Engl J Med.* 1996;335: 533–9.

berry, *Serenoa repens*. It has been a popular herbal remedy and has been embraced by those who are inherently skittish of traditional medicine and more willing to put their faith in "natural" herbal remedies. It is likely that saw palmetto has weak 5-alpha reductase-like activity and is considered by some as nature's finasteride (Proscar). Saw palmetto has been enthusiastically endorsed by many who are leery of the known side effects of medications such as Hytrin, Cardura, and Proscar. *The side-effect profile of saw palmetto has not been established.* Most of the buzz surrounding saw palmetto has come from word of mouth and testimonials. There are, however, some medical journal reports in which both urinary symptoms and urinary flow measurements were determined before and after saw palmetto treatment. Fifty men signed up for and forty-six completed one six-month study, which had several components:

- Urinary symptoms were assessed by a self-administered questionnaire, the International Prostate Symptom Score (IPSS) to establish severity of symptoms.
- Urinary flow rates, residual bladder volume, and PSA were measured with conventional standardized diagnostic tests.

Initially, men answered questions to assess their IPSS. This questionnaire is set up to determine how often men have a problem urinating and is scored on a 0–5 scale, with lower scores indicating no and higher scores revealing urinary problems of mild, moderate, or severe intensity. The scale is self-graded, and men answer questions such as: "Over the past month how often have you had to urinate again less than two hours after you finished urinating?" For "not at all," score 0; for "less than one time in 5," score 1; for "less than half the time," score 2; and so on, up to "almost always," which earns a score of 5. The six questions relating to ease of urination, steadiness and/or vigor of urinary stream, and need to strain to start urinating, are all part of the questionnaire. After men answer all questions, their scores are tallied. Men with a score of more than 10 are considered to have significant lower-urinary-tract (prostate) symptoms. As prostate symptoms improve, IPSS scores decline.

This study demonstrated a progressive improvement in IPSS scores in men who took commercially available 160 mg of saw palmetto per day for six months. In this group of forty-six men who completed the six-month study, overall IPSS score was 19.5 before and fell to 12.5 after saw palmetto treatment. However, not all men had equivalent responses. Some men had more symptomatic relief of urinary symptoms than others. A 50 percent or better improvement in individual symptom scores was apparent in 21 percent of men at two months, 30 percent at four months, and 46 percent at six months. Although symptom scores improved, urinary flow rates, prostate size, and prostate specific antigen (PSA) levels remained unchanged. This was only a relatively short-term preliminary study, and it is possible that when longer placebo-controlled studies are completed, more compelling evidence of saw palmetto's effectiveness or lack thereof will emerge.

Dr. Timothy Wilt, a physician at the Veteran's Administration Hospital in Minneapolis, has searched diligently for any medical articles that would allow him to decide if saw palmetto was effective in alleviating symptoms of BPH. He only included those studies that fulfilled certain criteria, such as measurements of urine flow rates and symptom score before and after treatment. He found eighteen separate medical articles that had sufficient data for analysis.

In short-term studies averaging nine weeks, saw palmetto was superior to placebo and about as effective as finasteride in improving peak urine flow. Men who started saw palmetto usually stayed with this form of treatment. Dropout rates, that is, men who discontinued treatment, were: placebo 7.0 percent, saw palmetto 9.1 percent, and finasteride 11.2 percent. Side effects of erectile dysfunction were reported in 0.7 percent of placebo-treated, 1.1 percent of saw palmetto–treated, and 4.9 percent of finasteride-treated men. Men who used saw palmetto reported no other significant side effects. Saw palmetto did not reduce prostate size, and the studies were not long enough to determine whether extended use of saw palmetto prevented long-term complications or decreased the need for prostate surgery.

PROSTATE SURGERY FOR
BENIGN PROSTATIC HYPERPLASIA (BPH)

When obstructive and/or irritative symptoms of BPH persist despite medical therapy with finasteride, terazosin, doxazosin, or saw palmetto, surgery to chisel down prostate size and reestablish a channel for freer urine flow must be considered. Inserting a probe into the urethra to visualize the area of obstruction allows the urologist to perform an operation called a transurethral prostatectomy (TURP). The doctor then shaves away prostatic tissue to reopen communication between bladder and urethra.

Men who have had a TURP experience no decrease in sexual desire and often, but not invariably, retain the ability to have erections, engage in sexual intercourse, and ejaculate. Unfortunately, the surgical procedure may cause damage to the internal bladder sphincter, the valve responsible for forward ejaculation of semen. A damaged bladder sphincter cannot close prior to ejaculation, resulting in retrograde ejaculation of semen backward into the bladder. Some men also have difficulty with bladder control and become incontinent after prostate surgery.

Retrograde ejaculation is clearly a major issue for men who want to produce their own offspring. Fortunately, BPH tends to affect older men. Although it is occasionally possible to retrieve semen that has been ejaculated backward into the bladder and use it for insemination, the procedure is onerous and time-consuming, with only a limited success rate.

COST OF TREATING BPH

Now that men with symptomatic BPH have at their disposal four treatment options—the alpha-blockers terazosin (Hytrin) and doxazosin (Cardura), the 5-alpha reductase inhibitor finasteride (Proscar), the herbal option saw palmetto, and surgery to decrease prostate bulk—they are literally awash in therapies and may have a difficult time deciding which of these remedies best suits their individual needs.

One possibility is called "watchful waiting," and is particularly appealing to those whose primary concern is cost. In Great Britain for example, where the National Health Service (NHS) picks up the tab for both medications and surgical treatment, the reasoning goes as follows: Drug treatment with finasteride (Proscar) does significantly decrease both the numbers of men who develop acute urinary retention and require either hospitalization for emergency catheter drainage of a blocked bladder or emergency prostate surgery to alleviate obstruction. However, the cost to the NHS is high, about $3.5 million for two years' treatment with finasteride (Proscar). The cost of emergency hospitalization and surgery for those men who had acute urinary obstruction was only $750,000, so that for those paying the bills, it makes more fiscal sense to allow men to experience the pain and suffering associated with acute urinary obstruction.

In a more comprehensive analysis comparing the cost of finasteride (Proscar), terazosin (Hytrin), and surgery, physicians at St. Luke's Hospital in New York City arrived at a different conclusion. They analyzed:

- Total cost of treatment, using a private-insurance and Medicare model
- Days lost from work
- Numbers of men who had relief of symptoms

The chances of achieving improved urinary flow during the first year of treatment were 88 percent for surgery, 67 percent with finasteride, and 74 percent with terazosin. The estimated total twenty-four-month cost is shown in Table 23.3 on the next page.

Another advantage of medical over surgical therapy was seen in an estimate of the days lost from work: twenty-two days after surgery and only eight days each with either terazosin or finasteride treatment. These au-

---

The Prostate and Its Problems

TABLE 23.3   Cost of Medical and Surgical Treatment of BPH

Treatment Cost–24 month per Individual	Private	Medicare
Surgery	$6,411	$3,874
Finasteride	$2,860	$2,161
Terazosin	$2,422	$1,820

SOURCE: Modified from Lowe FC, McDaniel RL, Chmiel JJ and Hillman AL. "Economic modeling to assess the costs of treatment with finasteride, terazosin and transurethral resection of the prostate for men with moderate to severe symptoms of benign prostatic hyperplasia." *Urology* 1995; 46:477–483

thors concluded that primary treatment for symptoms of BPH medical therapy is less expensive than surgical therapy over the first two years of treatment.

CONCLUSION

Prostate gland enlargement due to BPH is likely to occur in most men as they age. Though unavoidable, BPH, and the urinary symptoms it causes, may be held in check with either prescription or over-the-counter herbal medications. The most extensive experience is with the prescription medications terazosin (Hytrin), doxazosin (Cardura), and finasteride (Proscar). Short-term studies with saw palmetto indicate that this herbal medication may also provide relief of the symptoms caused by BPH. However, only finasteride (Proscar) can actually reduce prostate size and decrease the need for emergency prostate surgery.

Most men rely on their doctors to check prostate gland size during their annual physical exam. However, symptoms of prostate gland enlargement are readily apparent, and men who are having trouble urinating, find they have an urge to urinate, or are scurrying to the bathroom more often than usual should not wait for their annual exam but should pick up the phone and contact their physician to discuss treatment options sooner rather than later.

24

Prostate Cancer: The PSA Controversy

Prostate cancer is a fickle malignancy causing death in some men but allowing others to live long lives even without treatment. This chapter is devoted to helping you understand the issues and controversies surrounding the diagnosis and treatment of prostate cancer. If you do have prostate cancer, which treatment—surgery, radiotherapy, hormones, or no treatment—is best for you? What can be done to overcome the sexual side effects associated with prostate cancer treatment? The issues covered in this chapter include:

1. How common is prostate cancer?
2. The PSA test
3. Adjusting the PSA for age and race
4. What causes high PSA levels in men who do not have prostate cancer?
5. Improving the PSA: What is the Gleason score?
6. What happens when prostate cancer is not treated?
7. Testosterone and prostate cancer
8. Why does prostate cancer treatment cause hot flashes in men?
9. Difficult choices for men with an elevated PSA
10. Treatment of impotence following prostate cancer surgery

THE PROSTATE CANCER ENIGMA

Prostatic enlargement is not always benign. Sometimes the cells within the prostate gland turn ugly, undergo a malignant transformation, and a cancer begins to fester in a man's prostate. Today, there is a simple blood test called the PSA (prostate specific antigen) that allows doctors to detect prostate cancer at its earliest stage. A man and his doctor are often inclined to think of an elevated PSA level as an early warning signal requiring immediate action. Early treatment to either expunge the cancer from a man's body or at least neutralize and prevent this malignancy from advancing should then allow men with elevated PSA levels to live longer, more productive lives.

Sometimes that is exactly what happens. But on occasion, prostate cancer is so aggressive that it does not respond well or at all to any treatment.

There are also times when a man is better off left untreated, either because his prostate cancer though present is slow growing and not likely to represent a threat to their survival. Alternatively therapies intended to purge prostate cancer from a man's body may backfire and cause medical complications so stunning as to result in a rapid deterioration in the quality of a man's life.

The following vignettes of men with prostate cancer illustrate the range of possible outcomes.

Bill

I am usually not asked for medical advice at funerals, but Bill wanted to make sure he caught me before I returned to Boston. He had been my parents' friend and had known me since I was a child. After the service, eulogies, and internment, this jovial, balding, bespectacled man scoured the reception, slipped in behind me in line at the coffee urn, and then ushered me into a private space. Never one to mince words, he started with:

"They want to chop my nuts off."

"I beg your pardon."

"Look, my PSA is still elevated because they couldn't get all of the prostate cancer during surgery, so now they want to . . . you know . . . castrate me. To tell you the truth, at my age (he was seventy-one), my testicles are little more than ornamental, if you know what I mean, but I've grown sort of fond of them.

"I'm no fool," he went on. "If it has to be done to save, or at least extend my life, a few years, I'll agree, but if there were only some other way . . . "

There was another way.

At this time in mid-1985, doctors were starting to experiment with a novel hormone treatment to extend the lives of men with prostate cancer without resorting to surgery. I explained the nature of the hormone treatment to Bill and told him that it was then still considered experimental (today it is standard care), but if he wanted, I would try to link him up with one of the New York programs that was accepting new patients. He nodded. I made some calls on his behalf, then went back to chat with others who had come to pay their respects.

Twelve years later, another funeral, and I am back in New York.

"How do I look—terrific, huh?" Bill beamed.

He did. As a matter of fact, he looked much more fit than he had at the earlier funeral more than a decade earlier, when the prospect of surgical cas-

---

tration loomed large. He told me he was active, busy reading, writing, and planning travel and vacations with his wife.

"I just show up every three months and they give me a shot. That's all I have to do. I don't have any sex drive, but that has been a small price to pay. I feel strong and am really enjoying life. Frankly, I never felt better."

For the next thirteen years, Bill and his wife continued to travel together and had their lives further enriched, delighted by the time they could spend with their children and grandchildren.

When Bill eventually passed away at age eighty-nine, it was not because of prostate cancer, but, like many of his age, it was his heart that gave out one night, and he died quietly in his sleep.

Sam

He lived one more year than Bill did, but overall, Sam was not as fortunate.

"I should have never let them talk me into having that X-ray treatment for my prostate cancer," he moaned.

Nine years ago, diabetes mellitus was Sam's problem. He was a hulking, amiable man with a wardrobe of plaid suits, striped shirts, loud ties, and pale loafers. At first, all we needed to do to help him control his diabetes was to contain his prodigious appetite so that he could lose a few pounds. This was not at all easy for a man who had spent his entire adult life in the restaurant business. He struggled to alter his eating habits, but before long, he was starting to show some progress. Pills were added to help lower his blood-sugar levels; then when that was not enough, insulin injections began. One day, looking for something to do, he decided to attend a health fair for a "free blood pressure, blood sugar, cholesterol, and PSA test." Ten days later, a letter arrived congratulating him on his normal blood pressure, blood sugar, and cholesterol levels; but in that same letter, he learned for the first time that his PSA was elevated. For more information, he should call a number at the hospital for yet another free consultation. He was eighty-five years old.

"This nice young doctor told me that the PSA test was not normal, which meant I could have a cancer in my prostate, but they would only know for sure if they did a prostate biopsy. When the biopsy showed cancer, they said I could have prostate surgery or X-ray treatment (radiotherapy). Well, I didn't want to be cut so I told them to go ahead with the X-ray treatment."

"It was the dumbest thing I ever did."

"Now every time I sit down to go to the toilet the blood just keeps gushing out, always bright red, and the cramps, they are awful." He was telling me this once again in the emergency room while his nurse struggled to thread an IV needle into a tiny vein on his frail arm so that he could get another blood transfusion.

"I should never have allowed them to talk me into it," he muttered again.

Sam was upset because he had a complication of treatment. The X-ray beams aimed at his prostate cancer must pass through and occasionally irritate part of the lower bowel. As a result, Sam's bowel became fragile and never healed properly and would, at the slightest provocation, ooze blood. Then whenever he had to strain during a bowel movement, bright red blood would fill the toilet bowl, and Sam would end up in the hospital emergency ward for another transfusion. The bleeding was so severe that it caused him to become anemic. Over the ensuing years, he was rushed to the hospital at least forty-one separate times to staunch the bleeding and receive blood transfusions. His health deteriorated further. Weight peeled off his previously bulky frame, and as his muscles wasted away, there seemed to be nothing between his skin and his skeleton. He became progressively weaker.

At age ninety, a stroke left Sam unconscious and mute. The family, aware of his suffering, honored his wishes, decided against any more aggressive treatment, and Sam passed away quietly.

Knowing what we know today, many doctors would pause before ordering a PSA in an octogenarian or offering treatment to Sam or any other eighty-five-year-old man with prostate cancer out of concern that treatment-induced side effects might minimize the quality of life of a man who was not expected to live another ten or fifteen years. This remains an area of great controversy and concern among all who care for men with prostate cancer.

Cecil

Like Sam, Cecil had diabetes mellitus, which was discovered just before his first prostate cancer surgery. He had been losing weight, urinating a great deal, and was always thirsty but had chalked this up to his fondness for salty foods. In reality, high blood-sugar levels, and not salty food, were responsible for his unquenchable thirst, frequent urination, and loss of weight. With diet and insulin, blood-sugar values normalized, and he started to regain much of the weight he had lost.

Then without warning, he started losing weight once again. This time it was not due to diabetes. His prostate cancer had spread. Unlike Sam and Bill, who were well into their retirement years when their prostate cancer was diagnosed, Cecil was only fifty-one and still working when his prostate cancer was first diagnosed. He was also black. When prostate cancer strikes at an early age in African-American men, it can be particularly aggressive and difficult to contain. Even with the most up-to-date treatments available, nothing could slow down the relentless progression of his prostate cancer. Cecil was only fifty-four when he passed away.

Prostate cancer is unaccountably destructive in African-Americans, appearing early and spreading with uncommon ferocity. Unfortunately, cancers this aggressive tend to be resistant to all efforts to contain them, so these cancers bully their way through the body with infuriating speed, cutting short the life of Cecil and other young black men.

Charles

When he was sixty-four, Charles, a busy and vigorous, ruddy contractor with a fondness for flannel shirts and blue jeans, started to have difficulty getting an erection. At first he tried to ignore this new problem and ascribed his sexual problems to the pressures of work. Then at the urging of his wife, he went to see his urologist, who was already treating him with terazosin (Hytrin) for urinary symptoms caused by an enlarged prostate. Routine blood tests also revealed a low serum testosterone level, and he was referred to me for hormone treatment. Testosterone therapy was started, erections improved, and he was able to have sexual intercourse again, satisfying both him and his wife.

All was well for a while, but on one of his routine visits, I noted that his PSA level was starting to inch upward. A rising PSA always raises the possibility of underlying prostate cancer, but repeated prostate biopsies performed over several years had failed to reveal any cancerous cells within the prostate. Charles continues to rely on periodic testosterone injections to maintain sexual potency and daily Hytrin to control urinary symptoms. At seventy-four, he is thinking of retiring.

Urologists are convinced of a causal connection between testosterone treatment and prostate cancer. Endocrinologists are not. The linkage is actually rather difficult to prove. PSA levels may increase during testosterone treatment, but often, as was the case with Charles, the PSA elevation is not always associated with prostate cancer. Endocrinologists who use androgens to treat their testosterone-deficient men have no more instances of prostate cancer among their patients than do primary-care doctors who rarely, if ever, use testosterone treatment. The only uncontested facts are that men known to have prostate cancer should not receive testosterone supplements and that for some men, eliminating testosterone (by medical or surgical castration) will slow the spread of entrenched prostate cancer.

Watchful waiting—individualized attention tailored to each man's needs— is often the best approach. Some men like Charles will have just an elevated PSA but no evidence of prostate cancer. For them, continued careful follow-up may be all that is needed.

THE PROMISE AND PROBLEMS OF THE PSA

The cases described above illustrate how lethal a disease prostate cancer can be for some men like Cecil. Many like Bill respond well and live long lives with proper therapy, whereas others like Sam live long but tortured lives as a result of complications of prostate cancer treatment. There are even some men like Charles who have elevated PSAs and live long productive lives even without any treatment at all. That is why deciding what to do about prostate cancer is so complex.

HOW COMMON IS PROSTATE CANCER?

We have known for some time that prostate cancer is the most commonly diagnosed male malignancy and the second leading cause of cancer death in men. In recent years, prostate cancer has been on the front burner because several prominent men, General Norman Schwarzkopf, former senator Robert Dole, French president François Mitterand, Louis Farrakhan, and Harry Belafonte, to name a few, have either been diagnosed with or have died from this malignancy. No man, no matter how powerful he is, can ignore this disease.

This much is not in dispute. Prostate cancer was responsible for the deaths of 40,400 men in 1995, a figure not dissimilar to the 46,000 women who lost their lives to breast cancer in the same year.

Prostate cancer, however, differs from breast cancer in several important ways. Few women with breast cancer can expect to live long lives without treatment, whereas many men with prostate cancer can. Women rely on periodic breast self-examination and annual mammograms to identify breast cancers at their earliest possible stage, making prompt, frequently curative surgery feasible.

Men cannot do self-examinations of their own prostate glands. They must rely on their personal physicians to perform a digital rectal exam (DRE) (Figure 24.1) and arrange for prostate specific antigen (PSA) blood tests. Both the DRE and the PSA are now a routine part of every man's annual preventive health physical exam. Combining the two tests is believed to be the most efficient way to detect prostate cancer at its earliest, and theoretically most treatable, stage. The result of this intensive surveillance is that the *number of men bearing a prostate cancer diagnosis has reached epidemic proportions.*

In recent years, the number of prostate cancer deaths has remained fairly constant at about 40,000 per year. During the same time frame, the number of men diagnosed with prostate cancer has more than tripled, escalating from 100,000 in 1990 to 350,000 in 1997. The widespread use of the prostate specific antigen (PSA) test is responsible for the increased numbers of men diagnosed with prostate cancer.

THE PSA TEST

Initially the PSA test was greeted with great enthusiasm. Both the American Cancer Society and the American Urological Association encouraged doc-

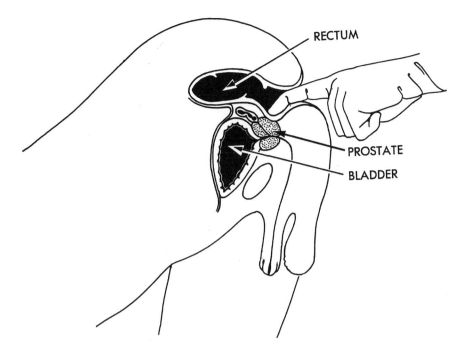

FIGURE 24.1   Digital Rectal Exam (DRE) of the Prostate Gland.

tors to include the PSA as part of the annual exam for all men over the age of fifty. However, as experience and disappointment with the PSA increased, others like the U.S. Preventive Services Task Force, the Canadian Task Force on the Periodic Health Exam, and the Canadian Urologic Associations have issued stern warnings opposing routine PSA screening. Many are now questioning whether the PSA test does more harm than good.

How could a test to detect cancer at its earliest, most curable stage be harmful?

- The PSA is not specific—many men with elevated PSAs do not have prostate cancer at all, whereas some men with "normal" PSAs do.
- An elevated PSA invariably triggers a chain reaction of additional costly diagnostic tests, including prostate ultrasound, prostate biopsy, and if the biopsy shows prostate cancer cells, it is decision time.
- When a man has an elevated PSA level and his prostate biopsy shows cancerous cells, treatment is usually recommended. Prostate surgery, radiotherapy, and/or surgical and medical castration may be considered.

Prostate Cancer: The PSA Controversy

But we are getting ahead of ourselves. First, some basic principles are in order.

To be useful, any diagnostic test must *have a high degree of specificity*. This means that when abnormal results occur, the test must identify a specific problem. If a man's blood pressure is consistently elevated, he has *high blood pressure, or hypertension*. If his red blood cell count is low, he has *anemia*. Both the blood pressure test and the red blood cell count *have a high degree of specificity*. An elevated blood pressure always indicates the presence of high blood pressure, or hypertension, just as a low red blood cell count indicates the presence of anemia. But a high PSA level does not always indicate the presence of a prostate cancer, and a low PSA level is no guarantee that there are no cancerous cells within a man's prostate gland.

- Thus, the PSA lacks specificity.

ADJUSTING THE PSA FOR AGE AND RACE

From extensive studies performed before the PSA was pressed into use, it was determined that normal healthy men had PSA levels of between 0 and 4 ng/ml (nanograms per milliliter). Men whose PSA levels are over 4.0 ng/ml are considered to be at risk for prostate cancer. It turns out that about 15 percent of men over the age of fifty do have a PSA over 4 ng/ml, yet only a handful, about one-fifth of that 15 percent, actually have prostate cancer. Further, a small number of men have prostate cancer even though their PSA levels are less than 4 ng/ml.

A man's prostate gland starts to enlarge as he ages, and when it does, more PSA is produced and released. This is why the majority (80 percent) of men age fifty to sixty-nine have elevated PSA values in the 4–10 ng/ml range yet do not have prostate cancer. That means that only 20 percent of men with PSAs between 4 and 10 ng/ml do have prostate cancer. However, if the PSA value is greater than 10 ng/ml, the chance of finding a prostate cancer increases to between 42 and 64 percent.

As we learn more about prostate cancer and the PSA, it becomes apparent that some men are more susceptible than others to the ravages of this malignancy. Prostate cancer is particularly brutal in blacks, occurring at an earlier age and often in a more advanced stage than in comparably aged white or Asian men. Doctors do not understand why this cancer is so vicious in blacks, but because it is, policies have been altered. Doctors now recommend that black men be screened for prostate cancer starting at age forty (or even younger in those black men with a family history of prostate cancer), whereas for men of other races, prostate cancer screening usually begins at age fifty.

WHAT CAUSES THE PSA LEVEL TO INCREASE IN
MEN WHO DO NOT HAVE PROSTATE CANCER?

Benign prostatic hyperplasia (BPH), which is simple age-related prostate enlargement, and prostate inflammation, or prostatitis, can cause the prostate to squirt larger than normal amounts of PSA into the bloodstream.

HOW DOES A MAN KNOW WHETHER
HIS ELEVATED PSA MEANS HE HAS
PROSTATE CANCER OR PROSTATITIS?

Men who have PSA values greater than 4 ng/ml invariably have additional diagnostic studies. Most have already had a careful digital rectal exam to check for prostate lumps. Those men with both prostate lumps and elevated PSAs are the ones most likely to have prostate cancer. If a man has prostate lumps (nodules) and/or an elevated PSA level, prostate biopsy is usually the next step. If the prostate biopsy reveals the presence of prostate cancer cells, then the diagnosis of prostate cancer is secure.

The next step is to decide on whether the prostate cancer should or should not be treated.

Whaddaya mean not treat my prostate cancer? I don't wanna die. Get rid of my cancer!

Of course! Nobody wants to know that he has a cancer—a time bomb—lurking in his body. Logic would lead us to believe that for prostate cancer as for all malignancies, early detection and prompt treatment should increase the chance of survival. But on occasion, logic and reality clash. The diagnosis and treatment of prostate cancer is one of those occasions.

The problem is that prostate cancer is not like other cancers. Prostate cancer is a mercurial malignancy, totally innocuous in some men, devastating in others—spreading rapidly beyond the confines of the prostate bed to ravage local lymph nodes, the spine, and beyond, eventually causing death. The majority of men, however, harbor slow-growing cancers that remain within and do not spread beyond the prostate area.

Often the appearance of the prostate cancer cell provides a clue to indicate if it is programmed to be slow growing and relatively harmless or more aggressive and lethal.

Those who press for treatment of *all men* with any cancerous cells in their prostate believe that the slow-growing cells invariably progress to aggressive cells. Others argue that if this transformation occurs, it does so slowly and over many years.

Exactly how many men actually have prostate cancer is not a matter of conjecture. We also know that the chance of discovering this specific cancer increases with age. Thus, men who die from heart disease, accidents, strokes, and any illness other than prostate cancer may also have a touch of cancer in their prostate glands. Cancerous cells are likely to be found in the prostates of 22 percent of those age 50–59, in 37 percent of men 60–79, and in more than half (53 percent) of those living to 80 and older. Applying these percentages to current U.S. census data tells us that more than 9 million men age 50 and older have prostate cancer. Working with these figures and knowing that there are about 40,000 prostate cancer deaths each year indicates to some that more men *have and live with prostate cancer than die from this malignancy.*

WHAT HAPPENS WHEN
PROSTATE CANCER IS NOT TREATED?

Physicians in Scandinavia have had the courage, or temerity, to have left untreated 223 men with early prostate cancer and to have followed their progress for 12.5 years. Men who participated in this study were elderly, with 138 over age 70 and 85 under that age. After 12.5 years of no treatment, 23 (10 percent) had died of prostate cancer, whereas many more men, 148 (66 percent) had died of heart diseases during the same time frame. The impression left by this oft-quoted study is that *not all men who have prostate cancer die from prostate cancer.* Others have found similar results, noting that without treatment, many men with early prostate cancer will live many years and die from some other disease.

A similar conclusion was reached in a Connecticut report on the fate of men age 65–75 whose prostate cancer was diagnosed between 1971 and 1976 and not treated. Those who had "low-grade" prostate tumors lived as long as other men their age, but those with more advanced prostate cancer had their life span shortened by four to eight years.

Others have echoed these findings, noting that 87 percent of men with certain types of prostate cancer can live for ten years even without surgery or radiotherapy. However, at ten years there was evidence of prostate cancer spread in 19 percent, 42 percent, and 74 percent of those who had respectively low-grade, moderately advanced, or very advanced prostate cancers on their original prostate biopsy.

Although none of these men had prostate surgery or radiotherapy, their prostate cancers were not totally ignored. Hormonal therapy, that is, treatment to deprive their cancer of testosterone, was often initiated at the first sign of prostate cancer spread. (See "Testosterone and Prostate Cancer" on page 338.)

Almost all of these long-term studies evaluating the effect of no treatment or minimal treatment began before doctors started using the prostate specific antigen (PSA) to diagnose prostate cancer. It is generally believed that the widespread use of the PSA is primarily responsible for the increasing numbers of men who are diagnosed with prostate cancer today. Information we have from the autopsy studies cited above indicated that the chance of finding prostate cancer on a biopsy increases in direct proportion to a man's age. There is a better than 50-50 chance of the prostate cancer cell being detected in any eighty-year-old man. Should all octogenarians have PSA tests followed by prostate biopsies and then surgery for their prostate cancer?

IMPROVING THE PSA: WHAT IS THE GLEASON SCORE?

Since the advent of the PSA as a routine screening test, others have sought to devise some way to improve its specificity. One way was to look for clues to cancer severity in the prostate biopsy. The Gleason score looks at the cancerous cells in the prostate biopsy and ranks them according to their malignant potential. In one such study, 767 men age 55–74 with elevated PSAs and prostate biopsies were graded according to the microscopic appearance of the prostate cancer (Gleason score). This scale rates prostate cancers according to certain characteristics that pathologists have associated with more or less chance of spread. More-aggressive-looking tumors are assigned a score of 8–10, whereas less-nasty-looking tumors are scored as 2–4, with scores of 5–7 being reserved for tumors of intermediate aggressiveness.

Men with Gleason scores of 2–4 faced a minimum (4–7 percent) chance of dying from prostate cancer in the next fifteen years, whereas for men with Gleason scores of 8–10, the risk of dying within that time frame increased to 60–87 percent. So now, in addition to knowing what their PSA levels are, men with prostate cancer have to be tuned into their Gleason score before they make any reasoned decision on what to do regarding treatment.

Still, cancer is such a terrifying word that the natural inclination is to want to do whatever is necessary to eliminate any, and all, cancerous cells. But what if the treatment does more harm than good?

How can ridding the body of cancer do any harm? Only if the method used to eliminate the cancer creates new problems, particularly those that affect a man's quality of life. Prostate surgery, radiation therapy, and medical or surgical castration, alone, or in combination, or no treatment at all are among the options available to men with prostate cancer. While either prostate surgery or radiation therapy may bring about a cure, there are side effects to these treatments. Impotence, incontinence, and bladder or lower-bowel irritation are common complications that create new problems often affecting men's quality of life. Further, to maximize the benefit of either prostate surgery or radiotherapy, other treatments are used to lower a man's testosterone level.

TESTOSTERONE AND PROSTATE CANCER

We have known for more than fifty years that prostate cancer is a testosterone-dependent malignancy. That does not mean that testosterone causes prostate cancer but that prostate cancer, once present, needs a constant source of testosterone, or other androgens (male hormones), to continue growing. Testosterone is, in a very real sense, an essential nutrient for prostate cancer. Remove testosterone and prostate cancer cells shrivel, a finding that has led to the enthusiastic endorsement of, first, surgical and, more recently, medical castration to slow the growth and spread of cancerous prostate tissue. As odd as it sounds, men with prostate cancer live longer, more productive lives without testosterone.

The linkage between testosterone and prostate cancer was discovered by accident and led to the Nobel Prize in medicine for Dr. Charles Huggins, a Chicago urologist who first recognized the relationship between testosterone and prostate cancer. In the early 1940s, Huggins and his associates in Chicago were trying to understand what causes prostate glands to grow. They knew that although all mammals have prostate glands, only man, the dog, and perhaps the African lion have the misfortune to develop prostate enlargement and prostate cancer. Dr. Huggins was, at first, interested in benign prostate hyperplasia (BPH), the most common prostate problem experienced by men and dogs. He had already demonstrated that large canine prostate glands stopped growing and actually decreased in size after dogs had their testicles removed. This observation established a role for testosterone in maintaining prostate growth but was too harsh a treatment to ever consider for healthy men with enlarged prostate glands.

One of Dr. Huggins' dogs had a cancer-filled prostate. Following castration, this dog's testosterone level fell and its prostate cancer disappeared! This discovery was soon transferred to Dr. Huggins's clinical practice.

Despite the most meticulous prostate surgery, his prostate cancer patients were dying at an alarming rate. Something had to be done and based on his experience with the dog with the cancerous prostate, Dr. Huggins was soon able to persuade his own prostate cancer patients to have their testicles removed in an effort to save their lives. Patients with prostate cancer who were castrated lost their ability to make testosterone and other male hormones (androgens). As grim as this treatment might sound, those men who agreed to have their testicles removed seemed to live longer than those who insisted on retaining their testicles. This was the start of what is now known as hormonal

---

338   SEXUAL HEALTH FOR MEN

or androgen ablative therapy for prostate cancer. Today, we are also able to use a clever hormonal treatment as medical therapy to eliminate testosterone production in men with prostate cancer without resorting to surgical castration.

Surgical castration, that is, removal of a man's testicles, causes blood testosterone levels to plummet promptly. Medical therapy (with either Lupron or Zoladex) spares a man the risk of surgery as well as the indignity of having his testicles removed. But with this form of androgen ablative therapy, blood testosterone levels do not fall quite as rapidly as after surgical castration. Indeed, blood testosterone levels first increase briefly before plunging to very low levels with both Lupron and Zoladex, the two most popular medical treatments currently used to contain the spread of prostate cancer.

Since prostate cancer cells need testosterone for continued growth, the elimination of testosterone deprives the prostate cancer of what is essential nourishment. Without testosterone, there is a stultifying effect, and the growth of these malignant cells is held in check. Either surgical or medical castration, though effective in slowing or arresting the spread of prostate cancer, consistently leaves in its wake the dual side effects of impotence and hot flashes.

MEDICAL THERAPY TO ELIMINATE TESTOSTERONE

Until recently, the only way to nullify testosterone's influence on prostate cancer cells was to remove the testicles with surgery (castration). There is now an alternative to surgery. The hormone in charge of regulating the testicle's testosterone output is luteinizing hormone (LH). The testicle is fastidious and will only make testosterone in response to a rhythmic episodic pattern of LH in the bloodstream. Eliminate the normal pulsatile LH rhythm and testosterone production stops cold!

Disabling pituitary LH secretion can be accomplished by shutting down the hypothalamic generator that controls pituitary LH pulses (see Chapter 12). Medications like gosserelin (Zoladex) and leuprolide (Lupron) do just that. Initially, both cause a brief final spasm of testosterone release, which is followed by a permanent suppression of male hormone production. Lupron or gosserelin injections, given once every three months, effectively eliminates testosterone release and nullifies the influence of this androgen on further prostate cancer growth. This form of treatment, known as *androgen (male hormone) ablative* therapy, is often recommended when prostate cancer persists after initial radiotherapy and is initiated immediately after radical prostate cancer surgery. (See Figure 24.2 on the next page.)

We know this because ninety-eight prostate cancer patients, men with an average age of about sixty-five, needed extensive prostate cancer surgery (radical prostatectomy). Following surgery, about half had routine care and were seen at regular intervals for follow-up visits. The remaining men had

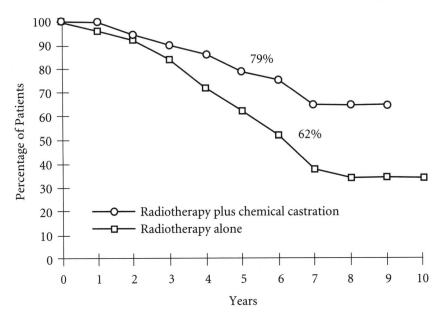

FIGURE 24.2   Survival of men with prostate cancer treated with radiotherapy alone or radiotherapy plus chemical castration. SOURCE: Adapted from M. Bolla, D. Gonzalez, P. Warde et al., "Improved Survival in Patients with Locally Advanced Prostate Cancer Treated with Radiotherapy and Goserelin," *N. Engl. J. Med.* 337 (1997): 295–300.

treatment designed to eliminate their ability to produce testosterone—androgen ablative therapy. The outcome for all men was tracked over the next 7.1 years. Those who had androgen ablative therapy lived longer free of prostate cancer than those who were followed carefully with observation and routine care. (See Table 24.1.)

In some cases, long-term androgen ablative therapy is all that is needed to keep the cancer at bay. Unfortunately, some prostate cancers eventually lose their ability to be influenced by testosterone. The prostate cancer becomes *androgen independent*. When that happens, further prostate cancer growth is possible and other nonhormonal treatments are needed to rein in further prostate cancer spread.

Removing the testicles by surgical castration or using medical androgen ablative therapy to stifle testosterone output are equally effective in slowing down the spread of prostate cancer. Deprived of testosterone, men invariably become impotent and, like menopausal women, frequently develop hot flashes.

HOT FLASHES IN MEN?

A sudden hot sensation, often apparent first in the head, then diffusing rapidly like a blazing intruder engulfing the neck, chest, and limbs in an unre-

TABLE 24.1   Comparison of Survival 7.1 Years After Prostate Cancer Surgery
With and Without Androgen Ablative Therapy

Outcome	Routine Care (51 men)	Androgen Ablation (47 men)
Died from prostate cancer	18	7
Died from other causes	16	3
Recurrent prostate cancer	42	7

SOURCE: Adapted from E.M. Messing, J. Manola, M. Saradsky, G. Wilding et al., "Immediate Hormonal Therapy Compared with Observation After Radical Prostatectomy and Pelvic Lymphadenopathy in Men with Node-Positive Prostate Cancer," *N. Engl. J. Med.* 341 (1999):1781-1788.

lenting inferno, followed by a drenching perspiration, characterize the constellation of symptoms known as hot flashes, or hot flushes. Intense, clearly visible, facial redness (the flush) heralds the onset of symptoms, often provoking comment from concerned onlookers. Hot flashes are experienced by at least 80 percent of menopausal women but not, as a rule, by older men.

When a woman reaches menopause, her ovaries stop making estrogens, causing serum estrogen levels to fall precipitously. It is the sudden decline in female hormone levels that seems to coincide with the onset of symptoms. Hot flashes cease when estrogen treatments replenish the body's estrogen stores.

Until recently, it was believed that hot flashes were the unique and exclusive burden of postmenopausal women. Now it appears that a select group of men can, and do, suffer from hot flashes.

The most common cause of hot flashes in men is surgical or medical castration, a treatment designed to control the advance of prostate cancer. Restoring sex hormone levels to normal should alleviate symptoms in men, as estrogen does in women, but unfortunately, sex hormone therapy is not provided because of concern that additional testosterone might provide the fuel to accelerate the growth and facilitate the spread of prostate cancer.

WHAT, IF ANYTHING, CAN BE DONE
FOR MEN WITH HOT FLASHES?

First it has been noted, particularly by those not suffering from hot flashes, that flashes, though troublesome, are not life-threatening. Others would disagree, for with newer treatments for prostate cancer, the numbers of men susceptible to hot flashes is increasing. About 76 percent of men will start to experience unrelenting hot flashes beginning within one to twelve months after castration. Once entrenched, flashes persist for an average of two and one-half years. Men with a flush-induced beet-red face often feel embarrassed while interacting with friends and at a competitive disadvantage in business negotiations. For them, flushes insinuate themselves as a major disruptive influence on their quality of life, and treatment to reverse the redness would be welcome.

TREATMENT OF HOT FLASHES IN MEN

Four totally different medications—an antihypertensive (clonidine), an estrogen (diethylstilbesterol, or DES), an androgen antagonist (cyproterone acetate), and the progesterone surrogate megestrol acetate—have all been used to control hot flashes in men. Because the actual process of the flush seems to involve the spasmodic redistribution of blood flow to the skin, clonidine, a medication that could stabilize that blood-flow pattern, was considered to be an ideal candidate to minimize the flushing process. Indeed, initial studies with clonidine reported considerable success in alleviating flushing symptoms, but this was soon refuted. In a recent double-blind study with one-half of the patients receiving clonidine and the other half a placebo, clonidine was no better than a placebo in decreasing hot flashes.

Curiously, men given female hormones, specifically the estrogen diethylstilbesterol (DES) did have a prompt cessation of hot flashes, but breast enlargement occurred so consistently with prolonged estrogen use that most men opted to put up with the flashes rather than grow breasts. Cyproterone acetate is not an androgen, but an anti-androgen, vitiating the impact of testosterone and other androgens. Androgen antagonists effectively nullify sex drive and for this reason have found favor in Europe as a court-mandated treatment to tone down what is perceived to be the inappropriate libido of habitual sexual predators. Cyproterone acetate also minimizes postcastration hot flashes because, in addition to its anti-androgen effect, this medication acts like another reproductive hormone, progesterone. Cyproterone acetate is not available in this country, but megestrol acetate (Megace), a medication with only progesterone-like activity, is.

In one recent study, megestrol was used to treat hot flashes in two groups of patients, menopausal women who could not take estrogens because they had estrogen-receptor-positive breast cancer, and men who had surgical or medical castration as treatment for prostate cancer. The onset and persistence of flashing was somewhat more intense in the males, with 61 percent of men and only 38 percent of women reporting more than ten flashes per day.

Once again, this was a placebo-controlled study, so megestrol 20 mg per day was pitted against placebo. After four weeks of treatment, hot flashes decreased by 21 percent in placebo-treated patients and 85 percent in those who received megestrol, a statistically significant advantage favoring this small dose of megestrol. Side effects were not a problem in this short-term study. Increased appetite and weight gain have been the dominant side effects when higher doses of megestrol were used for other purposes. For the moment, it appears that megestrol is a safe and effective treatment for prostate cancer patients who experience hot flashes.

For those men who do not have prostate cancer but do have hot flashes because of a spontaneous acute pituitary or testicular failure, hormone replacement with testosterone is safe and effective in alleviating symptoms.

DIFFICULT CHOICES FOR MEN WITH AN ELEVATED PSA

Primary-care physicians and internists have become disillusioned with the PSA. This is no doubt due to inappropriate expectations regarding the usefulness of this test as a first-strike weapon in the war against prostate cancer. Still, the man who wants to tilt the odds in his favor in the fight against prostate cancer has to do something. He should expect to have a digital rectal exam (DRE) as well as a PSA test as part of his annual physical. No harm is done as long as the DRE and PSA is normal, but an elevated PSA sets in motion a cascade of events that will inevitably lead to a prostate biopsy.

Once an elevated PSA suggests, and a prostate biopsy confirms, that a man has cancerous cells within his prostate, that man is faced with a troublesome dilemma involving one of three treatment options.

1. The man who chooses "no treatment" is gambling that he has one of the indolent nonaggressive prostate cancers that will stay within the prostate's boundaries and not spread.
2. The man who is older and has coexistent medical problems like severe heart disease, emphysema, or other chronic medical illnesses and is not expected to live more than ten years may opt to forgo prostate cancer surgery or radiotherapy to avoid unpleasant consequences of aggressive prostate cancer therapy. Before making any decision, this man should be able to have as much information as possible. Not only should he know his PSA level, but he should also inquire about his Gleason score.

    If he has a low Gleason score and is already at an advanced age, encumbered by other medical problems, he may not be expected to live for another ten years. In that case, he may choose to forgo prostate cancer surgery. But what man, at any age, wants to think his days are numbered?

3. If he is not plagued by any other medical problems, he may very well opt to go ahead with prostate cancer treatment, which may be either surgery with radical prostatectomy or one of several forms of prostate radiation therapy. It would be in his best interest to obtain more than one opinion regarding the treatment that is most likely to meet his needs. Any therapy does carry a potential risk of complications for some men. However small, there is always the chance of having post-treatment bowel or bladder control problems (incontinence) or loss of erectile function (impotence).

TABLE 24.2 Physician-Reported Percentages of Problems Developing Following Radical Prostatectomy or Radiation-Therapy Treatment of Prostate Cancer

Radical Prostatectomy	% Problems Reported
Impotence	20–85
Incontinence	1–27
Urethral stricture	10–18
Radiation Therapy	
Impotence	40–67
Anorectal complications	2–23
Urethral or bladder problems	3–17

WHY DO MEN BECOME IMPOTENT AFTER PROSTATE CANCER SURGERY?

Adjacent to the prostate are vital collections of blood vessels and nerves critical for erection. In the early 1980s, Dr. Patrick Walsh of Johns Hopkins Medical School focused his energies on these neurovascular bundles. He found that they are intimately involved in the transmission of vital signals to the spongy structures in the penis that must become engorged with blood for a fully rigid erection. If the neurovascular bodies were removed during surgery, erections would not occur.

Many urologists have not been able to duplicate the potency-preserving procedure developed by Dr. Walsh. The net result is that impotence and occasionally incontinence are common problems after prostate surgery or radiotherapy for prostate cancer. The information in Table 24.2, a compilation of results from many different centers, reflects doctors' perceptions of post-treatment problems, whereas Table 24.3 reflects the patients' perceptions of problems developing after radical prostatectomy. It could be argued that these distressing symptoms are a small price to pay to live longer. But not every man who has been treated for prostate cancer is comfortable with this fatalistic approach.

TABLE 24.3   Patient-Reported Percentages of Problems Developing Following
Radical Prostatectomy or Radiation-Therapy Treatment of Prostate Cancer

Problem	% Men Affected
Incontinence	
Requiring pads or other treatment	31
Dripping daily	23
Surgery for incontinence control	6
Impotence	
Had erections before surgery	90
No full erections after surgery	61
Able to have intercourse in past month	11

TREATMENT OPTIONS FOR MEN WHO BECOME IMPOTENT FOLLOWING PROSTATE CANCER SURGERY

Men become impotent after prostate cancer treatment because:

1. Surgery or radiotherapy damages the nerves or blood vessels vital for normal erections.
2. The prostate cancer diagnosis and treatment causes them to become despondent and experience a form of psychogenic impotence.
3. Androgen ablative medical therapy with Lupron or Zoladex or surgical castration has obliterated their capacity to produce testosterone.

Restoration of sexual potency is possible for many but not all men following prostate cancer treatment. A man's post-treatment sexual life is entirely dependent on the integrity of his vital sexual response systems.

For example, testosterone-deprived men like those described in the third category above will have little or no libido and are more concerned with survival than sex. For all others who have survived the initial phase of prostate cancer treatment, sexual thoughts and an interest in resuming a normal sex life assume great importance. Four types of treatment are available to help them overcome their erectile dysfunction. These include:

1. Viagra
2. Intrapenile injection or MUSE
3. Vacuum erection devices
4. Penile prosthesis implantation

Deciding which treatment best suits the individual man is entirely up to him. All of the four treatment options listed above can and often do increase the chance that a man will once again experience erections and be able to engage in sexual intercourse, but none are entirely foolproof.

1. Viagra improves erections and allows for satisfactory sexual intercourse in about 50 percent of men following prostate cancer treatment (Chapter 11).
2. Inrapenile injection or MUSE may be effective even when Viagra fails (Chapter 19).
3. Vacuum devices require somewhat more skill than either Viagra or MUSE, but when used properly, they can allow a man to have an on-demand erection that will make satisfactory sex possible (Chapter 20).
4. Implantation of a penile prosthesis is always an option, but a man who has recently had prostate cancer surgery may feel a little bit skittish about returning to the operating room again for insertion of the penile prosthesis (Chapter 18).

As with all of a man's choices, a chat with those who care about him the most—his partner and his doctor—is the first step before embarking on any treatment. A sexual life is definitely possible for the man who has had prostate cancer treatment.

25

The Fertile and the Infertile Man

The most accurate recent surveys indicate that 8.6 million couples in the United States would like to have children but cannot. They are said to be *involuntarily infertile*. In 40 to 50 percent of the cases, a *"male factor"* is considered to be wholly or partially responsible for the couple's sterility. The term "male factor" is appropriately vague, for it encompasses a range of problems from abnormal sperm development to lack of the spontaneous sperm-ovum fusion required for fertilization to occur.

To understand why problems might occur, it is necessary to review the reproductive process so that you and your partner understand the details of what makes it possible for men and women to have babies. Then we can outline the whole range of treatments now available for infertile couples to first identify and then correct their own problem and start a family.

NORMAL FERTILITY AND FERTILIZATION

During ovulation, a woman releases one egg (ovum), which then drifts into her fallopian tube. It is there in the fallopian tube that a single sperm will penetrate that ovum to achieve fertilization.

A man's fertility depends upon his ability to generate not just one but millions of sperm daily. Although only one sperm is needed for fertilization, the odds against this single sperm meeting up with that one ovum are formidable. To improve chances for natural conception, the system is flooded with sperm. During sexual intercourse, several million sperm are deposited in the vagina. Many perish immediately in the hostile acid environment of vaginal fluids. Others die at the cervix, the entrance to the womb.

Freshly ejaculated sperm can swim, but they cannot fertilize. They are buffeted by a sea of fertility-impeding chemicals called *decapacitating agents*. To acquire full fertilizing capability, sperm must be transformed, or *capacitated*. Normally this occurs as sperm pass through the uterine cervix.

Capacitated sperm then swim through the uterus at a steady pace, destined for the woman's fallopian tube. The sperm must arrive in time to fertilize her recently ovulated ovum. There is only a limited window of opportunity for fertilization, thirty-six hours each month.

When sperm enter the fallopian tube, they veer like a heat-seeking missile, aiming for the ovum. Immediately prior to the moment of fertilization, sperm go through yet another transformation, referred to as *hyperactivated motility*, in which they shift from a smooth-gliding swimming pattern to a frenzied, corkscrew-flailing motion with high spinning-speed torque. More work has to be done before the sperm enters the ovum.

Enzymes contained within the sperm head must disperse the shroud of cells (cumulus oophorus) surrounding the woman's ovum. This brings the sperm in direct contact with the outer lining of the ovum (zona pellucida). Now additional sperm enzymes allow the sperm to burrow into the body of the ovum (ooplasm). It is there within the ooplasm that the union of sperm and ovum nucleus takes place, finalizing the act of fertilization.

WHAT IS A NORMAL FERTILITY RATE?

The process of fertilization, though intricate and complex, functions quite satisfactorily for the majority of men and women. Healthy couples conceive at a predictable rate of 20 percent per month. After one year of "unprotected" intercourse (that is, intercourse without contraception), 86 to 90 percent of all normal couples will have initiated a pregnancy. Those who are unable to conceive after one year are considered to be infertile.

Invariably, it is the woman who first seeks help to determine why she cannot bear children. When an evaluation indicates that she is ovulating normally, has normal female anatomy, and has no obvious impediment to conception, suspicion is cast on the male partner.

The man is considered responsible for the infertility if the sperm he produces are few in number, unable to swim with proper velocity, immobilized by his partner's cervical mucus (and unable to enter her womb), or incapable of surviving the trek from vagina to fallopian tube.

NORMAL SPERM PRODUCTION

There is a division of labor within a man's testicles. One area is responsible for generating testosterone and another for producing sperm. Leydig cells produce testosterone, and Sertoli cells manufacture sperm. Two different pituitary hormones oversee testosterone and sperm production. Luteinizing hormone (LH) activates Leydig-cell testosterone production, whereas follicle stimulating hormone (FSH) supervises sperm production. The relationship between the pituitary hormones and the testicle is one of mutual dependence. The testicle relies on the pituitary to provide LH and FSH. The pituitary, in turn, releases these hormones in response to the productivity of the cells of the testicle.

When testosterone output lags, blood testosterone values fall. These low testosterone levels goad the pituitary into dispatching additional LH to increase the supply of testosterone. In addition to sperm, the Sertoli cells manufacture a protein called inhibin. If sperm production fails, inhibin levels decline. In response to low inhibin levels, the pituitary releases more FSH in hopes of revitalizing sperm output.

There is, unfortunately, a point of no return. Occasionally, the testicles are so wracked by infection or inflammation that they cannot mobilize enough healthy Sertoli cells to rejuvenate sperm production even in response to a surge in FSH. Then sperm counts remain low and FSH levels high. The level of FSH circulating in the blood is a reliable index of the extent of damage suffered by the sperm-producing Sertoli cells. A combination of a low sperm count and an elevated serum FSH level bespeaks a poor prognosis for resurrecting sperm development. In contrast, low sperm count with normal or low FSH levels indicates opportunities for improving sperm output with hormone therapy.

Because of the prodigious obstacles to fertilization, nature has provided man with the ability to produce millions of sperm. Exactly how many millions are needed to guarantee fertility has been a subject of some debate. Scientists have recently learned that it is not merely the total number but also the shape, swimming velocity, and maturity of sperm that determine fertility. These vital properties of sperm are revealed by an examination of the semen.

SEMEN ANALYSIS

The semen analysis is the linchpin in the evaluation of the infertile man. This microscopic study, performed after men provide semen by masturbating, provides valuable information about the total number of sperm present, how many are freely moving (the motility index), and how long their active swimming motion persists.

By convention, sperm counts are recorded as millions of sperm per one cubic centimeter (cc) of semen. Normal fertile men have a sperm count of between 20 and 80 million sperm per cc. Although some men with sperm counts as low as 5 to 10 million per cc have been able to impregnate their partners, *20 million sperm per cc* is considered the minimal number required for fertilization.

Some men have no sperm in their ejaculate, a condition referred to as *azoospermia*. The problem usually results from testicular failure due to either viral injury such as mumps or genetic disorders such as Klinefelter's syndrome. (See Chapter 12.) Occasionally, the testicle produces a normal amount of sperm, but none appears in the ejaculate because the ducts carrying sperm from the testicle to the urethra are blocked. This condition is called *obstructive azoospermia*.

Some men produce some but not enough sperm and are said to have *oligospermia*. This problem can be a consequence of an intrinsically imperfect testicle or an impairment in the pituitary stimulus to sperm development. Differentiating testicular (primary) from pituitary (secondary) causes of oligospermia is of paramount importance. When the testicle's sperm-producing cells are scarred, sperm production cannot proceed or be activated. However, if these cells are not producing sperm only because of the lack of proper hormonal stimulation, opportunities exist for increasing the testicle's sperm output.

A substantial number of infertile men have normal numbers of sperm and are thus referred to as "normal but infertile." Immunologic factors, antisperm antibodies, or sperm-cervical mucus incompatibility are thought to be responsible for their infertility.

Curiously, one group of infertile men makes too many sperm, a condition known as *polyzoospermia*. Infertile polyzoospermic men have mind-boggling sperm counts of 250 million per cc. Approximately 38 percent of them can initiate a pregnancy, but unfortunately, the sperm-ovum union is often blighted. The partners of polyzoospermic men suffer a high incidence of first-trimester miscarriage; the factors responsible remain obscure.

Routine semen analysis also provides information regarding the swimming velocity of sperm. Sperm have a tail that moves back and forth to propel the sperm in seminal fluid and through the vagina, womb, and ultimately into the fallopian tubes. Some sperm are simply better swimmers than others. Examined under the microscope, healthy sperm exhibit an effortless swimming (or motility) pattern that ordinarily persists for several hours. Defective sperm have a languorous or sluggish swimming motion. They lack the vigor to make the journey to inseminate an egg. Men whose sperm concentration is dominated by a high percentage of languid sperm are infertile. The technical name for this condition is *asthenospermia*.

Infections of the prostate gland, seminal vesicles, or urethra cause bacteria and pus (white blood cells) to mingle with sperm. Bacteria and pus disrupt sperm motility and diminish fertilizing capacity. This condition, called *pyospermia*, can be treated with antibiotics. Once the infection is cleared up, sperm swim more freely, and opportunities for fertility are enhanced.

TREATMENT OF INFERTILITY

The treatment of male infertility is, in principle, simple; first pinpoint and then correct the impediment to fertility. Scientists have devised a legion of medical and surgical programs to encourage a man's testicles: to increase their output of sperm, to enhance and invigorate sperm's fertilizing capability, to counteract the immunologic barriers to conception, to unclog channels blocking the unrestrained flow of sperm from the testicle to the urethra, and to bypass anatomic obstacles to insemination.

NO SPERM: AZOOSPERMIA

If repeated semen analyses fail to show sperm in semen, the diagnosis of azoospermia is secure. The outlook for the azoospermic man is not hopeful unless the cause can be traced to a defect in pituitary gland stimulation to the testicle or an obstruction in one of the ducts responsible for transporting sperm from the testicle to the seminal fluid.

Men whose testicles are understimulated by the pituitary can be treated with synthetic pituitary hormones. In cases of obstructive azoospermia, microsurgery can alleviate the obstruction and allow sperm to flow freely from the testicle to the urethra.

Unfortunately, the majority of men with azoospermia have irreparable damage to their testicles. Included in this group are men whose Leydig cells (testosterone secretion) and Sertoli cells (sperm output) never functioned properly because of genetic disorders. They are impotent as well as infertile. Another group of men has suffered a selective injury to their sperm-producing Sertoli cells. Since their Leydig cells churn out normal amounts of testosterone, these men remain potent. But they are infertile because viral infections, chemotherapy, or X-ray treatments harmed their Sertoli cells. There is no way to revive sperm production once the Sertoli cells are fatally injured.

LOW SPERM COUNT: OLIGOSPERMIA

Men with low sperm counts (oligospermia) may not be, strictly speaking, infertile, but *subfertile*. Fertility is not always an either-or phenomenon. Some subfertile men are capable of initiating a pregnancy, but not within the same standard one-year time frame; it takes two to three years of unprotected intercourse.

In many cases, the number and quality of sperm produced by a man's testicles can be improved either by varicocele surgery or by the administration of hormones or drugs.

THE VARICOCELE AND VARICOCELE SURGERY

Surgical treatment is predicated on the assumption that the testicles are intrinsically capable of normal sperm production but are restrained from do-

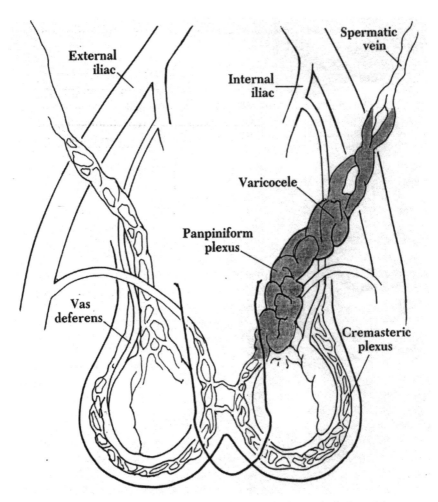

FIGURE 25.1   A varicocele (in black) and its proximity to the left testicle.

ing so by a local structural abnormality. A tangle of veins, a varicocele, may surround the testicle (usually the left one). Most varicoceles are readily apparent to sight and touch. (See Figure 25.1.) Men with varicoceles frequently have semen analyses characterized by low sperm counts or a disproportionate number of poorly swimming sperm.

The current thinking is that the heat generated by blood in the varicocele has a negative impact on the testicle's ability to produce sperm. Varicocele surgery allows testicular temperatures to return to normal, and if there are no other obstacles, normal sperm production and fertility should be the outcome.

Several studies have compared the pregnancy rates of women whose partners had varicocele surgery with those of women whose partners did not have surgery to correct the problem. The results are inconclusive. Men who do not have varicocele surgery may be no less fertile than men who undergo surgery. Since these men are not truly infertile but merely subfertile, their partners would likely conceive eventually without surgery.

Men considered the best candidates for varicocele surgery are under thirty years old, have reductions in sperm count to no less than 10 to 15 million per cc, may have a decrease in testicular size (but only in one testicle), have no evidence of pus in their semen, and have normal or only slightly elevated FSH levels. Men unlikely to benefit from surgery are over thirty-eight years of age, have sperm counts lower than 5 million per cc, frequently have decreased volume of both testicles or pus in their semen, and have a markedly elevated serum FSH value indicating severe damage to the sperm-producing Sertoli cells.

HORMONE AND DRUG TREATMENTS

Hormone and drug treatments are designed to provide supplemental stimulation to the sperm-producing Sertoli cells in the testicles. Serum FSH levels before treatment provide a useful index of subsequent success. Only men with normal or just slightly elevated serum FSH levels are appropriate candidates.

Several forms of treatment—all of them arduous—are available. The most elaborate option is reserved for men with idiopathic hypogonadotropic hypogonadism. (See Chapter 12.) A pump, identical to an insulin pump, links up with a tube and needle placed under the skin to deliver intermittent pulses of gonadotropin-releasing hormone (GnRH) into the bloodstream. This stimulates pituitary release of both LH and FSH. The impact of LH is seen immediately; pulses of LH invigorate testosterone production. Serum testosterone, libido, and potency increase, although sperm production initially remains low. With time, the sperm-producing cells start to respond and sperm counts increase after nine to twelve months of therapy.

Increasing the pulsatile release of LH and FSH can also be accomplished with clomiphene (Clomid, Serophene), an oral medication commonly used to treat infertility in women. Clomiphene increases the frequency and amplitude of LH and FSH pulses and stimulates testosterone and sperm production in some men. Sperm count does not increase until the patient has had six to nine months of therapy. Although clomiphene has been employed for many years to increase sperm output, it has not yet been sanctioned for this use by the Food and Drug Administration.

Oddly enough, two female hormones have proved effective in increasing sperm production. A substance normally produced during pregnancy—human growth chorionic gonadotropin (hCG)—has LH-like properties and stimulates testosterone production. Human menopausal gonadotropin (hMG) (found in an equally unlikely source: the urine of menopausal women), has potent FSH-like properties and can also increase sperm output.

Both hCG and hMG must be administered by injection. The usual procedure is to start treatment with hCG to increase the testicles' output of testosterone. The resulting high testosterone levels can reawaken dormant sperm-producing cells. This alone may be a sufficient stimulus to start up sperm production again. In other instances, men may need additional hormonal stimulus in the form of the FSH surrogate hMG.

Injections of hCG are given twice a week for three to six months. If sperm counts show no improvement, hMG injections are added to the treatment schedule. Patience and forbearance are required. Improvements in sperm output can be provoked with this form of therapy, but they occur only after nine to fifteen months of therapy.

INCOMPATIBILITY OF SPERM AND CERVICAL MUCUS

Men with normal sperm counts, the "normal but infertile" group, require investigation beyond the semen analysis. If a man's sperm output is adequate and his sperm motility is vigorous, additional studies must be performed to address the specific issue of why his apparently healthy sperm do not inseminate.

In many cases, it is the inability of sperm to penetrate cervical mucus that is causing the infertility. The mucus produced by a woman's cervix is, for most of the month, impervious to sperm. The character of the mucus changes—it becomes pliant to allow sperm to gain safe passage into the uterus—only in the middle of the menstrual cycle, during ovulation. Swimming sperm linger for a time in the cervical mucus before they tunnel through into the uterus. This temporary stopover has provided investigators with another research tool, the postcoital test.

This test has now become an important component of the evaluation of infertile couples with unexplained infertility. Two to four hours after intercourse, the woman comes to the doctor's office. The physician takes a sample of her cervical mucus and examines it under the microscope. The presence of actively swimming sperm is normal. If sperm are present but not actively swimming, a "sperm-cervical mucus incompatibility" is thought to be the cause of the infertility.

Once the postcoital test determines that sperm are present but immobilized by cervical mucus, further sophisticated tests are required to resolve whether the cervical mucus or the sperm is causing the problem.

Samples of the cervical mucus are exposed to sperm from a male known to be fertile. (The test is done on a slide in the physician's laboratory.) If the stranger's sperm swim easily through the cervical mucus, the mucus is not the source of the problem. If, on the other hand, the foreign sperm make no headway or are immobilized by the cervical mucus, a "cervical factor" must contribute to the couple's infertility.

In the second experiment, the man's sperm and cervical mucus from a woman known to be fertile are combined. If the sperm are incapable of making progress through the cervical mucus, it is presumed that the sperm possess antibodies that preclude penetration of any cervical mucus. This condition, known as "immunologic infertility," occurs in about 8 percent of infertile men.

Immunologic barriers to fertility are found more frequently in men who have had vasectomies. Vasectomized men who divorce or lose their wives to illness may remarry and wish to reconsider the wisdom of their self-imposed sterility. A vasectomy reversal operation (vasovasotomy) is possible. Following vasovasotomy, normal numbers of sperm appear in the semen, but in 60 to 80 percent of cases, the sperm are coated with an antibody and neither penetrate cervical mucus nor fertilize ova. Neutralizing the fertility-impeding impact of this antibody is essential if fertility is to be restored.

TREATMENT OF IMMUNOLOGIC INFERTILITY

The cortisonelike medications prednisolone and prednisone, with their potent antibody-neutralizing effects, are the mainstay of treatment of immunologic infertility.

Intensive prednisolone therapy (about 96 mg daily) is prescribed for the man during the two weeks preceding his partner's ovulation. The prednisolone should neutralize or inhibit all the antibodies residing on the surface of the sperm head. Sexual intercourse is timed to coincide with ovulation, at which time prednisolone is discontinued. If the woman does not become pregnant with the first course of prednisolone therapy, subsequent cycles can be initiated.

On the average, 35 percent of couples infertile because of immunologic infertility can expect to initiate a pregnancy after prednisolone or prednisone treatment. Some men respond more satisfactorily to treatment than others. Men who have been infertile for two years or less are more likely to respond to prednisolone than those with long-standing infertility. The treatment achieves optimum results when the woman's physiology offers no impediment to fertilization. Women who have anatomical abnormalities of the uterus or fallopian tubes or a "cervical factor" that impairs the passage of sperm into the uterus must be treated along with their partners.

This form of therapy is not benign. Prednisolone and prednisone can cause acne, weight gain, headaches, upset stomach, and especially mood swings. Men taking high doses of prednisolone have insomnia and are irritable, aggressive, and argumentative. These consistent and predictable side effects reverse fully when treatment ends.

NONCOITAL REPRODUCTION

It is now possible for men and women to initiate a pregnancy without even engaging in sexual intercourse. This is referred to as noncoital reproduction. Two generic classes of noncoital reproduction are currently available: artificial insemination of the women with either her partner's or a donor's sperm and assisted reproduction such as in vitro fertilization and gamete intrafallopian tube transfer.

ARTIFICIAL INSEMINATION

Artificial insemination is a viable treatment option for some infertile couples. The man's sperm can be collected and infused directly into the woman's vagina. To improve opportunities for insemination, the collected sperm can be processed and treated (capacitated) so that only the most actively swimming and viable sperm are used. In cases of cervical factor infertility, the physician can bypass the cervix by instilling the sperm directly into the uterus.

Artificial insemination with the partner's sperm is successful in inducing a pregnancy in only about 18 percent of infertile couples. Researchers believe the low success rate is due to the fact that the sperm are most likely flawed and burdened by an inherent defect in fertilizing potential. Current methods of sperm enrichment enhance the fertilizing capability of these sperm only to a limited degree.

Statistics improve if artificial insemination is performed with normal sperm. Young men with certain types of malignancies such as lymphoma, Hodgkin's disease, and testicular cancer often have normal sperm production. Remarkable advances in medicine have allowed many of these men to be cured. However, as noted, the drugs and X-ray treatment commonly used invariably cause irreparable damage to sperm-producing cells. Prior to treatment, men can collect semen by masturbation, deposit it in a sperm bank, and preserve it for future use.

After the cancer victim has been successfully treated, he now has the opportunity to start a family. Young men with cancer who make a "deposit" in the sperm bank prior to chemotherapy can anticipate a 45 to 60 percent chance of pregnancy when they make a "withdrawal" and use their own sperm to inseminate their partners.

Insemination with donor sperm has produced successful pregnancies in 250,000 Americans. The sperm donor, usually a healthy young medical or graduate student, provides semen for a fee and is guaranteed anonymity. He will not know the woman to be inseminated, and she in turn will be unable to determine his identity. The doctor performing the insemination attempts to match general physical appearance between the donor and the woman's husband.

Insemination coincides with the women's ovulation. Several monthly inseminations are often required before pregnancy is established. Donor insemination succeeds 60 to 75 percent of the time, depending on the woman's age and regularity of ovulation. Age is a critical factor. In one large study performed in France, pregnancy rates were 74 percent in women under thirty, 61 percent in women between thirty-one and thirty-five, but only 53 percent in women over thirty-five.

Inseminated pregnancies are indistinguishable from spontaneous pregnancies in terms of rates of miscarriage (15 to 18 percent) and birth defects (4 to 5 percent).

IN VITRO FERTILIZATION

In women with blocked fallopian tubes, the egg cannot migrate into the fallopian tube to be available for insemination. A procedure has been developed to overcome this anatomic obstacle. The woman takes medication to encourage ovulation of multiple eggs (ova), and then a physician removes the ripened ova directly from the woman's ovary. The ova are placed in a laboratory dish (a petri dish, not a test tube).

The man provides sperm by masturbating. Sperm are first capacitated and then added to the ova. Fertilization and early embryonic development take place in the laboratory dish while hormone treatment prepares the lining of the woman's uterus. Ordinarily, several of the growing embryos are implanted in the uterus in the hopes that one or two will survive to term. This procedure is known as in vitro fertilization (IVF).

The same methods have been useful in the treatment of certain infertile men as well. Men with low sperm counts, poor sperm mobility, or normal sperm counts but immunologic infertility have participated in IVF programs.

IVF is beneficial for these men for several reasons. The methods used in preparing sperm for IVF act as a gleaning process and salvage only the most motile and fertile sperm. Men with low sperm counts occasionally have limited numbers of perfectly normal sperm. These healthy sperm are usually overlooked in a semen analysis dominated by languid sperm. A medical laboratory can selectively segregate the handful of active sperm from their more inefficient brethren and then treat this elite corps further to allow them to undergo the process of capacitation, enhancing their fertilization potential.

The anatomic barriers to sperm-ovum interaction that may be present in men with immunologic infertility are obliterated by the simple expedient of placing the enriched sperm in direct contact with ova. The total number of sperm that must be present for IVF is only a fraction—one-tenth—of that required for insemination through intercourse. The success rate of pregnancy culminating in a live birth is 18 to 28 percent in couples with male-factor infertility.

GAMETE INTRAFALLOPIAN TUBE TRANSFER

Fertilization normally takes place not in a laboratory dish but in the fallopian tube. Some individuals have modified the fundamental techniques used in IVF to mimic the normal process of conception. This technique, referred to as gamete intrafallopian tube transfer (GIFT), has been especially useful in the treatment of infertile men.

As with in vitro fertilization, the woman is treated with hormones to maximize ovulation. Several ova are then removed from her ovary, mixed with the man's capacitated sperm, and inserted back into the fallopian tube. This allows conception to take place within the fallopian tube, mimicking the normal process. The embryo(s) then migrate into the uterus and develop normally. (See Figure 25.2.)

To date, 18 to 38 percent of couples considered infertile because of a male factor have been able to initiate a pregnancy with GIFT. Additional studies will have to be performed to determine whether this extraordinary success rate can be sustained.

INTRACYTOPLASMIC SPERM INJECTION (ICSI)

Everything we know about human reproduction would lead us to believe that a man who has inadequate sperm-producing capability and a below-normal sperm count with many abnormally shaped and/or poorly swimming sperm would be permanently and irrevocably infertile. However, doctors have now found a way to use a single imperfect sperm from this man to initiate a perfect pregnancy.

To do this, they circumvent all normal or assisted reproduction techniques, as illustrated in Figure 25.3. Life starts with the union of a single sperm and one ovum, an event that can be duplicated in the laboratory. This revolutionary technique is referred to as *intracytoplasmic sperm injection (ICSI)*. The ICSI process is fascinating to some but disturbing to others, for more so than any other method of assisted reproduction, ICSI utilizes human sperm and ova as if they were little more than reproductive spare parts.

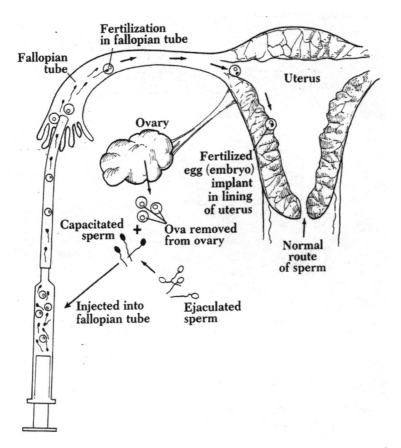

FIGURE 25.2   Illustration of the steps involved in the assisted reproduction technique known as gamete intrafallopian tube transfer GIFT.

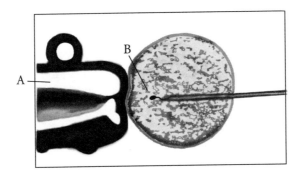

FIGURE 25.3   Intracytoplasmic sperm injection (ICSI). Microclamp (A) steadies ovum for direct insertion of sperm (B) from micro pipette.
SOURCE: Adapted from Randy S. Morris and Norbert Gleicher, "Genetic Abnormalities, Male Infertility, and ICSI," *Lancet* 347 (1996): 1277.

It is not enough to bring sperm and ova together, since fertilization occurs only when a sperm enters the body, or *cytoplasm,* of the woman's ovum. To do this, the sperm must penetrate the ovum's dense outer shell, the *zona pellucida.* Normally, the zona acts as a protective barrier for the ovum, yielding to allow only the fittest and most vigorously swimming sperm access, while simultaneously fending off the sluggish and misshapen sperm, considering them unfit for entry.

However, it turns out that a woman's ovum is not totally impervious to these cast-off sperm rejects. Under certain circumstances, the ovum can be coaxed into accepting less-than-perfect sperm. That is only one of the unique features of ICSI. Although it shares many of the preparatory steps of other forms of assisted reproduction, ICSI differs because it uses what are called micromanipulation techniques to insert a single designated sperm through the zona pellucida and directly into the body (cytoplasm) of the ovum.

Those couples contemplating ICSI should be prepared for the superovulation techniques used to force the female partner to produce, and then release, multiple eggs (ova) for fertilization. Men produce a semen sample by masturbation, or in some instances have sperm extracted from the sperm-transporting ducts (epididymis, vas deferens) or directly from the testicle. In IVF, thousands of sperm circle several ova in the hopes that a few will penetrate and fertilize several ova. In contrast, ICSI is a one sperm–one ovum joint venture. As illustrated in Figure 25.3, one ovum is isolated and steadied so that a *single sperm* can be injected directly into the ovum's *cytoplasm* to begin the process of fertilization.

WHEN IS ICSI APPROPRIATE?

ICSI is not likely to be the first treatment option offered to couples experiencing difficulty initiating a pregnancy. Other more traditional techniques of ovulation enhancement as a prelude to in vitro fertilization (IVF) or gamete intrafallopian tube transfer (GIFT) are considered more mainstream. ICSI appears to be uniquely suited for men who release less, in some cases considerably less, than the 20 million sperm per cc ejaculated by fertile men. We know that as numbers of sperm ejaculated decline, so do opportunities for conception. One group of men has such limited sperm production that the amount they ejaculate is no more than a fraction of the fertile man's sperm output. These men have sperm counts of less than .5 million (500,000) forward-moving sperm in their ejaculated seminal fluid and are considered to have severe oligospermia. Even with all of the sophisticated methods commonly used to improve sperm quality during IVF, the chances of initiating a pregnancy with such a low sperm count are virtually nil. With ICSI, however, fertilization rates, followed by embryo implantation, have been almost 39 percent, compared to the 18–20 percent achieved with IVF.

TABLE 25.1 Number of Major and Minor Congenital Abnormalities Seen in Babies Born in New York State After Spontaneous Pregnancies and After IVF and ICSI

Number of Babies	Spontaneous	IVF	ICSI
Delivered	>30,000	653	177
Major malformations	1,080 (3.6%)	23 (3.5%)	1 (0.6%)
Minor malformations	840 (2.8%)	20 (3.1%)	2 (1.1%)
Total	1,920 (6.4%)	43 (6.6%)	3 (1.7%)

This figure is even more impressive when one considers that most IVF successes are the result of insemination with thousands of high-quality normal sperm, whereas the single sperm used for ICSI need not be. Low in number, abnormal in appearance, unable to move properly, the sperm used for ICSI are by all criteria totally inadequate for initiating a pregnancy.

This is what frightens critics most about ICSI. Is it violating some intended natural plan to take sperm that under normal circumstances would be incapable of initiating a pregnancy and inject that unhealthy, unfit sperm into a human ovum to help someone have a baby? If these sperm are so inadequate, the argument goes, perhaps they should not be used to make childless couples parents. What about the possibility of these sperm creating children with severe birth defects?

So far this has not proven to be true. A recent survey of babies born in New York state from spontaneous pregnancies, after IVF or after ICSI, demonstrated no difference in major or minor birth defects (congenital malformations). (See Table 25.1)

However, ICSI is still a "frontier treatment," in use only since 1992, and several questions remain. For example, it is too early to know whether children born of ICSI will themselves be fertile or infertile. Will abnormalities not noted at birth emerge in adult life? Physicians using ICSI are concerned about these very issues and often seek out the latest genetic techniques to determine whether embryos conceived during this process are carrying any incapacitating or lethal genes prior to implanting the embryo in the mother's uterus. The system in place, while careful and thorough, is not yet perfect, nor is it ever likely to be. Infertile men and their partners considering ICSI should be fully informed about the advantages as well as the unknown aspects of this exciting, still clearly investigational treatment for male-factor infertility.

ETHICAL ISSUES

Advances in assisted or noncoital reproduction have proceeded at a dizzying pace. The arena, once the exclusive domain of infertile couples and their physicians, has now attracted the attention of religious leaders, laypersons, legislators, and ethicists.

There is, to be sure, something eerie about how facile we have become in tinkering with sperm and ova, as if they were little more than reproductive spare parts. The new technology has offered scientists unprecedented opportunities to examine nuances of reproduction in exquisite detail but has also created unimagined moral dilemmas.

No one quibbles with the propriety of using a husband's sperm to inseminate his wife. Even the use of donor sperm for insemination has now been accepted. But what about donor ova?

The woman participating in an IVF program knows that the hormone treatment she receives will force her ovaries to release up to eight to ten mature ova. This is more than enough for her immediate needs. Ordinarily, only three or four ova will be inseminated, allowed to develop into embryos, and then implanted in her uterus. What is the proper disposition of her "surplus" ova? Should they be discarded? Is it preferable to have them fertilized by her husband's sperm, allowed to develop as embryos, and then frozen to be retrieved for use by the couple at a later date? Should unfertilized ova or embryos be donated to other infertile couples?

The American Fertility Society (AFS) has grappled with many of these ethical concerns and has proposed a set of guidelines for donor insemination and IVF. The guidelines suggest that ova and embryos be considered the property of the genetic parents, who alone may decide on their disposition. The donation of unused, unfertilized ova as well as early embryos is acknowledged as an acceptable and ethical practice.

Not everyone is comfortable with this formulation. Some religious groups are uneasy with the entire process of assisted reproduction, which they perceive to be "unnatural." Others, willing to accept the principles of IVF, are troubled by unforeseen difficulties that are implicit, if not explicit, in the document as drafted.

The stipulation that the embryos are the "property of the donors" sounds admirable, but what if a husband and wife divorce? Who owns the embryo—the husband or the wife? What happens if both husband and wife die? Who determines the fate of the orphan embryo? Judges have already been pressed into service to resolve these thorny issues.

IVF and GIFT programs, once restricted to academic centers, are now sprouting as self-contained outpatient facilities. The proliferation of IVF units, some more successful than others, has brought this new reproductive technology within reach of most infertile men and women in this country. Now is the time to reflect on these vexing questions and decide how the new reproductive technology can best be used to the benefit of infertile couples and society.

26

Is There a
Male Menopause?

The notion that the older man must inevitably fall prey to a condition analogous to the female menopause has been bandied about for decades. The terms "male climacteric" and "male menopause" have found favor as the man's counterpart to a woman's menopause. Male climacteric has been vigorously championed, as if some cosmic-fairness doctrine demanded that both men and women experience equal-opportunity afflictions of aging. Others have been just as ardent in insisting that there is no evidence for the existence of either a male climacteric or a male menopause. What is the truth?

WHY QUIBBLE OVER
CLIMACTERIC AND MENOPAUSE?

Menopause and climacteric are words of Greco-Roman origin. The words *mens* (Greek) or *mensis* (Latin), meaning "month," serve as the root used to designate different stages in a *woman's* first menstrual period *(menarche)*. The same root *mens* serves to characterize either a continuation *(menstruation)* or cessation *(menopause)* of monthly cycles of vaginal bleeding.

The word "climacteric" has an equally intriguing linguistic history, dating back to the sixth-century Greek philosopher Pythagoras. He considered the first climacteric, or critical life stage, of a *man's* life to be at age seven; with additional climacterics or pivotal events occurring at ages twenty-one, forty-nine, fifty-six, and eighty-one.

Today, "climacteric" is used to designate physical changes at different ages in either sex, or in the female as a synonym for menopause. Physicians groping for a succinct phrase to describe the impact of aging on older men initially found the term "male menopause" unwieldy and biologically silly. Therefore, they resurrected the gender-neutral term "climacteric."

Dr. August Werner, a St. Louis internist, introduced the term "male climacteric" in a medical paper published in 1939 in the *Journal of the American Medical Association*. He thought it was "reasonable to believe that many if not all men passed through a climacteric period somewhat similar to that of women." He described two middle-aged men, both of whom we would today recognize as having hormonal deficiencies. Treatment with testosterone injections was said to be beneficial.

Five years later, a growing medical literature on the male climacteric had been amassed. Two physicians, Dr. Carl Heller of Vancouver and Dr. Gordon Myers of Detroit, pooled their collective experience and catalogued the symptoms thought to be characteristic of the male climacteric: "nervousness, psychic depression, impaired memory, inability to concentrate, easy fatigability, insomnia, hot flashes, periodic sweating, and loss of sexual vigor." (These symptoms often accompany menopause in women.) They also observed that in contrast to women, older men remained fertile.

Drs. Heller and Myers sensed that psychologic factors might be responsible for climacteric symptoms in some men, whereas other men clearly had a reduction in testosterone secretion function as they aged. Their postulate was not fully explored at the time because only primitive diagnostic methods were available in 1944. It was, for example, not possible to measure a man's testosterone level reliably until the 1970s.

Today we can measure testosterone with some facility, and this has afforded us a greater appreciation of when a man's testosterone production surges and ebbs and how these hormone fluxes govern a man's physical well-being and sexual function throughout his life.

THE ROLE OF HORMONES IN SEXUAL AND REPRODUCTIVE FUNCTION

From the moment of conception to senescence, a single remarkable system, the hypothalamic-pituitary-gonadal axis, masterminds the sexual and reproductive destiny of both men and women. (See Chapter 12.) Individual components of this system must function in a tightly coordinated pattern to ensure the efficient evolution of the human race. This hormone-driven system works throughout life but functions at different levels of intensity in the developing fetus and during childhood, adolescence, the peak adult reproductive years, and old age. Hormones start to influence sexual destiny shortly after conception and then sustain dynamic function, albeit with variable vigor, throughout our lives.

EFFECTS OF AGING ON HORMONE PRODUCTION IN WOMEN

As women age, their ovaries fail and can neither release ova nor produce their full female ration of estrogens. In an effort to resuscitate flagging ovarian function and restore estrogen levels to normal, the hypothalamus becomes wildly active, sending bursts of pituitary hormones in a last-ditch effort to resurrect the failing ovary.

A normal ovary would respond to these stimuli by increasing estrogen output. The aging ovary is, alas, not capable of responding to these pituitary signals by doling out additional hormones. Thus, serum estrogen levels remain low in older women. The bursts of pituitary hormones are believed by some to be responsible for the flushing and sweating that are so characteristic of menopausal hot flashes.

Hot flashes cease when estrogen pills or patches reestablish normal, or near normal, blood estrogen levels. Until recently, it was believed that hot flashes were the unique, and exclusive, burden of postmenopausal women. Now it appears that a select group of men can, and does, suffer from hot flashes. A man's hot flashes are every bit as disconcerting and troublesome as a woman's, but, unfortunately, somewhat more difficult to treat.

The most common cause of hot flashes in men is surgical or medical castration, a treatment designed to restrain the advance of prostate cancer. Restoring sex hormone levels to normal should alleviate symptoms in men, as estrogen does in women, but unfortunately, sex hormone therapy is not provided because of concern that additional testosterone might provide the fuel to accelerate the growth and facilitate the spread of prostate cancer. There are, however, other options for men who have hot flashes. (See Chapter 24.)

However, the majority of aging men do not experience hot flashes because even though their hormone output falters, they do not have the sudden and abrupt declines in hormone levels needed to trigger a hot flash. Nonetheless, no man escapes unscathed from the aging process.

IMPACT OF AGING ON A MAN'S
TESTOSTERONE PRODUCTION

When scientists first looked into the effect of aging on male hormones, their studies yielded conflicting results. One group found that older men, like older women, experienced a form of gonadal failure. Their testes did not function adequately and were unable to produce normal amounts of either testosterone or sperm. Other investigators presented compelling evidence to prove that aging impairs neither testosterone secretion nor sperm production. There is a reason for this contradiction. Although investigators from both camps set out to examine the same problem, they did not study precisely similar groups of men.

Dr. Alexander Vermeulen, a Belgian scientist, was one of the first to report that a progressive decrease in serum testosterone levels occurred in men after age 50. He found that men age 20–50 had roughly comparable serum testosterone levels. Between ages 50 and 60, levels fell, but only slightly. Then, with each subsequent decade, levels fell markedly. Dr. Vermeulen was careful to note, however, that although serum testosterone levels declined, they didn't reach clinically significant subnormal values until after age 80.

These observations were supported by a large study of 466 Australian males, ranging in age from 2 to 101. Again, a progressive decline in serum testosterone levels seemed to be a natural consequence of advancing age, and the report confirmed that older men maintained their serum testosterone levels in the normal range until the eighth decade.

Both studies, as well as comparable reports from the United States, were completed in the mid-1970s, just before gerontology became a full-fledged medical specialty.

When gerontologists began to study the impact of aging on serum testosterone levels, they found quite different results. One group based in Baltimore and another in Boston found that serum testosterone levels did not change with age. Indeed, the values of men age 64–88 were indistinguishable from those of men age 31–44.

The gerontologists had recruited and studied only *extraordinarily healthy older men* and women. They charged that the earlier reports showing a decrease in the aging man's serum testosterone levels with age were flawed because the older men who were the basis of these reports were not well. Many illnesses common to older men can cause their serum testosterone levels to fall.

Whenever the conventional wisdom established by one group of researchers is challenged, we all benefit. A new flock of scientists have now focused their efforts on exploring the impact of aging on male sexual and reproductive function. Dr. Vermeulen, too, extended and expanded his research activities.

Stung by criticism that his earlier observation that decreasing testosterone levels were due to either environmental factors or unrecognized medical problems in the men he studied, Dr. Vermeulen now studied Trappist and Benedictine monks. Once again, he found a difference in serum testosterone levels between men under 60 (average age, 37) and men over 60 (average age, 71), but this time the variation was less pronounced. Although the difference was statistically significant, both values fell well within the normal range for healthy men.

Dr. Vermeulen extended his studies to a larger group and compared the hormone levels of younger and older men living in different environments. His younger group included military draftees and medical workers. Older men were either retired and living at home or were less vigorous nursing-home residents. This time, less dramatic decreases in serum testosterone levels were noted. Even men with an average age of 93 had testosterone levels in the normal range!

This impressively documented report demonstrated that as men age, their *testosterone production ebbs but does not cease.* Thus, from a sex-hormone standpoint, the situation in the aging male is not analogous to the hormone changes a woman experiences as she goes through menopause.

HOW THE BRAIN, PITUITARY GLAND, AND TESTICLE (HYPOTHALAMIC-PITUITARY-GONADAL AXIS) INFLUENCE HORMONE OUTPUT IN OLDER MEN

In the mid-1980s, scientists started to tease apart the elements of the driving force behind a man's sexual and reproductive life and examined the impact of aging on a man's hypothalamic-pituitary-gonadal axis.

1. The hypothalamus, the pituitary, and the testicle do not work with the same degree of vigor and efficiency in aging men. The differences are subtle and can be discerned only with elaborate and intricate research techniques.
2. The rhythms governing male sexual function originate in the hypothalamus. A young man's hypothalamus releases GnRH in a brilliant burst, and small blood vessels carry it to the pituitary in a dramatic fanfare. The older man's hypothalamus retains the ability to manufacture and secrete GnRH, but the pulses seem more measured and somewhat less urgent, so that the GnRH signal received by the pituitary is best described as *sotto voce.*

In younger men, testosterone levels show a distinct rhythmic pattern, with highest values in the morning and significantly lower levels in the evening. Older men lose this rhythm, maintaining a constant level of circulating serum testosterone throughout the day. It is as if the driving force regulating sexual function has shifted from high to low gear.

The pituitary can function only when it receives the appropriate GnRH signals from the hypothalamus. As one might anticipate, the dampened pulses of GnRH evoke suboptimal release of pituitary hormones.

The testicle has two biologic functions: to produce the hormone testosterone and to manufacture and release sperm. Different cells in the testis regulate these individual functions. It has been known for some time that the total number of cells producing testosterone decreases with age. The testicles of older men have at least 44 percent fewer testosterone-producing cells than the testicles of younger men. Older men also have a selective scarring of the sperm-producing cells. Nevertheless, the testicles have an extraordinary reserve capacity and do not need their full complement of sperm-producing or testosterone-releasing cells to function normally. Men who have lost one testicle to surgery maintain testosterone production and full potency and fertility as well.

Does increasing age alone cause a meaningful impairment in testosterone- and sperm-producing capabilities? One obvious way to answer this question is to study these specific components of testicular function in men of advanced age.

A group of physicians from the Max Planck Institute in Germany compared the testicular function of 23 men age 60–88 with that of 20 men age 24–37. First, they examined blood samples to determine the levels of the critical hormones testosterone, LH, and FSH. In both groups, the levels were normal—and virtually identical. Next, they performed sperm counts. The semen analyses of young and old men were similar; both groups' values fell in the normal range considered acceptable for fertility. Finally, they examined the fertility potential of these sperm. They found that the sperm of men in the older group (average age, 67) had a fertilizing effect equivalent to that of the sperm of men in the younger group (average age, 29).

A REAPPRAISAL OF MALE MENOPAUSE

Probably the best way to understand the impact of aging is to reexamine the symptoms originally thought to be characteristic of the "male climacteric syndrome," or male menopause: nervousness, psychic depression, impaired memory, inability to concentrate, easy fatigability, insomnia, hot flashes, periodic sweating, and loss of sexual vigor.

- Nervousness and depression are most likely a reflection of a bona fide depression that commonly occurs in older men. Treatment is available.
- Memory and concentration problems are probably indications of the mild memory deficit (dementia) that is seen in some, though not all, aging men. Treatment is not yet fully effective.
- Insomnia is also common. The reasons for altered sleep habits are not entirely clear, but it appears that with aging, men and women establish different sleep patterns and require less sleep than they did in their youth. Here another hormone deficiency—inadequate *melatonin*—may be a factor. (See Chapter 27.) A more specific type of insomnia, the *inability to stay asleep*, may also be a sign of an underlying *depression*.
- Hot flashes and sweating are uncommon in older men. However, men may experience hot flashes after surgical removal of their testicles or medical treatment to inhibit prostate cancer growth. (See Chapter 24.)

- Loss of sexual vigor is a common problem for men as they age. The diminution in sexual desire and potency is only occasionally the result of hormone failure. More often, a sexual slowing down can be attributed to a combination of physical problems that occur as a natural consequence of aging.

Although all systems required for normal male sexual function remain operational in older men, these systems function with decidedly less verve. With aging, blood flows less briskly to the genitals. Nerves that carry signals to allow erections to occur transmit their impulses with less velocity. The hormonal system that propels male sexual and reproductive function continues to chug along at an adequate, if not ideal, pace. For many older men, the function of vascular, neurologic, and hormonal systems, though suboptimal, is still sufficient for enjoyment of sex.

Thus, it is not the collapse of any single system but rather the collective impact of "adequate but suboptimal" functioning of all that explains the decline in sexual activity of the aging man. Unlike the situation in menopause in which a single organ, the ovary, fails, no single organ or system failure can be identified in the aging male. Therefore, strictly speaking, men do not experience anything comparable to menopause; there is no hormonal evidence of *male menopause.*

For the majority of healthy older men, sexual function persists, but with some limitations:

- Men's ability to experience an erection in response to visual images or fantasy declines with age. Men retain their interest in, and can experience pleasure from, sexual activity but are dependent on more primitive reflexes to acquire an erection.
- The older man retains the ability to have reflex erections in response to manual or oral stimulation. This implies that the local nerves and arteries responsible for providing increased blood flow to the penis are preserved.
- Older men find that their reflex erections do not have the same staying power as the erections they had when they were younger. Continued genital stimulation can extend the duration of the erection.
- Diminished ejaculatory volume is a natural consequence of aging and should not be a cause for concern. Actually, the sperm concentration increases as the volume of fluid declines.

A new term, "presbyrectia," has been coined by Dr. Helen S. Kaplan of Cornell Medical School in New York to describe the modifications in penile erectile response now accepted as normal for aging men. As "presbyopia" describes aging men's visual alterations and "presbycussis" their decrease in hearing, so "presbyrectia" characterizes the changing pattern of erectile capability.

It is not possible to assign a precise date for the onset of presbyrectia for all men. The earliest signs probably surface sometime after the age of sixty. The process accelerates during the seventies and is firmly entrenched after the age of eighty.

No one has yet identified a scheme or treatment program to stave off the inevitable and universal impact of different stages in the evolution of presbyrectia.

Older men can anticipate that aging will impose some limitations in sexual capacity. Patterns of sexual activity will have to be realigned to compensate for these limitations. Increasing, almost exclusive, reliance on genital stimulation to initiate reflex erections is necessary. Local genital stimulation also enhances the effectiveness of Viagra at all ages. But Viagra, alas, is not a safe option for men receiving nitrate therapy for heart problems.

Aging itself does not obliterate sexual urges or the ability to derive pleasure from sex. Couples who work within the boundaries of sexual functioning imposed by the effects of aging can continue to experience a satisfying sexual life.

WHAT ABOUT "ANDROPAUSE" OR THE ADAM (ANDROGEN DEFICIENCY OF AGING MALE) SYNDROME?

Just as presbyrectia has been coined to describe the persistent, albeit occasionally sluggish erectile function of older men, two new terms—"andropause" and the "ADAM (androgen deficiency of aging male) syndrome"—have been introduced to embrace a wide constellation of physical and psychologic experiences common to older men. The andropause concept has caught on in Europe, whereas urologists have been more intrigued with the "first man" appeal of the ADAM syndrome.

Several dedicated andropause clinics have emerged in European countries to offer nutritional information, advice on vitamins, and more often than not androgen supplementation. All of the injections, pills, and patches used in this country are accessible, and used without hesitation, in these clinics.

However, other androgen supplements such as safe testosterone pills—testosterone undecanoate—as well as rub-on testosterone and dihydrotestosterone gels, not available in the United States, figure prominently in the treatment of andropause abroad.

Testosterone undecanoate is a pill that is not plagued by the liver-damaging side effects of oral androgen preparations currently used on this side of the Atlantic.

Dihydrotestosterone gel (DHT Gel) is a male hormone that is rubbed on and absorbed through the skin, raising blood DHT levels. We have had encouraging experience with this medication. Investigators in the United States are just now starting to evaluate the effect of increasing blood DHT levels on the health and well-being of older men. Recent evidence suggests that DHT may play a significant role in maintaining libido and stabilizing erectile function and possibly protecting the prostate in men of all ages.

The possible benefits and adverse effects of these newer male hormones are being explored with great fervor. So far, no increase in prostate hyperplasia, prostate cancer, or PSA levels has been evident from the use of any of these novel androgen preparations. DHT Gel may be the ideal androgen for man in the millennium. (See Chapter 15.)

We will have to wait and see.

27

Restoring Youthful Hormone Levels in Mature Men

Every one has to, but no one wants to, grow old.

The process of aging strips men and women of the youthful vitality all wish was still part of their lives. As our years increase in number, our hormones decrease in quantity. Is this just a coincidence, or is the age-related decline in hormone levels responsible for all, or at least some of, the senior slowdown? What would happen if we rejuvenated our hormone supplies? This chapter provides answers to the common questions about men and testosterone, DHEA, growth hormone, and melatonin.

HORMONES AND THE AGING (MATURE) MAN

Today, all of us are living longer than ever. Even before Congress ordained that those living to age sixty-five would be considered "old" and qualify for Medicare, the numbers of men in and above this age had been increasing exponentially. (When Medicare was enacted, a man's life expectancy was only sixty-seven, making it a safe bet that no man would linger for too many years at the Medicare trough. But when Medicare was conceived, the actuaries advising Congress must have been looking at *absolute numbers* and *ignoring trends*.)

In 1900, only 3.1 million men were sixty-five years or older, whereas by 1997, the number of men in this age group was 33.9 million, an elevenfold increase. This trend is expected to continue, and it is likely that by 2030, there will be more than 70 million men in the sixty-five-plus age group! (Figure 27.1 on page 374.)

But the numbers of men living longer and longer doesn't just stop at age sixty-five. Men currently in the 65–74 age group have increased eightfold since the turn of the century. Even the group of men classified as "old old" is adding to its roster. Today, the absolute numbers of men age eighty-five and older is now thirty-one times greater than in 1900.

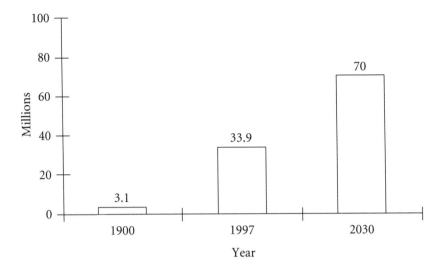

FIGURE 27.1 Numbers of American men age 65 and older in 1900, 1997, and projected to be alive in 2030. SOURCE: Adapted from S. Bhasin, C. J. Bagatell, W. J. Bremner, S. R. Plymate et al., "Issues in Testosterone Replacement in Older Men," *J. Clin. Endocrinol. Metab.* 83 (1998): 435–438.

While it is gratifying to know that men can live longer, the process of aging does have its drawbacks. Some are inevitable and irrevocable, whereas others are more pliable and amenable to change.

Only one aspect of aging, the passage of years, is inexorable. Other consequences of a man's maturing are not quite so immutable. For example, those who are discontent with age-related graying of the hair need not be. An array of hair-coloring products is no farther away than the local hairdresser or drugstore. Local papers and magazines bristle with promotions from cosmetic surgeons all eager to help you look years younger.

The same desire to reject aging and recapture youth, or, at least, *the appearance of youth,* has led medical researchers, curious by nature, to wonder: *What would happen if older men had the hormone levels of younger men?*

After all, it was reasoned, we do not hesitate to offer supplemental estrogens to women when they enter menopause. Why not provide older men with a testosterone booster or jack up levels of other hormones plentiful in youth but scarce in aging?

Until recently, physicians have balked at the concept of offering testosterone therapy because although aging men may be relatively *testosterone impoverished, they are not absolutely testosterone deficient.* Since hormone replacement therapy has been reserved for those men and women with *bona fide hormone deficiencies,* that is, hormone levels that are well below the recognized normal range, doctors have not been eager to offer testosterone to men with normal, albeit low-normal, testosterone levels.

It is true that as men age, their testosterone production is not as efficient as it was when they were younger, but the amount of testosterone produced is sufficient to allow circulating total testosterone levels to cling tenaciously to the "normal range" for many years. Because doctors have an abiding faith in normality, they are disinclined to meddle when blood-test values caress the "normal range." They would not, for example, order blood transfusions for a patient whose blood count is barely below normal any more than they would prescribe insulin injections for someone with a "high-normal" blood-sugar level. By the same reasoning, they have, until recently, been disinterested in offering hormone supplements to aging men with low-normal testosterone values.

Now that thinking is starting to change, and doctors are taking the first tentative steps to evaluate the impact of testosterone and other supplemental hormone treatments on the health and well-being of elderly men.

WHEN YEARS ADVANCE, HORMONES RETREAT

No man at seventy has the same hormonal profile he did when he was twenty-five. (See Figure 27.2 on page 376.) Although serum testosterone levels may remain "normal" in older men, this normality is deceptive, for as the numbers of men in each succeeding decade increase, the percentages of those with low testosterone levels also swell (See Figure 27.3 on page 377).

WHAT EFFECT DOES AGE HAVE ON
A MAN'S OTHER HORMONES?

Testosterone is not the only hormone that drifts downward as a man's years increase. At least three other important hormones—the pituitary's growth hormone, the pineal gland's melatonin, and the adrenal gland's androgen DHEA (dehydroepiandrosterone)—all decline after age fifty in men as well as women. Until recently. this was not a cause for concern because the significance of dwindling levels of these obscure hormones was not appreciated.

The recent recognition that a decline in growth hormone may be linked to the loss of muscle mass in aging and the possibility of below-normal melatonin levels accounting for the insomnia of the elderly have resurrected interest in these arcane hormones. Further, the surprising correlation between very low DHEA levels and premature cardiovascular death has also caused doctors to reexamine the precise role of these hormones in men's health and well-being. Researchers use the time-honored techniques of evaluating strength, sleep, and survival before, during, and after restoring

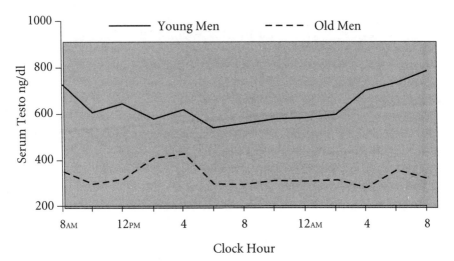

FIGURE 27.2 Differences between serum testosterone levels throughout a 24-hour period in men with an average age of 25 and 71. SOURCE: Adapted from W. J. Bremner, M. V. Vitiello, and P. N. Prinz, "Loss of Circadian Rhythmicity in Blood Testosterone Levels with Aging in Normal Men," *J. Clin. Endocrinol. Metab.* 56 (1983): 1278–1281.

youthful hormone levels in older men and women. But before plunging into an automatic regimen of supplying youthful hormone levels to older men and women, they must address several critical issues.

HORMONES AND AGING: CRITICAL QUESTIONS

1. What are the causes of:
    A. Age-related declines in hormone levels?
2. What are the consequences of:
    A. Insinuating twenty-year-old hormone levels into *sixty-five-plus-year-old bodies*?
    B. Sacrificing the protective effect of low hormone levels?
3. Is there any downside to boosting hormone levels in aging men? Will hormone supplements adversely affect men's:
    A. Prostate-specific antigen (PSA) levels?
    B. Blood cholesterol and lipid values?
    C. Blood pressure?
    D. Red blood cell count (hematocrit)?
    E. Body hair?
    F. Chances of becoming bald?
    G. Acne?
    H. Water retention?

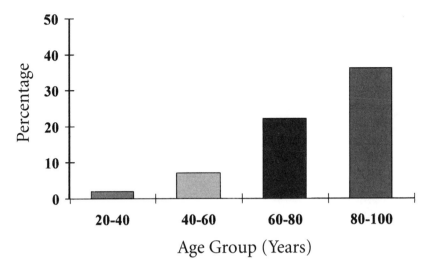

Age Group (Years)

FIGURE 27.3   Percentages of healthy men in different age groups with below normal testosterone levels. (Adapted from Tenover JL. "Aging and male sexual function." Chapter 8 in *The Handbook of Sexual Function*, 1999. The American Society of Andrology, San Francisco, CA.)

TESTOSTERONE REPLACEMENT THERAPY IN OLDER MEN

The age-associated decline in men's testosterone output is due to two factors. First, the total number of testosterone-producing Leydig cells declines with age, so the testicle's testosterone-producing capacity is diminished to some degree. Second, weaker signals from the pituitary gland also limit testosterone output by the testicle. It is this combination of fewer cells with testosterone-producing capability and less incentive for the remaining cells to make male hormone that is responsible for an aging man's diminished testosterone output. What happens when doctors reverse the course of nature and go ahead and buff up the testosterone levels of older men?

Dr. J. Lisa Tenover of Emory University School of Medicine and Dr. John Morley of St. Louis University School of Medicine have given older men with low or low-normal serum testosterone levels testosterone injections in a dose (100 mg of testosterone per week) sufficient to mimic levels seen in men half their age. Men in Dr. Tenover's group were on average sixty-seven years old, whereas Dr. Morley studied men a decade older with a mean age of seventy-seven. But age was not the only difference. Dr. Tenover performed a double-blind placebo crossover trial. Each man received either testosterone or placebo injections for the first three months and then for the next three months was given what he did not receive in the first three-month bloc. The sequence of testosterone-placebo administration was kept a secret. In contrast, Dr. Morley compared the effect of testosterone to no treatment in a group of seventy-seven-year-old men.

In both reports, raising serum testosterone levels caused lean body (muscle) mass to increase. Bone growth, red blood cell count, and oxygen-carrying capacity of blood was also augmented, but total and low-density lipoprotein (LDL) cholesterol levels decreased. There was a small but significant increase in the prostate specific antigen (PSA) in testosterone-treated men. Prostate size, however, did not appear to change significantly.

Although the doctors performing the study and the participating volunteers were not told in advance the testosterone-placebo sequence, all men knew when they had received testosterone injections. During the three months of testosterone treatment, men reported increased sex drive, greater effectiveness, and more confidence in business transactions, as well as an overall improvement in their sense of well-being.

Both doctors cautioned against widespread use of testosterone supplements in aging men until more long-term studies are performed. All in the medical profession are chastened by the *primum non nocere* ("first do no harm") doctrine. Some older men undoubtedly feel better after fleeting (three-month) boosts in testosterone levels, but will long-term testosterone treatment:

1. Increase a man's prostate size?
2. Stimulate the growth of dormant prostate cancer cells?
3. Increase the risk for heart disease?
4. Shorten a man's life span?
5. Create some other unanticipated health risk?
6. Provide men with an improved sense of physical well-being?

In another study, testosterone supplements were given to two groups of men: those who had very low blood testosterone levels—the *truly testosterone deficient*—and those whose blood testosterone levels would still be considered normal, but *low normal*. Ordinarily, testosterone supplements would be offered only to those men with bona fide testosterone deficiency, but Dr. Peter Snyder of Philadelphia decided to offer testosterone treatment to those men with borderline low testosterone values. The goal was to see how men over the age of sixty-five would respond if they suddenly had the male hormone levels of healthy young men.

The study lasted three years! Men over the age of sixty-five were divided into two groups—treatment and placebo. Half of the men wore a testosterone patch and the other half a placebo patch every day for three years. This was an extensive research project, and men had their strength, muscle mass, bone density, sexuality, sense of well-being, and perception of health status evaluated before and after treatment.

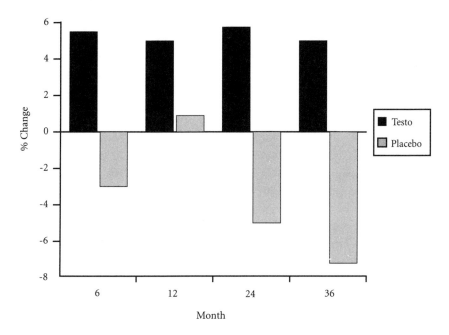

FIGURE 27.4   Men's perception of their physical function during treatment with testosterone or placebo. Positive numbers indicate improvement and negative numbers reflect a decline in physical condition. (Adapted from Snyder P.J., Peachey H, Hannoush P, Loh L et al. Effect of testosterone treatment on body composition and muscle strength in men over 65 years of age. *J Clin Endocrinal Metab* 1999; 84:2647-53.

At the conclusion of the thirty-six-month-long study, the following was clear for men with very low and slightly low or *lowish testosterone* levels:

- Testosterone therapy has its greatest impact when given to men with very low testosterone levels. For these genuinely testosterone-deficient men, building up blood testosterone levels is more likely to result in an improvement in strength, muscle mass, bone density, sexuality, and sense of well-being.
- Boosting the testosterone levels of sixty-five-year-old men who start out with *lowish testosterone* values has a less dramatic effect. They will, for example, experience an increase in muscle bulk but no measurable improvement in strength or bone density. However, testosterone-treated men tend to feel better than comparably aged placebo-treated men.
- Before the study, the men were questioned about their own estimates of their physical function. After establishing baseline answers,

the same questions were asked at periodic intervals throughout the thirty-six months of the study. Placebo-treated men had a progressive decline in physical capabilities, whereas testosterone-treated men experienced an immediate and sustained increase in sense of well-being and physical function for as long as they continued testosterone supplements (see Figure 27.3).

To date, none of the theoretical concerns about possible health risks associated with testosterone supplements have proved to be a problem, but another testosterone-mediated side effect has surfaced and given physicians pause. In one long-term (one-year) study of testosterone supplementation, worrisome increases in red blood cell count and hematocrit did occur. Ordinarily, we think of a vigorous red blood cell count as beneficial because oxygen carried in red blood cells helps every cell in the body. There is, however, a point at which having too many red blood cells is counterproductive and harmful. Then blood must be drained from a man's body to restore the proper blood count. This complication has occurred only rarely and to date has been limited to one form of testosterone supplementation—*testosterone injections*. No similar problems have been reported when testosterone patches were used to increase serum testosterone levels in testosterone-deficient men.

WHAT ABOUT CORRECTING OTHER AGE-ASSOCIATED HORMONE DEFICIENCIES?

As noted above, testosterone is not the only hormone that wanes with aging. Other androgens (male hormones) as well as growth hormone, abundant during youth, and melatonin all dwindle to token levels as we age. What if we could reverse the clock and provide all men and women with a "hormonal face-lift" so that not just testosterone but all the vigorous hormones of youth would persist forever within the aging body?

Would insinuating a young man's hormone profile in an older man's body resurrect youthful passions and power or merely reactivate acne and all the agonies of adolescence? Is there any downside to meddling in what appears to be an orderly and programmed diminution of anabolic hormone production?

Two terms, "anabolism" (building up) and "catabolism" (breaking down), distinguish the primary metabolic events of youth and aging. The anabolic hormones—testosterone and human growth hormone—and an adrenal androgen (dehydroepiandrosterone sulfate) produced in abundance during our youth all decline as we age. The age-related decrease in anabolic hormone production coincides with loss of muscle mass (catabolism) and diminished vigor, stamina, and sexual function. Is there is a cause-and-effect relationship between the decrease in anabolic hormones and the natural consequences of aging? If the diminution in anabolic hormone level was indeed responsible for any, or all, of the frailties of aging, then restoring youthful hormone levels should materially improve the sense of well-being and improve the quality of life of older men and women. This is precisely the premise behind the new wave of anti-aging clinics.

Sensing the concern of men and women about growing old, the clinics' directors have seized upon fragments of what is known about hormones and aging and have promoted treatment with DHEA, growth hormone, and melatonin to stave off the aging process. They publish monographs and cite what appears to be persuasive evidence of the rejuvenating properties of different hormone combinations and attract many followers. How well do these hormones really work?

DHEA

The jawbreaker-named hormones dehydroepiandrosterone (DHEA) and dehydroepiandrosterone sulfate (DHEA-S) exhibit remarkable variability throughout life. DHEA-S is produced in the adrenal glands of both men and women, but not all the time. DHEA does not make an appearance in the bloodstream until just before puberty. Then a veritable torrent of this adrenal androgen quite suddenly appears. DHEA acts as the hormonal harbinger of adolescence, and is the hormone responsible for stimulating the growth of axillary (armpit) and pubic (groin) hair. Any man or woman whose memory is good enough to summon up those preteen years may recall faint wisps of hair appearing under their arms and groin at an early age. This early sexual hair makes its appearance before girls have their first menstrual periods and before young boys start to shave. Those latter events rely on estrogen in young women and testosterone in young men. When these gonadal hormones or estrogen burst on the scene, they herald the onset of reproductive life.

Once they appear in the bloodstream, levels of DHEA-S remain fairly steady and constant until about age fifty. After that age, DHEA-S levels decline precipitously, a phenomenon that was, until recently, considered to be a natural, innocuous consequence of aging not materially altering the well-being of older men and women. Newer studies have challenged that premise, and there is now great enthusiasm among some groups for using medication to reinstate and maintain young-adult DHEA-S levels for all men and women over the age of fifty.

---

[1]Years later, Congress would pass the Dietary Supplement and Health Care Act, allowing many health-care products like DHEA to be marketed with little or no need to prove that they do what they are purported to do. (See Chapter 21, "The Lure of Alternative Medicine," for more details.)

TABLE 27.1   Average Initial Plasma DHEA-S Level and Twelve Year Mortality.

Age Group	DHEA-S mcg/dl (level of those still living)	DHEA-S mcg/dl (level of those who died)
50–54	277	102
55–59	213	129
65–69	156	114
70–74	136	120
75–79	100	79

The enthusiasm for increasing DHEA and DHEA-S levels can be traced to a 1986 report linking very low DHEA-S levels with premature death. Researchers in California obtained blood samples from 242 healthy men who were 50–79 years old at the outset and then traced their progress for the next twelve years. During that time period, 76 men died. Those who were destined to expire had the very lowest DHEA-S levels, creating the impression that like *high* cholesterol values, *low* DHEA-S levels were a harbinger of ill health. The association of unusually low DHEA-S levels with early death from heart disease was independent of the men's age at the start of the study. (See Table 27.1.) Since then, men have eagerly sought to normalize DHEA-S levels as a means of avoiding premature death.

DHEA has had a checkered history, and its benefits, if any, remain an area of intense scientific controversy and debate. For example, the FDA had, at one time, discouraged over-the-counter sales of DHEA because of the lack of evidence attesting to that hormone's safety and efficacy. But that decision was made in 1985, just one year prior to the publication of the article linking low DHEA-S levels with shortened life span.[1]

Doctors asked a simple question. If low DHEA levels are so menacing, why not increase DHEA levels and see what happens? That is precisely what Dr. Samuel Yen and his colleagues have been doing for years. Their early attempts to increase DHEA levels overshot the mark and created untoward metabolic problems. Recently, however they have been using lower, more physiologic doses, designed to replicate the DHEA levels of young adult men and women and targeting middle-aged men and women for their initial research efforts.

In one recent study, thirteen men and seventeen women with an average age of fifty-five received either three months of DHEA or placebo in random order. The most remarkable finding was an improved sense of well-being by both men and women who received DHEA. Individuals commented that they had "improved quality of sleep, were more relaxed, had increased energy, and a better ability to handle stress" when they were receiving DHEA, but not placebo. Libido did not change during treatment, leading the authors to conclude that the benefits achieved were specific for DHEA and distinct from those observed with testosterone.

Another curious finding was an increase in the blood level of a growth hormone–related protein, but unlike growth hormone itself (see below), DHEA did not alter the proportions of muscle and fat in these middle-aged men and women. Thus, to date the benefits achieved with DHEA therapy have been predominantly on the psychologic well-being of men and women. However, other studies have suggested that raising DHEA levels may have subtler benefits, including improved immune responses and a favorable impact on blood-sugar levels in older men.

One troublesome aspect of the DHEA puzzle is that cigarette smoking seems to be associated with increased DHEA-S levels. Between 1982 and 1984, a group of 543 healthy doctors volunteered to participate in a study to determine what aspects of their daily activity, diet, habits, family history, and so on would have a beneficial or adverse effect on their subsequent health. Blood samples collected as part of that study were frozen and analyzed for the cholesterol content initially, and more recently for DHEA and DHEA-S. The highest DHEA-S levels were seen in the doctors who in 1982 were then-current smokers, followed in sequence by past smokers, with those who had never smoked having the lowest DHEA-S levels. The paradox of finding the most-favorable DHEA-S levels in men who engage in the least-favorable health practices is exactly opposite of what would be expected. It is clear that the DHEA story is still evolving. The only uncontested fact is that with age, there is an inevitable downward trend in DHEA and DHEA-S levels. What remains unresolved is whether reversing that trend with DHEA pills will be worthwhile for anyone other than those who are marketing this hormone.

It is easy to find DHEA. Corner pharmacies and vitamin and nutritional-supplement purveyors keep their store shelves stocked with ample supplies of DHEA in assorted doses. The cult of DHEA enthusiasts continues to grow. Spurred on by articles appearing in popular magazines, this adrenal androgen is increasingly being thought of as a rejuvenating hormone. We have woefully little information to justify that conclusion. More substantial research is required before we can accurately assess exactly what can be anticipated or feared from increasing DHEA levels in older men and women. (See Chapter 22.)

HUMAN GROWTH HORMONE

As its name implies, growth hormone is needed for normal growth and development. The pituitary gland doles out appropriate amounts of growth hormone from childhood to support our growth and development. Some children are unable to make growth hormone and fail to grow properly. This can be corrected by providing these youngsters with the hormone they are lacking.

Children with pituitary problems, however, are not the only ones who have low growth-hormone levels. Normal men and women also experience a significant decline in growth hormone output as they age. This has prompted some to think of aging as a growth-hormone deficiency state requiring treatment.

In addition to its growth-promoting capability, growth hormone can act as an anabolic hormone and build muscle, a fact that has not escaped the attention of bodybuilders and other athletes. Casual perusal of the men who are used to model for the covers of muscle and fitness magazines will reveal that some of these men have developed the jutting jaw, wide-spaced teeth, and distorted skull that is characteristic of those who may have overindulged in the use of growth-hormone supplements to beef up their muscles.

A loss of muscle and increase in fat mass is characteristic of aging. Could growth-hormone treatment reverse that trend and improve the lot of older men and women?

Occasional articles in the popular press have individual seniors flexing their muscles and egos to offer testimony to the remarkable changes they experienced once they started growth-hormone injections. Those familiar with the actions of growth hormone would suspect that these anecdotal claims of benefits that are little more than outlandish bravado. To know for sure whether growth-hormone treatment is beneficial and not harmful, more detailed measurements are required.

The first major research in this area was performed by Dr. Daniel Rudman and his colleagues in Milwaukee who gave growth-hormone injections to a group of men between the ages of sixty-one and eighty-one to determine the effect of this medication on their body composition. They knew that for growth hormone to work, it must first stimulate production of a growth factor called IGF-1. When IGF-1 levels are low, growth does not occur. Low IGF-1 levels occur not only in growth-hormone deficient children but are also common in older men. Dr. Rudman gave twelve men enough growth hormone to increase their IGF-1 levels to a "youthful range" and left another group of comparably aged men untreated and followed their progress for six months. During this time, the growth-hormone treated men had a remarkable 8.8 percent increase in lean body mass, a 14.4 percent decrease in body fat, a 7.1 percent increase in skin thickness, and a 1.6 percent increase in spine bone density. Untreated patients had no change in body composition over the same period. This seminal report stimulated considerable enthusiasm for the use of growth hormone as a palliative treatment to reverse the age-related trend toward more fat and less muscle. Sub-

TABLE 27.2   Adverse Effects After 6 Months of Growth Hormone or Placebo Treatment

Side Effect Reported	From those on Growth Hormone	From those on Placebo
Hand Stiffness	10 (38%)	1 (4%)
Fatigue	5 (19%)	2 (8%)
Joint pains	14 (54%)	3 (11%)
Edema	17 (65%)	6 (23%)

sequent research revealed that increasing growth-hormone levels in elderly men was not entirely benign. Dr. Rudman did not continue to promote this treatment without cautioning men about the significant adverse effects that accompanied this treatment.

Six years later, Dr. Maxine Papadakis performed a similar study and gave growth hormone or placebo to fifty-two somewhat older (average age, 75) men with low growth-hormone and IGF-1 levels. Treatment lasted six months. Men were evaluated before and after treatment not only with respect to their body composition but also to see if they were, in any measurable way, improved physically or mentally.

For these septuagenarians, growth-hormone treatment did increase lean body mass by 4.3 percent (half of that achieved by the sixty-year-old men in Dr. Rudman's study) and decreased fat by about 13.1 percent. These changes were significantly greater than those seen in the men receiving placebo injections, who continued their steady loss of lean muscle mass during the six months of the study.

However, this increase in lean muscle and decrease in fat distribution in growth-hormone treated men was not translated into any particular advantage in physical strength as measured by hand grip, knee extension, or endurance. Nor was any other improvement in physical or mental function apparent following treatment. Growth-hormone treated men could be readily distinguished from their placebo-treated counterparts by their side-effect profile. Stiffness, aches, arthritis-like pains, edema, and fatigue were common. (See Table 27.2.)

In addition to the frequency with which serious side effects occur, another cause for concern is the financial burden of treatment. Growth-hormone therapy costs about $12,000–14,000 per year, an expense grudgingly borne by managed-care companies for the relatively small numbers of growth-hormone-deficient children. Similar largesse is unlikely to be extended to older men, for whom benefits are marginal at best. Those men who remain eager to dabble in growth-hormone therapy will have to contend with both the $12,000–14,000 annual expense as well as the often grotesque side effects caused by growth-hormone injections. At present, daily injections are the only way to increase growth-hormone levels.

One drug company did develop a pill to stimulate more growth-hormone secretion in older men. Treatment raised growth hormone and IGF-1 values to youthful levels, leading many to think that this would be another blockbuster medication with an enormous market. But the drug company that had developed the drug soon abandoned this project because of inadequate benefits and worrisome side effects.

MELATONIN

Tucked away dead center in the middle of the brain is an obscure structure called the pineal gland, which churns out a hormone called melatonin. Not to be confused with the similar-sounding but totally different skin pigment, melanin, melatonin helps control our sleeping and waking. Melatonin levels are very low during our daytime waking hours but then start their ascent about 9:00 P.M., increase steadily throughout the evening hours, and are at their peak between 2 and 4 A.M. when most of us are fast asleep. Since blood levels of this hormone are almost undetectable during the day when we need to be awake and alert and then start to appear in the bloodstream when our workday is winding down, it is likely that that we need melatonin to fall asleep and stay asleep.

Each of us has within our pineal gland a unique internal biologic clock keyed to light and dark cycles throughout the day. The pineal gland seems to respond to cues sent from our eyes to suppress melatonin production during daylight hours and then allow increased melatonin output as evening descends. For reasons that we still do not fully understand, our ability to maintain this orderly cycle is not constant, and serum melatonin levels decline with aging. Some older men and women are plagued by insomnia, are unable to either fall asleep or stay asleep, and do not feel refreshed when they wake in the morning. These elderly insomniacs tend to have lower melatonin levels than comparably aged men and women who sleep well, leading to the theory that a deficiency of this pineal hormone is responsible for their restless nights.

If inadequate amounts of melatonin are responsible for their sleeplessness, then normalizing melatonin levels should help. Indeed, this is precisely what happens. In studies of both young and old men and women, sleep efficiency, defined as the time it takes to fall asleep as well as the total duration of restful sleep, improves as melatonin levels are increased. Regular melatonin pills have a rapid effect, helping people fall asleep promptly but do not necessarily last through the night. A longer-acting so called controlled-release form of melatonin seems to be more reliable in extending the duration of sleep through the night.

Fallout from melatonin research has extended from the plight of the sleepless elderly to the harried business traveler who must grapple with the inevitable "jet lag" that comes with traveling through multiple time zones. The businessman who journeys from New York to Los Angeles will find himself awakening at 4:00 A.M. Los Angeles time, which is equivalent to his usual New York wake-up time of 7:00 A.M., because despite the time zone difference, his pineal gland's internal clock is still set to release melatonin as if he were still in New York. After a few days in Los Angeles, his pineal will reset to adjust to West Coast time. Judicious use of melatonin pills before he travels seems to make the transition in between time zones much easier.

The hypnotic, that is, sleep-inducing actions, of melatonin appear to be well established, but like many of the other hormones discussed in this section, this pineal hormone has been imbued with a rich folklore. Claims that melatonin is a miracle drug with properties to reverse aging, extend life, and fend off fearsome illnesses such as AIDS and Alzheimer's disease are unsubstantiated. Activists in this area are now engaged in a pitched battle. One group is hawking a book called *The Melatonin Miracle*. Other more sober-minded researchers refute what they perceive to be the egregious, scientifically inaccurate, and preposterous statements made in that book.

WHY MESS WITH MOTHER NATURE?

The age-associated downward drift of hormones has been, for the most part, accepted as part of the natural sequence of events, coinciding with the ratcheting down of other faculties such as endurance, mental acuity, and sexual function. The isolation of specific hormone deficiencies and the ease with which they can be corrected has been too tempting to ignore. After all, today we have the pills, patches, and injections at hand to turn back the hormonal clock and replicate the hormonal pattern of the young in those who are, if not old, at least not so young anymore. No easy answers exist, but with the knowledge currently available, we can say the following about specific hormone supplements:

Testosterone

Short-term (meaning three-year) treatment seems to be well tolerated and improves energy, stamina, and confidence. Consequences of longer-term treatment, particularly as it relates to its effect on prostate size and activating latent prostate cancer cells, will have to await the results of studies currently in progress. Unexpected problems have developed in some men who have an inordinate increase in their red blood cell count. These men have either had to have periodic drainage of blood from their veins (phlebotomy) or abandon testosterone treatment altogether. Periodic checks of blood counts are probably worthwhile in men receiving supplemental testosterone therapy. To date, this has been more of a problem in men receiving testosterone injections and has not been observed as often in men using testosterone-impregnated patches.

DHEA

Evidence for beneficial effects of this adrenal androgen is intriguing but limited and far from proven by the scientific evidence at hand. As additional information on benefits and possible toxicity surface, DHEA may prove to be a useful energizing medication for the elderly, but it is still too early to recommend widespread use of this hormone. Fortunately, DHEA has proven to be remarkably benign and people who are curious about its effects can probably take it for a month or two to see if it makes a difference in their lives. Women who use high DHEA doses for long periods of time do run the risk of developing extra facial hair in their beard and mustache area.

Growth Hormone

The increase in lean body mass and decrease in fat mass observed consistently with thrice-weekly growth-hormone injections seems to be real, with greater effects seen in men in their sixties than those over age seventy-five. However, no improvement in function or thinking seems to occur with this improvement in body composition. Frequent side effects and extraordinary expense cloud the future use of this medication in the elderly.

Melatonin

This obscure pineal hormone has been a pleasant surprise, for it seems to provide a relatively safe treatment for the insomnia and sleeplessness so common in elderly men and women.

28

What's Next for Men in the Millennium?

Where you go from this point on really depends on you and your partner. Allow some time and work together to provide honest answers to specific questions:

1. Is your sex life everything you want it to be?
2. Do you want to know if you need Viagra?
3. Would a little more testosterone help or harm?
4. Are there really anti-aging hormones that will change your life?
5. Are urinary problems caused by a large prostate gland disrupting your life?
6. Do you worry about prostate cancer?
7. Are you concerned about your fertility?
8. Have changes in health materially affected the quality of your life?

Chapters 1 through 27 provide answers to the first seven questions. This chapter addresses the relationship between a man's sexuality and his quality of life.

QUALITY OF LIFE

In recent years, an entirely new dimension has been added to the health-care equation. As more and more men and women live longer lives, their ability to enjoy their extended longevity has emerged as a major priority. Within the medical profession, we physicians are now starting to look at what are now termed quality of life (QOL) issues. A man's ability to enjoy sex is an important component of his QOL, and doctors are no longer writing off a man's lost sexual function as an inevitable consequence of treatment for high blood pressure, benign prostatic hyperplasia, and prostate cancer.

More than fifty years ago, the World Health Organization defined health not only as the *absence* of disease but also as the *presence* of physical, mental, and social well-being. Since then, quality of life and health-related qual-

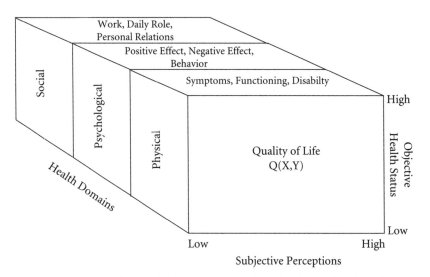

FIGURE 28.1 Evaluating multiple objective and subjective health domains to assess quality of life. Modified from Testa, M.A. and Simonson, D.C. "Assement of Quality of Life Outcomes," *N Engl J. Med* 1996; 334: 835–40.

ity of life (HRQOL) research has helped to define the impact of both illnesses and their treatments on the QOL of men and women. Questionnaires now probe a man's overall health as well as his physical, psychologic, and social capabilities. Data from QOL questionnaires provide a more complete picture of the impact of illnesses and their treatment on overall well-being. (See Figure 28.1.) Scores derived from QOL questionnaires are often used in conjunction with ongoing research. For example, studies comparing blood-pressure-lowering medications or prostate cancer treatments may show equivalent blood pressure reduction or cancer-free survival but a difference in the number of side effects (adverse events). Sexual side effects are now among the adverse events receiving increased attention for very good reason.

A man's zest for sex persists as his lifespan increases. At all ages, sexuality remains an important factor in the fabric and overall quality of his life. We can chart a man's lifetime patterns of sexual intercourse (coital activity). First-time sexual encounters occasionally start in the teenage years, but for the average man, serious sex starts when he is in his twenties and intensifies during his mid-thirties. Thereafter, sex tends to plateau. For the normal man, sexual desire persists but, alas, not always with the same passion as when he was younger and sex was a novelty. (See Figure 28.2.) Nonetheless, at any age, sex remains a major determinant of the quality of a man's life.

In men's second and third decades, sexual activity peaks and they may have intercourse daily or at least several times a week. Thereafter, with each advancing decade sexual intercourse frequency declines somewhat but does

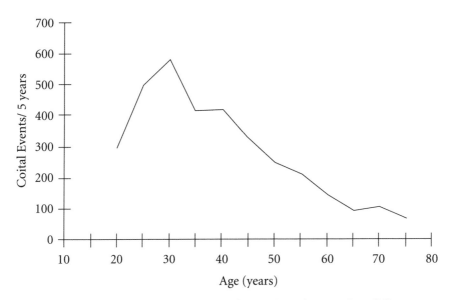

FIGURE 28.2   Charting a man's sexual behavior (coital activity) at different ages of his life. SOURCE: Adapted from J. L. Tenover, "Aging and Male Sexual Function," in *The Handbook of Sexual Dysfunction* (San Francisco: American Society of Andrology, 1998), chap. 8, pp. 39–42.

not stop. Men in their seventies still enjoy sexual intercourse, although sex for septuagenarians may be only once or twice a month. These figures should serve to dispel the popular notion that sex is only for the very young.

But there is a caveat here. The numbers cited above were culled from surveys performed many years before Viagra was available. It is likely that five years from now, results will be different. Within a few years, the numbers of men of all ages reporting satisfaction from sex will likely increase, especially for those generally healthy men who struggle to maintain their sexuality as they age.

The effectiveness of Viagra has delighted many but puzzled others because it has introduced a new health-care concept known as *lifestyle pharmacology*. The distinguished medical journal the *Lancet* defines lifestyle pharmacology as: "Drugs not to prevent death *but to enhance the quality of life*."

Implicit in this definition is the premise that quality of life issues are trivial concerns requiring little attention or resources. But that sort of thinking creates a problem. We have only a few genuinely life-saving medications—yet we are all living longer. If, as now seems to be the case, many of us are all destined to survive to advanced age, shouldn't we do everything possible to maximize the quality of life for our additional years?

The answer seems to be *not if it costs money*, especially somebody else's money. Thus, Viagra has been singled out as a "high-cost, high-volume drug capable of bankrupting drug budgets in order to improve the sexual capacity of the male." That statement issued in Great Britain *before Viagra was widely available* betrays two basic anxieties, one related to money and the other to sex.

Herein lies a major conundrum. Today's physicians are being asked to expand their horizon. Along with their traditional role in fending off disease and minimizing disability, doctors are now expected to incorporate concerns for QOL issues. This is an admirable goal, but one that has now run head on into fiscal reality.

The primary concern of Great Britain's National Health Service is to remain *solvent*, whereas most U.S. managed-care companies aim to be *profitable*. For either to achieve their objective, they must husband their resources: government subsidies for the NHS and patient premium dollars for managed-care companies. So they routinely disallow payment for what they perceive to be frivolous procedures like face-lifts and liposuction. But they have customarily covered the cost of treatment for many other non-life-threatening conditions.

Those responsible for paying the bills do not balk at covering the cost of prescription medications for other non-life-threatening ailments like acne or hay fever.

But sex is somehow different. Despite the suffering and disruption in the QOL that male sexual dysfunction causes to both men and women, insurers have been uneasy footing the bill for any treatment of male sexual problems. Citing a puritanical ethic, they point with pride to their denial of payments for women's birth control pills to justify their refusal to cover the cost of Viagra for men.

But the analogy is flawed. Birth control pills allow healthy women to have sex without fear of pregnancy. Impotence remedies allow sexually impaired men to enjoy sex without fear of failure.

Men do not always speak up for their rights, nor when asked directly are they likely to be candid about the importance of sex in their lives. Rather, they betray their concerns in more subtle ways by, for example, shunning products perceived to be threats to their sexuality. Impotence and decreased libido occur only rarely in men who use finasteride as Proscar to reduce prostate size or as Propecia to reverse male-pattern baldness. Impotence occurred in only 2.1 percent of 14,712 Proscar-treated men. Still, sexual dysfunction was the most frequently reported side effect and the major explanation offered by men who chose to discontinue Proscar therapy. When word leaked out that impotence occurred in less than 4 percent of men taking Propecia to reverse baldness, Propecia failed to meet sales expectations. Baldness is not life-threatening, so Propecia can be classified as

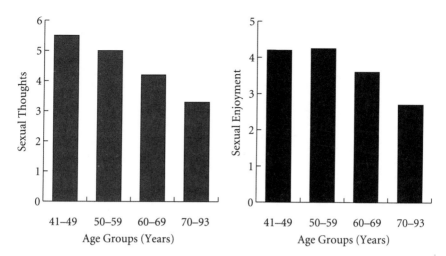

FIGURE 28.3   Sexual thoughts and enjoyment of men over time. SOURCE: Adapted from J. L. Tenover, "Aging and Male Sexual Function," in *The Handbook of Sexual Dysfunction* (San Francisco: American Society of Andrology, 1998), chap. 8, pp. 39–42.

yet another *lifestyle medication*—but curiously no one is seeking to limit its sales. Thus, drugs that may *disrupt male sexual function* are tolerated, whereas those designed to *enhance male sexuality* are perceived as a threat.

There are still other ways to learn how men and women rank the importance of sex in their lives. Ask them directly about their sexual thoughts and capacity for sexual enjoyment. In surveys of men age 40–90, sexual thoughts and pleasure persisted, although a gradual age-associated decline was apparent. Forty-year-old men were more sexually stirred than those in their nineties, but at all ages, men reported deriving some pleasure from sex. (See Figure 28.3.)

When both men and women were queried, most reported persistent pleasure in sexual activity. Until age seventy-nine, sexual satisfaction was an important part of life for 50 percent or more of men. Comparably aged women's interest in sex persists with only slightly less enthusiasm. (See Table 28.1.)

Not surprisingly, a man's ability to acquire and maintain an erection is one of the determinants of his ability to derive pleasure from sexual intercourse. An increasing number of men experience difficulty in this sexual sphere as they age. (See Table 28.2.)

The data reveal some important trends. Both men and women's interest in sex is sustained for many years beyond what we have been led to believe. The percentages of those enjoying sex at all ages are remarkable, especially considering that not everyone in this age group is 100-percent healthy.

TABLE 28.1   Sexual Activity of Married Men and Women

	Men		Women	
Age	Yes/Total	%	Yes/Total	%
60–64	83/95	87%	57/89	64%
65–69	64/81	79%	49/77	64%
70–74	18/31	58%	13/30	43%
75–79	13/26	50%	9/25	36%
80+	4/14	29%	1/4	25%

SOURCE: Modified from Diokno, *Arch. Intern. Med.* 1990.

TABLE 28.2   Numbers of Men Reporting Difficulty Acquiring or Maintaining an Erection

Age	Numbers /Total	% Having Difficulty
60–64	27/94	29%
65–69	27/78	35%
70–74	14/30	47%
75–79	25/24	63%
80+	9/14	64%

SOURCE: Modified from Diokno, *Arch. Intern. Med.* 1990.

But this study, published in 1990, was actually the result of interviews conducted in the late 1980s. Since then, the longevity of men and women has continued to increase, as has the overall health of all in this age group.

MALE SEXUALITY AND QUALITY OF LIFE

More recent surveys bring an added dimension to the arena by focusing not just on sex itself but on "life satisfaction" or quality of life of men with erectile dysfunction. It is by now axiomatic to acknowledge that a disrupted sex life not only hurts the man with erectile dysfunction but his sexual partner as well. However, other areas (domains) of his life also suffer when a man has erectile dysfunction. A remarkably concise questionnaire called the Short Form 36 (SF-36) elicits information about the quality of a man's life in sexual as well as nonsexual domains. It does not matter whether his sexual problems stem from physical or psychologic causes, the sexually marginalized man always scores low on SF-36 questions designed to determine his satisfaction with:

1. Life as a whole
2. Sexual life

3. Family life
4. Partnership relations
5. Business dealings

Questionnaires like the SF-36 and others are being used with increasing frequency to gauge the impact of treatment on a man's quality of life before and after treatment for common problems like prostate cancer.

QUALITY OF LIFE AFTER PROSTATE CANCER SURGERY

Renewed interest in health-related quality of life issues has prompted doctors to explore QOL issues in men who have had radical prostatectomy treatment for prostate cancer. In one Australian study of 140 men after successful surgical treatment, impotence was identified by 40 percent of men as the single most significant treatment-related problem affecting their lives. By way of comparison, only 12 percent listed concern about cancer, and even fewer (8 percent) felt their lives were seriously disrupted by post-surgical incontinence. Those men troubled by impotence had the lowest QOL scores in all domains. The authors concluded, "loss of sexual function and its effect on QOL needs to be given greater emphasis in counseling before radical prostatectomy."

These findings were echoed in another report on men's quality of life after treatment for prostate cancer. Unlike the earlier Australian study, this Denver study questioned wives about their husband's QOL after surgery. Impotence occurred in 70 percent of men after surgery, resulting in low QOL scores.

Those quality of life domains that suffer in men with erectile dysfunction improve promptly when sexual function is restored with penile injection therapy. Discomfort and inconvenience as well as the queasy feeling a man gets sticking a needle into his penis have contributed to the high dropout rate with this treatment. The jury is still out on whether Viagra will be as useful in improving the QOL in men who have had radical prostatectomy for prostate cancer. Dropouts have not been a problem with Viagra, for men who start usually stay with this form of treatment. Preliminary surveys indicate that life satisfaction improves in about 65 percent of men who use Viagra, but detailed evaluation of the long-term impact of this novel medication on a man's quality of life have not yet been completed. Regrettably, Viagra is not always effective in men who develop impotence after prostate cancer surgery, and for those men who fail with Viagra, penile injection still remains a viable option.

Interest in Viagra persists, not only for men but for women as well. Some women do not enjoy sex because they cannot get sexually aroused. Studies to learn whether the woman with diminished sexual arousal will benefit from Viagra are currently underway.

ARE WE MESMERIZED BY SEX, AND IF SO, IS THAT A PROBLEM?

One of the enduring legacies of the late 1990s is that despite our protestations to the contrary, we are still intrigued by sex. Men and women alike griped about the endless media coverage of the President Clinton–Monica Lewinsky sex scandal. They told pollsters they absolutely *did not want to hear one more word* about this subject. Still, record numbers clicked on their TV sets and tuned in to the Barbara Walters interview of Monica Lewinsky.

Then, books by Ms. Lewinsky, reporter Dan Isikoff, and Clinton confidant George Stephanopolous, all describing different perspectives of the same sexual escapade, became best-sellers. We claim to, but should not be, taken aback by our own and the public's interest—no, obsession—with sex. Are we embarrassed about our interest in prurient subjects? We shouldn't be. Maintaining a healthy interest in sex is vital.

There is nothing about our fascination with sex that should cause us any shame. From biblical times to the present, vigorous sex has been an integral component of a full life. There is a sense among mature men and women that since we are no longer children, we should have outgrown our preoccupation with sex, but we will not. A man's sexuality and fertility are too important to all men as well as to those who love them.

Fortunately, for men and women, medical science now has many methods for dealing with male sexual dysfunction. Impotence—erectile dysfunction—need not be a lifelong sentence to celibacy; difficulty with conceiving need not condemn a couple to childlessness. Certainly no treatment is foolproof. Nevertheless, if you have a sexual problem and are willing take that difficult first step to seek help, you will most likely be rewarded. With proper diagnosis, a specific treatment plan tailored to your specific needs can be devised. The results—restoration of sexual potency, a more satisfying sex life, and, if desired, fertility—can improve health and well-being and allow you to enjoy an improved quality of life.

Let us continue.

References

CHAPTER 5. YOU ARE NOT ALONE

Feldman, H. A., B. Goldstein, D. G. Hatzichristou et al. Impotence and its medical and psychosocial correlates: Results of the Massachusetts Male Aging Study. *J. Urol.* 151 (1994): 54–61.

Frank, E., C. Anderson, and D. Rubinstein. Frequency of sexual dysfunction in "normal" couples. *N. Engl. J. Med.* 299 (1978): 111–115.

Kinsey, A. C., W. B. Pomeroy, and C. E. Martin. *Sexual behavior in the human male.* Philadelphia: Saunders, 1948.

Moore, J. T., and Y. Goldstein. Sexual problems among family medicine patients. *J. Fam. Pract.* 10 (1980): 243–247.

Reading, A. E., and W. M. Wiest. An analysis of self-reported sexual behavior in a sample of normal males. *Archives of Sexual Behavior* 13 (1984): 69–83.

Slag, M. F., J. E. Morley, M. K. Elson et al. Impotence in medical clinic outpatients. *JAMA* 249 (1983): 1736–1740.

Spector, K. R., and M. Boyle. The prevalence and perceived aetiology of male sexual problems in a non-clinical sample. *Br. J. Med. Psychol.* 59 (1986): 351–358.

Werner, A. Sexual dysfunction in college men and women. *Am. J. Psychiatry* 123 (1975): 164–168.

CHAPTER 6. THE SIX PHASES OF NORMAL MALE SEXUAL FUNCTION

Cole, T. M. Sexuality in the spinal cord injured. In R. Green, ed., *Human sexuality: A health practitioner's text.* Baltimore: Williams and Wilkins, 1975.

deGroat, W. C., and A. M. Booth. Physiology of male sexual function. *Ann. Int. Med.* 92 (1980): 329–331.

Friedman, M. Success phobia and retarded ejaculation. *Am. J. Psychother.* 27 (1973): 78–84.

Levine, S. B. Marital sexual dysfunction: Ejaculation disturbances. *Ann. Int. Med.* 84 (1976): 575–579.

Ovesey, L., and H. Meyers. Retarded ejaculation: Psychodynamics and psychotherapy. *Am. J. Psychother.* 22 (1968): 185–201.

Sadock, V. A. Normal human sexuality and psychosexual disorders. In H. I. Kaplan and B. J. Sadock, eds., *Comprehensive textbook of psychiatry.* 4th ed. Baltimore: Williams and Wilkins, 1985.

Silver, J. R. Sexual problems in disorders of the nervous system. Part 1: Anatomical and physiological aspects. *Br. Med. J.* 3 (1975): 480–482.

CHAPTER 10. RECENT ADVANCES IN MALE SEXUALITY

Girding for Sex

Allen, R. P., and C. B. Brendler. Nocturnal penile tumescence predicting response to intracorporeal pharmacological erection testing. *J. Urol.* 140 (1988): 518–522.

Benson, G. S., J. McConnell, and L. I. Lipshultz. Neuromorphology and neuropharmacology of the human penis. *J. Clin. Invest.* 65 (1980): 506–513.

Brindley, G. S. Physiology of erection and management of paraplegic infertility. In T. B. Hargreave, ed., *Male infertility.* Berlin: Springer-Verlag, 1983.

Condra, M., A. Morales, D. H. Surridge, J. A. Owen, P. Marshall, and J. Fenemore. The unreliability of nocturnal penile tumescence recording as an outcome measurement in the treatment of organic impotence. *J. Urol.* 135 (1986): 280–282.

Doman, J., and D. J. Kupfer. Computer analysis of EEG, FOG, and NPT activity during sleep. *Int. J. Biomed. Comput.* 23 (1988): 191–200.

Ellis, D. J., K. Doghramji, and D. H. Bagley. Snap-gauge band versus penile rigidity in impotence assessment. *J. Urol.* 140 (1988): 61–63.

Goldstein, I., M. B. Siroky, D. S. Sax, and R. J. Krane. Neurourologic abnormalities in multiple sclerosis. *J. Urol.* 128 (1982): 541–545.

Kaiser, F. E., and S. G. Korenman. Impotence in diabetic men. *Am. J. Med.* 85 (1988): 147–152.

Kaneko, S., and W. E. Bradley. Penile electrodiagnosis: Value of bulbocavernosus reflex latency versus nerve conduction velocity of the dorsal nerve of the penis in diagnosis of diabetic impotence. *J. Urol.* 137 (1987): 933–935.

Karacan, I., P. J. Salis, M. Hirshkowitz, R. E. Borreson, E. Narter, and R. L. Williams. Erectile dysfunction in hypertensive men: Sleep-related erections, penile blood flow and musculovascular events. *J. Urol.* 142 (1989): 56–61.

Karacan, I., R. L. Williams, J. I. Thornby, and P. J. Salis. Sleep-related penile tumescence as a function of age. *Am. J. Psychiatry* 132 (1975): 932–937.

Lavoisier, P., J. Proulx, F. Courtois, and F. de Carufel. Bulbocavernosus reflex: Its validity as a diagnostic test of neurogenic impotence. *J. Urol.* 141 (1989): 311–314.

Lehman, T. P., and J. J. Jacobs. Etiology of diabetic impotence. *J. Urol.* 129 (1983): 291–294.

Lipson, L. L. Special problems in treatment of hypertension in the patient with diabetes mellitus. *Arch. Intern. Med.* 144 (1984): 1829–1831.

Marshall, P., D. Surridge, and N. Delva. The role of nocturnal penile tumescence in differentiating between organic and psychogenic impotence: The first stage of validation. *Arch. Sex. Behav.* 10 (1981): 1–10.

Phelps, G., M. Brown, J. Chen et al. Sexual experience and plasma testosterone levels in male veterans after spinal cord injury. *Arch. Phys. Med. Rehabil.* 64 (1983): 47–52.

Reynolds, C. F., III, M. E. Thase, R. Jennings et al. Nocturnal penile tumescence in healthy 20- to 59-year-olds: A revisit. *Sleep* 12 (1989): 368–372.

Schiavi, R. C., C. Fisher, D. White, P. Beers, and R. Szechter. Pituitary-gonadal function during sleep in men with erectile impotence and normal controls. *Psychosom. Med.* 46 (1984): 239–254.

Siroky, M. B., D. S. Sax, and R. J. Krane. Sacral signal tracing: The electrophysiology of the bulbocavernosus reflex. *J. Urol.* 122 (1979): 661–664.

Thase, M. E., C. F. Reynolds III, J. R. Jennings et al. Diagnostic performance of nocturnal penile tumescence studies in healthy, dysfunctional (impotent), and depressed men. *Psychiatry Research* 26 (1988): 79–87.

Valleroy, M. L., and G. H. Kraft. Sexual dysfunction in multiple sclerosis. *Arch. Phys. Med. Rehabil.* 65 (1984): 125–128.

Velcek, D. Discogenic impotence. *Int. J. Impotence Res.* 1 (1989): 95–113.

Wasserman, M. D., C. P. Pollak, A. J. Spielman, and E. D. Weitzman. The differential diagnosis of impotence: The measurement of nocturnal penile tumescence. *JAMA* 243 (1980): 2038–2042.

Wincze, J. P., S. Bansal, D. Malhotra, A. Balko, J. G. Susset, and M. Malmud. A comparison of nocturnal penile tumescence and penile response to erotic stimulation during waking states in comprehensively diagnosed groups of males experiencing erectile difficulties. *Arch. Sex. Behav.* 17 (1988): 333–348.

The Flow of Blood: Arteries and Veins

Abelson, D. Diagnostic value of the penile pulse and blood pressure: A Doppler study of impotence in diabetics. *J. Urol.* 113 (1975): 636–639.

Andersen, K. V., and G. Bovim. Impotence and nerve entrapment in long distance amateur cyclists. *Acta. Neurol. Scand.* 95 (1997): 233–240.

Bar-Moshe, O., and M. Vandendris. Treatment of impotence due to perineal venous leakage by ligation of crura penis. *J. Urol.* 139 (1988): 1217–1219.

Bond, R. E. Distance bicycling may cause ischemic neuropathy of the penis. *Physician Sportsmed.* 3 (1975): 54–56.

Bookstein, J. J., and A. L. Lurie. Selective penile venography: Anatomical and hemodynamic observations. *J. Urol.* 140 (1988): 55–60.

Buvat, J., A. Lemaire, M. Buvat-Herbaut, J. D. Guieu, J. P. Bailleul, and P. Fossati. Comparative investigations in 26 impotent and 26 nonimpotent diabetic patients. *J. Urol.* 133 (1985): 34–38.

Chin, R. C., D. Lidstone, and P. E. Blundell. Predictive power of penile/brachial index in diagnosing male sexual impotence. *J. Vasc. Surg.* 4 (1986): 251–256.

DePalma, R. G., H. A. Emsellem, C. M. Edwards et al. A screening sequence for vasculogenic impotence. *J. Vasc. Surg.* 5 (1987): 228–236.

Duchame, S. H., and K. M. Gill. *Sexuality after spinal cord injury: Answers to your questions.* Baltimore: Paul Brookes Publishing Co., 1997.

Engel, G., S. J. Burnham, and M. F. Carter. Penile blood pressure in the evaluation of erectile impotence. *Fertil. Steril.* 30 (1978): 687–690.

Goldstein, I., M. B. Siroky, R. L. Nath, T. N. McMillian, J. O. Menzoian, and R. J. Krane. Vasculogenic impotence: Role of the pelvic steal test. *J. Urol.* 128 (1982): 300–306.

Karacan, I., P. J. Salis, M. Hirshkowitz, R. E. Borreson, E. Narter, and R. L. Williams. Erectile dysfunction in hypertensive men: Sleep-related erections, penile blood flow and musculovascular events. *J. Urol.* 142 (1989): 56–61.

Kedia, K. R. Vasculogenic impotence: Diagnosis and objective evaluation using quantitative segmental pulse volume recorder. *Br. J. Urol.* 56 (1984): 516–520.

Kerstein, M. D., S. A. Gould, E. French-Sherry et al. Perineal trauma and vasculogenic impotence. *J. Urol.* 127 (1982): 57.

Lewis, R. W. Venous surgery for impotence. *Urol. Clin. North Am.* 15 (1988): 115–121.

Lugg, J. A., N. F. Gonzalez-Cadavid, and J. Rajfer. The role of nitric oxide in penile erection. *J. Androl.* 16 (1995): 2–4.

Michal, V., R. Kramar, and J. Pospichal. External iliac "steal syndrome." *J. Cardiovasc. Surg.* 19 (1978): 355–357.

Shaw, W. W., and A. W. Zorgniotti. Surgical techniques in penile revascularization. *Urology* 23 (1984): 76–78.

Virag, R. Pelvic steal syndrome: An appraisal illustrated by clinical and haemodynamic data on seven cases. *VASA* 10 (1980): 304–307.

Virag, R., P. Bouilly, and D. Frydman. Is impotence an arterial disorder? A study of risk factors in 440 impotent men. *Lancet* 1 (1985): 181–184.

Zorgniotti, A. W., G. Rossi, G. Padula, and R. D. Makovsky. Diagnosis and therapy of vasculogenic impotence. *J. Urol.* 123 (1980): 674–677.

CHAPTER 11. MALE SEXUAL CHEMISTRY AND VIAGRA

Becker, A. J., C. G. Stief, S. Machtens et al. Oral phentolamine as treatment for erectile dysfunction. *J. Urol.* 159 (1988): 1214–1216.

Boolell, M., S. Gepi-Atlee, C. Gingell, and M. Allen. UK-92480, a new oral treatment for erectile dysfunction: A double-blind placebo-controlled crossover study demonstrating dose response with RigiScan and Efficacy with outpatient diary. *Proceedings of the American Urologic Association* 155 (1996): 495, Abstract 739.

Bradbury, J. Viagra approved in Europe, but UK tells doctors not to prescribe. *Lancet* 352 (1998): 963.

Derry, F. A., W. W. Dinsmore, M. Fraser et al. Efficacy and safety of oral sildenafil (Viagra) in men with erectile dysfunction caused by spinal cord injury. *Neurology* 51 (1998): 1629–1633.

Eardley, I., R. J. Morgan, W. W. Dinsmore, J. Pearson et al. UK-92480, a new oral treatment for erectile dysfunction: A double-blind, placebo-controlled trial with treatment taken as required. *Proceedings of the American Urologic Association* 155 (1996): 495, Abstract 737.

Fallen taboo: Frank talk on Viagra is about cost. *New York Times*, July 11, 1998, pp. D1–D2.

Garg, R. K., A. Khaishgi, and P. Dandona. Is management of impotence with sildenafil changing clinical practice? *Lancet* 353 (1999): 375–376.

Gingell, C.J.C., A. Jardin, A. M. Olsson, W. W. Dinsmore et al. UK-92480, a new oral treatment for erectile dysfunction, placebo-controlled, once daily dose response study. *Proceedings of the American Urologic Association* 155 (1996): 495, Abstract 738.

Goldstein, I., T. F. Lue, H. Padma-Nathan, R. C. Rosen et al. Oral sildenafil in the treatment of erectile dysfunction: Sildenafil Study Group. *N. Engl. J. Med.* 338 (1998): 1397–1404.

Gwinup, G. Oral phentolamine in nonspecific erectile insufficiency. *Ann. Int. Med.* 109 (1988): 162–163.

New York and Wisconsin will defy federal directive to provide Viagra through Medicaid. *New York Times,* July 3, 1998, p. A12.

Rendell, M. S., J. Rajfer, P. A. Wicker et al. Sildenafil for treatment of erectile dysfunction in men with diabetes: A randomized controlled clinical trial. *JAMA* 281 (1999): 421–426.

Vobig, M. A., T. Klotz, M. Staak et al. Retinal side effects of sildenafil. *Lancet* 353 (1999): 375.

CHAPTER 12. HORMONES AND SEXUALITY

Baskin, H. J. Endocrinologic evaluation of impotence. *South. Med. J.* 82 (1989): 446–449.

Blackwell, R. E., and R. Guillemin. Hypothalamic control of adenohypophyseal secretions. *Ann. Rev. Physiol.* 35 (1973): 357–390.

Blumer, D., and A. E. Walker. Sexual behaviour in temporal lobe epilepsy. *Arch. Neurol.* 16 (1967): 37–43.

Bobrow, N. A., J. Money, and V. G. Lewis. Delayed puberty, eroticism, and sense of smell: A psychological study of hypogonadotropinism, osmatic and anosmatic (Kallmann's syndrome). *Arch. Sex. Behav.* 1 (1971): 329–344.

Carter, J. N., J. E. Tyson, G. Tolis, S. Van Vliet, C. Faiman, and H. G. Friesen. Prolactin-secreting tumors and hypogonadism in 22 men. *N. Engl. J. Med.* 299 (1978): 847–852.

Chopra, I. J., and D. Tulchinsky. Status of estrogen-androgen balance in hyperthyroid men with Graves' disease. *J. Clin. Endocrinol. Metab.* 38 (1974): 269–277.

Franks, S., H. S. Jacobs, N. Martin, and J. D. Nabarro. Hyperprolactinemia and impotence. *Clin. Endocrinol.* 8 (1978): 277–287.

Hierons, R., and M. Saunders. Impotence in patients with temporal lobe lesions. *Lancet* 2 (1966): 761–764.

Hill, T. C., A. L. Holman, R. Levett et al. Initial experience with SPECT (single photon computerized tomography) of the brain using N-isopropyl I-123 iodoamphetamine (concise communication). *J. Nucl. Med.* 23 (1982): 191–195.

Johnson, J. Sexual impotence and the limbic system. *Br. J. Psychiat.* 111 (1965): 300–303.

Kidd, G. S., A. R. Class, and R. A. Vigersky. The hypothalamicpituitary-testicular axis in thyrotoxicosis. *J. Clin. Endocrinol. Metab.* 48 (1979): 798–802.

Korenman, S. G., S. Viosca, D. Garza et al. Androgen therapy of hypogonadal men with transscrotal testosterone systems. *Am. J. Med.* 83 (1987): 471–478.

Linde, R., G. C. Doelle, N. Alexander et al. Reversible inhibition of testicular steroidogenesis and spermatogenesis by a potent gonadotropin-releasing hormone agonist in normal men: An approach toward the development of a male contraceptive. *N. Engl. J. Med.* 305 (1981): 663–667.

McBride, R. L., and J. Sutin. Amygdaloid and pontine projections to the ventromedial nucleus of the hypothalamus. *Comp. Neur.* 174 (1977): 377–396.

Meikle, A. W., N. A. Mazer, J. F. Moellmer et al. Enhanced transdermal delivery of testosterone across nonscrotal skin produces physiological concentrations of testosterone and its metabolites in hypogonadal men. *J. Clin. Endocrinol. Metab.* 74 (1992): 623–628.

Mills, T. M., V. T. Wiedmeier, and V. S. Stopper. Androgen maintenance of erectile function in the rat penis. *Biol. Reprod.* 46 (1992): 342–348.

Nagulesparen, M., V. Ang, and J. S. Jenkins. Bromocriptine treatment of males with pituitary tumours, hyperprolactinaemia, and hypogonadism. *Clin. Endocrinol.* 9 (1978): 73–79.

Prescott, R.W.G., P. Kendall-Taylor, K. Hall et al. Hyperprolactinaemia in men: Response to bromocriptine therapy. *Lancet* 1 (1982): 245–249.

Santen, R. J., and C. W. Bardin. Episodic luteinizing hormone secretion in man: Pulse analysis, clinical interpretation, physiologic mechanisms. *J. Clin. Invest.* 52 (1973): 2617–2628.

Slag, M. F., J. E. Morley, M. K. Elson et al. Impotence in medical clinic outpatients. *JAMA* 249 (1983): 1736–1740.

Spark, R. F. Neuroendocrinology and impotence. *Ann. Int. Med.* 98 (1983): 103–105.

Spark, R. F., C. A. Wills, and H. Royal. Hypogonadism, hyperprolactinaemia, and temporal lobe epilepsy in hyposexual men. *Lancet* 1 (1984): 413–417.

Spark, R. F., G. O'Reilly, C. A. Wills, B. J. Ransil, and R. Bergland. Hyperprolactinaemia in males with and without pituitary macroadenomas. *Lancet* 2 (1982): 129–132.

Spark, R. F., R. A. White, and P. B. Connolly. Impotence is not always psychogenic: Newer insights into hypothalamic-pituitary-gonadal dysfunction. *JAMA* 243 (1980): 750–755.

Veldhuis, J. D., A. D. Rogol, M. L. Johnson, and M. L. Dufau. Endogenous opiates modulate the pulsatile secretion of biologically active luteinizing hormone in man. *J. Clin. Invest.* 72 (1983): 2031–2040.

Winters, S. J., R. S. Mecklenburg, and R. J. Sherins. Hypothalamic function in men with hypogonadotrophic hypogonadism. *Clin. Endocrinol.* 8 (1978): 417–426.

Wortsman, J., W. Rosner, and M. L. Dufau. Abnormal testicular function in men with primary hypothyroidism. *Am. J. Med.* 82 (1987): 207–212.

Yamada, T., and M. A. Greer. The effect of bilateral ablation of the amygdala on endocrine function in the rat. *Endocrinology* 66 (1960): 565–574.

CHAPTER 13. THE TESTOSTERONE RENAISSANCE

Bhasin, S., T. W. Storer, N. Berman, C. Callegari et al. The effects of supraphysiologic doses of testosterone on muscle size and strength in normal men. *N. Engl. J. Med.* 355 (1996): 1–7.

Burger, H., J. Hailes, J. Nelson, and M. Menelaus. Effect of combined implants of oestradiol and testosterone on libido in postmenopausal women. *Lancet* 294 (1987): 936–937.

Coodley, G. O., M. K. Coodley, M. O. Loveless, and H. D. Nelson. Endocrine function in the HIV wasting syndrome. *J. Acquired Immune Defic. Syndromes* 7 (1994): 46–51.

Dobs, A. S., M. A. Dempsey, P. W. Ladenson, and B. F. Polk. Endocrine disorders in men infected with human immunodeficiency virus. *Am. J. Med.* 84 (1988): 611–616.

Durant, R. H., V. I. Rickert, C. S. Ashworth et al. Use of multiple drugs among adolescents who use anabolic steroids. *N. Engl. J. Med.* 328 (1993): 922–926.

Hardiman, P. J., P. D. Abel, and J. Ginsburg. Peripheral vascular effects of gonadotropin-releasing agonists in men. *J. North Am. Menopause Soc.* 2 (1995): 159–161.

Marder, H. K., L. S. Srivastava, and S. Burstein. Hypergonadotropism in peripubertal boys with chronic renal failure. *Pediatrics* 72 (1983): 384–389.

Rabkin, J. G., and R. Rabkin. Testosterone replacement therapy for HIV infected men. *AIDS Reader* 5 (1995): 136–144.

Rako, S. *The hormone of desire: The truth about sexuality, menopause, and testosterone.* New York: Harmony Books, 1996.

Sherwin, B., and M. Gelfand. Differential symptom response to parenteral estrogen and/or androgen administration in the surgical menopause. *Am. J. Obstet. & Gynecol.* 151 (1985): 153–160.

Terney, R., and L. G. McLain. The use of anabolic steroids in high school students. *Am. J. Dis. Child.* 144 (1990): 99–103.

World Health Organization Task Force on Methods for the Regulation of Male Fertility: Contraceptive efficacy of testosterone induced azoospermia in normal men. *Lancet* 336 (1990): 955–959.

CHAPTER 15. DIHYDROTESTOSTERONE (DHT)

Barrett-Connor, E., K. T. Khaw, and S.S.C. Yen. A prospective study of dehydroepiandrosterone sulfate, mortality and cardiovascular disease. *N. Engl. J. Med.* 315 (1986): 1519–1524.

Dallob, A. L., N. S. Sadick, W. Unger et al. The effect of finasteride a 5-alpha reductase inhibitor on scalp skin testosterone and dihydrotestosterone concentrations in patients with male pattern baldness. *J. Clin. Endocrinol. Metab.* 79 (1994): 703–706.

de Lignieres, B. Transdermal dihydrotestosterone treatment of "andropause." *Annals of Medicine* 25 (1993): 235–241.

Gormley, G. J., E. Stoner, R. G. Bruskewitz et al. The effect of finasteride on men with benign prostatic hyperplasia. *N. Engl. J. Med.* 327 (1992): 1185–1191.

Horton, R., I. Antonipillai, and F. Sattler. A defect in generating dihydrotestosterone in AIDS patients with wasting. Abstract P1-173, presented at the Tenth International Congress of Endocrinology, San Francisco, 1996.

Mantzoros, C. S., E. I. Georgiadis, and D. Trichpoulos. Contribution of dihydrotestosterone to male sexual behavior. *Brit. Med. J.* 310 (1995): 1289–1291.

Mills, T. M., C. M. Reilly, and R. Lewis. Androgens and penile erection: A review. *J. Androl.* 17 (1996): 633–638.

Morales, A. J., J. J. Nolan, J. C. Nelson, and S.S.C. Yen. Effects of replacement doses of dehydroepiandrosterone in men and women of advancing age. *J. Clin. Endocrinol. Metab.* 78 (1994): 1360–1367.

Nestler, J. E., N. A. Beer, D. J. Jakubowicz et al. Effects of insulin reduction with benfluorex on serum dehydroepiandrosterone (DHEA), DHEA sulfate and blood pressure in hypertensive middle aged and elderly men. *J. Clin. Endocrinol. Metab.* 80 (1995): 700–706.

Regelson, W., R. Loria, and M. Kalmi. Dehydroepiandrosterone (DHEA): The "mother steroid." Immunologic action. *Ann. N.Y. Acad. Sci.* 719 (1994): 553–563.

Rittmaster, R. Finasteride. *N. Engl. J. Med.* 330 (1994): 120–125.

Salvini, S., M. J. Stampfer, R. L. Barbieri, and C. H. Hennekens. Effects of age, smoking and vitamins on plasma DHEA-S levels: A cross-sectional study in men. *J. Clin. Endocrinol. Metab.* 74 (1992): 139–143.

Spark, R. F., L. Sanchez, B. J. Dezube, and H. Libman. Is dihydrotestosterone the preferred androgen for AIDS wasting? 1998 Abstract OR 43-6. Presented at ENDO 98, the Endocrine Society Eightieth Annual Meeting, New Orleans.

Tenover, J. S. Prostates, pates, and pimples: The potential use of steroid 5 alpha reductase inhibitors. *Endocrinology and Metabolism Clinics of North America* 20 (1991): 893–909.

Walsh, D. S., C. L. Dunn, W. D. James et al. Improvement in androgenetic alopecia (Stage V) using topical minoxidil in retinoid vehicle and oral finasteride. *Arch. Dermatol.* 131 (1995): 1373–1375.

CHAPTER 16. MEDICATIONS, CHEMICALS, AND SEXUAL POTENCY

Apter, A., Z. Dickerman, N. Gonen et al. Effect of chlorpromazine on hypothalamic-pituitary-gonadal function in 10 adolescent schizophrenic boys. *Am. J. Psychiatry* 140 (1983): 1586–1591.

Bain, S. C., M. Lemon, and A. F. Jones. Gemfibrozil-induced impotence. *Lancet* 336 (1990): 1389.

Balon, R., V. K. Yeragani, R. Pohl, and C. Ramesh. Sexual dysfunction during antidepressant therapy. *J. Clin. Psychiatry* 54 (1993): 209–212.

Bansal, S. Sexual dysfunction in hypertensive men: A critical review of the literature. *Hypertension* 12 (1988): 1–10.

Brenner, J., D. Vugrin, and W. F. Whitmore Jr. Effect of treatment on fertility and sexual function in males with metastatic nonseminomatous germ cell tumors of testis. *Am. J. Clin. Oncol.* 8 (1985): 178–182.

Carson, C. C., and R. D. Mino. Priapism associated with trazodone therapy. *J. Urol.* 139 (1988): 369–370.

Clonidine (Catapres) and other drugs causing sexual dysfunction. *Med. Lett. Drugs Ther.* 19 (1977): 81–82.

Cocores, J. A., N. S. Miller, A. C. Pottash, and M. S. Gold. Sexual dysfunction in abusers of cocaine and alcohol. *Am. J. Drug Alcohol Abuse* 14 (1988): 169–173.

Colin Jones, D. G., M. J. Langman, D. H. Lawson, and M. P. Vessey. Postmarketing surveillance of the safety of cimetidine: Twelve-month morbidity report. *Q. J. Med.* 54 (1985): 253–268.

Condra, M., A. Morales, J. A. Owen, D. H. Surridge, and J. Fenemore. Prevalence and significance of tobacco smoking in impotence. *Urology* 27 (1986): 495–498.

Cooper, A. J. Factors in male sexual inadequacy: A review. *J. Nerv. Ment. Dis.* 149 (1969): 337–359.

Croog, S. H., S. Levine, A. Sudilovsky, R. M. Baume, and J. Clive. Sexual symptoms in hypertensive patients: A clinical trial of antihypertensive medications. *Arch. Intern. Med.* 148 (1988): 788–794.

Croog, S. H., S. Levine, M. A. Testa et al. The effects of antihypertensive therapy on the quality of life. *N. Engl. J. Med.* 314 (1986): 1657–1664.

Cunningham, G. R., and M. Hirshkowitz. Inhibition of steroid 5 alpha-reductase with finasteride: sleep-related erections, potency, and libido in healthy men. *J. Clin. Endocrinol. Metab.* 80 (1995): 1934–1940.

Danesi, R., R. V. La Rocca, and M. R. Cooper et al. Clinical and experimental evidence of inhibition of testosterone production by suramin. *J. Clin Endocrinol. Metab.* 81 (1996): 2238–2246.

Dawley, H. H., Jr., D. K. Winstead, A. S. Baxter, and J. R. Gay. An attitude survey of the effects of marijuana on sexual enjoyment. *J. Clin. Psychol.* 35 (1979): 212–217.

Drugs and male sexual function. Editorial, *Br. Med. J.* 2 (1979): 883–884.

Forsberg, L., B. Gustavii, T. Hojerback, and A. M. Olsson. Impotence, smoking, and beta-blocking drugs. *Fertil. Steril.* 31 (1979): 589–591.

Fossa, S. D., S. Ous, T. Abyholm, and M. Loeb. Post-treatment fertility in patients with testicular cancer. Part 1: Influence of retroperitoneal lymph dissection on ejaculatory potency. *Br. J. Urol.* 57 (1985): 204–209.

Gardner, E. A., and J. A. Johnson. Bupropion: An antidepressant without sexual pathophysiologic action. *J. Clin. Psychopharmacol.* 5 (1985): 24–29.

Ghadirian, A. M., G. Chouinard, and L. Annable. Sexual dysfunction and plasma prolactin levels in neurolepic treated schizophrenic outpatients. *J. Nervous Mental Dis.* 170 (1982): 463–467.

Gilbert, D. G., R. L. Hagen, and J. A. D'Agostino. The effects of cigarette smoking on human sexual potency. *Addict. Behavior* 11 (1986): 431–434.

Glass, R. M. Ejaculatory impairment from both phenelzine and imipramine, with tinnitus from phenelzine. *J. Clin. Psychopharmacol.* 1 (1981): 152–154.

Goldstein, I., M. I. Feldman, P. J. Deckers, R. K. Babayan, and R. J. Krane. Radiation-associated impotence: A clinical study of its mechanism. *JAMA* 251 (1984): 903–910.

Goldwasser, B., I. Madgar, P. Jonas, B. Lunenfeld, and M. Many. Imipramine for the treatment of sterility in patients following retroperitoneal lymph node dissection. *Andrologia* 15 (1983): 588–591.

Gossop, M. R., R. Stern, and P. H. Connell. Drug dependence and sexual dysfunction: a comparison of intravenous users of narcotics and oral users of amphetamines. *Br. J. Psychiatry* 124 (1974): 431–434.

Gwee, M. C., and L. S. Cheah. Actions of cimetidine and ranitidine at some cholinergic sites: Implications in toxicolocy and anesthesia. *Life Sci.* 39 (1986): 383–388.

Harrison, W. M., J. G. Rabkin, A. A. Ehrhardt et al. Effects of antidepressant medication on sexual function: a controlled study. *J. Clin. Psychopharmacol.* 6 (1986): 144–149.

Herman, J. B., A. W. Brotman, M. H. Pollack, W. E. Falk, J. Biederman, and J. F. Rosenbaum. Fluoxetine-induced sexual dysfunction. *J. Clin. Psychiatry* 51 (1990): 25–27.

Jensen, R. T., M. J. Collen, K. E. McArthur et al. Comparison of the effectiveness of ranitidine and cimetidine in inhibiting acid secretion in patients with gastric hypersecretory states. *Am. J. Med.* 77 (1984): 90–105.

Jensen, R. T., M. J. Collen, S. J. Pandol et al. Cimetidine-induced impotence and breast changes in patients with gastric hypersecretory states. *N. Engl. J. Med.* 308 (1983): 883–887.

Juenemann, K. P., T. F. Lue, J. A. Luo, N. L. Benowitz, M. Abozeid, and E. A. Tanagho. The effect of cigarette smoking on penile erection. *J. Urol.* 138 (1987): 438–441.

Kline, M. D. Fluoxetine and anorgasmia. Letter, *Am. J. Psychiatry* 146 (1989): 804–805.

Korenman, S. G. Clinical assessment of drug-induced impairment of sexual function in men. *Chest* 83 (1983): 391–392.

Kowalski, A., R. O. Stanley, L. Dennerstein, G. Burrows, and K. P. Maguire. The sexual side effects of antidepressant medication: A double-blind comparison of two antidepressants in a nonpsychiatric population. *Br. J. Psychiatry* 147 (1985): 413–418.

Labbate, L. A., and M. H. Pollack. Treatment of fluoxetine induced sexual dysfunction with bupropion: A case report. *Ann. Clin. Psychiatry* 6 (1994): 13–15.

Lin, S. N., P. C. Yu, M. C. Yang, L. S. Chang, B. N. Chiang, and J. S. Kuo. Local suppressive effect of clonidine on penile erection in the dog. *J. Urol.* 139 (1988): 849–852.

Lipson, L. L. Special problems in treatment of hypertension in the patient with diabetes mellitus. *Arch. Intern. Med.* 144 (1984): 1829–1831.

_____. Treatment of hypertension in diabetic men: Problems with sexual dysfunction. *Am. J. Cardiol.* 53 (1984): 46A–50A.

McEwen, J., and R. H. B. Meyboom. Testicular pain caused by mazindol. *Br. Med. J.* 287 (1983): 1763–1764.

Melman, A., J. Fersel, and P. Weinstein. Further studies on the effect of chronic alpha-methyldopa administration upon the central nervous system and sexual function in male rats. *J. Urol.* 132 (1984): 804–808.

Mendelson, J. H., N. K. Mello, S. K. Teah, J. Ellingboe, and J. Cochin. Cocaine effects on pusatile secretion of anterior pituitary, gonadal, and adrenal hormones. *J. Clin. Endocrinol. Metab.* 69 (1989): 1256–1260.

Mitchell, J. E., and M. K. Popkin. Antidepressant drug therapy and sexual dysfunction in men: A review. *J. Clin. Psychopharmacol.* 3 (1983): 76–79.

_____. Antipsychotic drug therapy and sexual dysfunction in men. *Am. J. Psychiatry* 139 (1982): 633–637.

Moss, H. B., and W. R. Procci. Sexual dysfunction associated with oral antihypertensive medication: A critical survey of the literature. *Gen. Hosp. Psychiatry* 4 (1982): 121–129.

Newman, H. F., and H. Marcus. Erectile dysfunction in diabetes and hypertension. *Urology* 26 (1985): 135–137.

Nijman, J. M., S. Jager, P. W. Boer, J. Kremer, J. Oldhoff, and H. S. Koops. The treatment of ejaculation disorders after retroperitoneal lymph node dissection. *Cancer* 50 (1982): 2967–2971.

Peden, N. R., J. M. Cargill, M. C. Browning, J. H. Saunders, and K. G. Wormsley. Male sexual dysfunction during treatment with cimetidine. *Br. Med. J.* 1 (1979): 659.

Quirk, K. C., and T. R. Einarson. Sexual dysfunction and clomipramine. *Can. J. Psychiatry* 27 (1982): 228–231.

Rabkin, J. G., F. M. Quitkin, P. McGrath, W. Harrison, and E. Tricamo. Adverse reactions to monoamine oxidase inhibitors. Part 2: Treatment correlates and clinical management. *J. Clin. Psychopharmacol.* 5 (1985): 2–9.

Report of Medical Research Council Working Party on Mild to Moderate Hypertension. Adverse reactions to bendrofluazide and propranolol for the treatment of mild hypertension. *Lancet* 2 (1981): 539–543.

Reynolds, C. F., III, E. Frank, M. E. Thase et al. Assessment of sexual function in depressed, impotent, and healthy men: Factor analysis of a brief sexual function questionnaire for men. *Psychiatry Res.* 24 (1988): 231–250.

Rothschild, A. J. Selective serotonin reuptake inhibitor-induced sexual dysfunction: Efficacy of a drug holiday. *Am. J. Psychiatry* 152 (1995): 1514–1516.

Scharf, M. B., and D. W. Mayleben. Comparative effects of prazosin and hydrochlorothiazide on sexual function in hypertensive men. *Am. J. Med.* 86 (1989): 110–112.

Schneider, J., and H. Kaffarnik. Impotence in patients treated with elofibrate. *Atherosclerosis* 21 (1975): 455–457.

Segraves, R. T. Effects of psychotropic drugs on human erection and ejaculation. *Arch. Gen. Psychiatry* 46 (1989): 275–284.

Segraves, R. T., R. Madsen, C. S. Carter, and J. M. Davis. Erectile dysfunction associated with pharmacological agents. In R. T. Segraves and H. W. Schoenberg, eds., *Diagnosis and treatment of erectile disturbances: A guide for clinicians.* New York: Plenum, 1985.

Sjogren, K., and A. R. Fugl-Meyer. Some factors influencing quality of sexual life after myocardial infarction. *Int. Rehabil. Med.* 5 (1983): 197–201.

Smith, D. E., D. R. Wesson, and M. Apter-Marsh. Cocaine- and alcohol-induced sexual dysfunction in patients with addictive disease. *J. Psychoactive Drugs* 16 (1984): 359–361.

Stevenson, R.W.D., and L. Solyom. The aphrodisiac effect of fenfluramine: Two case reports of a possible side effect to the use of fenfluramine in the treatment of bulimia. *J. Clin. Psychopharmacol.* 10 (1990): 69–71.

Thase, M. E., C. F. Reynolds III, J. R. Jennings et al. Nocturnal penile tumescence is diminished in depressed men. *Biol. Psychiatry* 24 (1988): 33–46.

Van Thiel, D. H., J. S. Gavaler, P. K. Eagon, Y. B. Chiao, C. F. Cobb, and R. Lester. Alcohol and sexual function. *Pharmacol. Biochem. Behav.* 13 (1980): 125–129.

Walker, P. W., J. O. Cole, E. A. Gardner et al. Improvement in fluoxetine associated sexual dysfunction in patients switched to bupropion. *J. Clin. Psychiatry* 54 (1993): 459–465.

Wein, A. J., and K. N. Van Arsdalen. Drug-induced male sexual dysfunction. *Urol. Clin. North Am.* 15 (1988): 23–31.

Yager, J. Bethanechol chloride can reverse erectile and ejaculatory dysfunction induced by tricyclic antidepressants and mazindol: Case report. *J. Clin. Psychiatry* 47 (1986): 210–211.

CHAPTER 17. PSYCHOLOGIC FACTORS AFFECTING POTENCY AND EJACULATION

Beck, J. G., and D. H. Barlow. The effects of anxiety and attentional focus on sexual responding. Part 1: Cognitive and affective patterns in erectile dysfunction. *Behav. Res. Ther.* 24 (1986): 19–26.

Chesney, A. P., P. E. Blakeney, C. M. Cole, and R. A. Chan. A comparison of couples who have sought sex therapy with couples who have not. *J. Sex. Marital Ther.* 7 (1981): 131–140.

Daniel, D. G., V. Abernethy, and W. R. Oliver. Correlations between female sex roles and attitudes toward male sexual dysfunction in thirty women. *J. Sex. Marit. Ther.* 10 (1984): 160–169.

Dekker, J., W. Everaerd, and N. Verhelst. Attending to stimuli or to images of sexual feelings: Effects on sexual arousal. *Behav. Res. Ther.* 23 (1985): 139–149.

Derogatis, L. R., J. K. Meyer, and S. Kourlesis. Psychiatric diagnosis and psychological symptoms in impotence. *Hillside Journal of Clinical Psychiatry* 7 (1985): 120–133.

Farkas, G. M., L. F. Sine, and I. M. Evans. Personality, sexuality and demographc differences between volunteers and nonvolunteers for a laboratory study of male sexual behavior. *Arch. Sex. Behav.* 7 (1978): 513–520.

Geisser, M. E., F. T. Murray, M. S. Cohen, P. J. Shea, and R. R. Addeo. Use of the Florida sexual history questionnaire to differentiate primary organic from primary psychogenic impotence. *J. Androl.* 14 (1993): 298–303.

Geisser, M. E., T. W. Jefferson, M. Spevack, T. Boaz, R. G. Thomas, and F. T. Murray. Reliability and validity of the Florida sexual history questionnaire. *J. Clin. Psychol.* 47 (1991): 519–528.

Hall, K. S., Y. Binik, and E. Di Tomasso. Concordance between physiological and subjective measures of sexual arousal. *Behav. Res. Ther.* 23 (1985): 297–303.

Kaplan, H. S. *The new sex therapy: Active treatment of dysfunctions.* New York: Brunner/Mazel, 1974.

Kinsey, A. C., W. B. Pomeroy, and C. E. Martin. *Sexual behavior in the human male.* Philadelphia: Saunders, 1948.

Kockott, G., W. Feil, D. Revenstorf, J. Aldenhoff, and U. Besinger. Symptomatology and psychological aspects of male sexual inadequacy: Results of an experimental study. *Archives of Sexual Behavior* 9 (1980): 457–475.

Levine, S. B. The psychological evaluation and therapy of psychogenic impotence. In R. T. Segraves and H. W. Schoenberg, eds., *Diagnosis and treatment of erectile disturbances: A guide for clinicians.* New York: Plenum, 1985.

Masters, W., and V. Johnson. *Human sexual inadequacy.* Boston: Little, Brown, 1970.

_____. *Human sexual response.* Boston: Little, Brown, 1966.

Morse, W. I., and J. M. Morse. Erectile impotence precipitated by organic factors and perpetuated by performance anxiety. *CMA Journal* 127 (1982): 599–601.

Notzer, N., D. Levran, S. Mashiach, and S. Soffer. Effect of religiosity on sex attitudes, experience and contraception among university students. *J. Sex. Marital Ther.* 10 (1984): 57–62.

Reynolds, C. F., III, E. Frank, M. E. Thase et al. Assessment of sexual function in depressed, impotent, and healthy men: Factor analysis of a brief sexual function questionnaire for men. *Psychiatry Res.* 24 (1988): 231–250.

Roose, S. P., A. H. Glassman, B. T. Walsh, and K. Cullen. Reversible loss of nocturnal penile tumescence during depression: A preliminary report. *Neuropsychobiology* 8 (1982): 284–288.

Sakheim, D. K., D. H. Barlow, J. G. Beck, and D. J. Abrahamson. The effect of an increased awareness of erectile cues on sexual arousal. *Behav. Res. Ther.* 22 (1984): 151–158.

Schover, L. R., J. M. Friedman, S. J. Weiler, J. R. Heiman, and J. LoPiccolo. Multiaxial problem-oriented system for sexual dysfunctions: An alternative to DSM-III. *Arch. Gen. Psychiatry* 39 (1982): 614–619.

Segraves, R. T., H. W. Schoenberg, C. K. Zarins, P. Camic, and J. Knopf. Characteristics of erectile dysfunction as a function of medical care system entry point. *Psychosomatic Medicine* 43 (1981): 227–234.

Stief, C. G., W. Bahren, W. Scherb, and H. Gall. Primary erectile dysfunction. *J. Urol.* 141 (1989): 315–319.

Takanami, M., M. Matsuhashi, A. Maki et al. Evaluation of therapeutic efficacy in psychogenic impotence by means of logarithmic scoring. *Urology* 27 (1986): 309–317.

Weintraub, W., and H. Aronson. Patients in psychoanalysis: Some findings related to sex and religion. *Am. J. Orthopsychiatry* 44 (1974): 102–108.

CHAPTER 18. PENILE IMPLANTS

Apte, S. M., J. G. Gregory, and M. H. Purcell. The inflatable penile prosthesis, reoperation and patient satisfaction: A comparison of statistics obtained from patient record review with statistics obtained from intensive follow-up search. *J. Urol.* 131 (1984): 894–895.

Barrett, D. M., D. C. O'Sullivan, A. A. Malizia et al. Particle shedding and migration from silicone genitourinary prosthetic devices. *J. Urol.* 146 (1991): 319–322.

Barry, J. M. Clinical experience with hinged silicone penile implants for impotence. *J. Urol.* 123 (1980): 178–179.

Benson, R. C., Jr., D. M. Barrett, and D. E. Patterson. The Jonas prosthesis: Technical considerations and results. *J. Urol.* 130 (1983): 920–922.

Bertram, R. A., C. C. Carson, and L. F. Altaffer. Severe penile curvature after implantation of an inflatable penile prosthesis. *J. Urol.* 139 (1988): 743–745.

Beutler, L. E., F. B. Scott, R. R. Rogers Jr., I. Karacan, P. E. Baer, and J. A. Gaines. Inflatable and noninflatable penile prostheses: Comparative follow-up evaluation. *Urology* 27 (1986): 136–143.

Brooks, M. B. Forty-two months of experience with the Mentor inflatable penile prosthesis. *J. Urol.* 139 (1988): 48–49.

Carson, C. C., and C. N. Robertson. Late hematogenous infection of penile prostheses. *J. Urol.* 139 (1988): 50–52.

Collins, K. P., and R. H. Hackler. Complications of penile prostheses in the spinal cord injury population. *J. Urol.* 140 (1988): 984–985.

Fallon, B., S. Rosenberg, and D. A. Culp. Long-term followup in patients with an inflatable penile prosthesis. *J. Urol.* 132 (1984): 270–271.

Finney, R. P., J. R. Sharpe, and R. W. Sadlowski. Finney hinged penile implant: Experience with 100 cases. *J. Urol.* 124 (1980): 205–207.

Furlow, W. L., and B. Goldwasser. Salvage of the eroded inflatable penile prosthesis: A new concept. *J. Urol.* 138 (1987): 312–314.

Furlow, W. L., and R. C. Motley. The inflatable penile prosthesis: Clinical experience with a new controlled expansion cyclinder. *J. Urol.* 139 (1988): 945–946.

Furlow, W. L., B. Goldwasser, and J. C. Gundian. Implantation of model AMS 700 penile prosthesis: Long-term results. *J. Urol.* 139 (1988): 741–742.

Gerstenberger, D. L., D. Osborne, and W. L. Furlow. Inflatable penile prosthesis: Follow-up study of patient-partner satisfaction. *Urology* 14 (1979): 583–587.

Gregory, J. G., and M. H. Purcell. Scott's inflatable penile prosthesis: Evaluation of mechanical survival in the series 700 model. *J. Urol.* 137 (1987): 676–677.

Hollander, J. B., and A. C. Diokno. Success with penile prosthesis from patient's viewpoint. *Urology* 23 (1984): 141–143.

Joseph, D. B., R. C. Bruskewitz, and R. C. Benson Jr. Long-term evaluation of the inflatable penile prosthesis. *J. Urol.* 131 (1984): 670–673.

Kabalin, J. N., and R. Kessler. Experience with the hydroflex penile prosthesis. *J. Urol.* 141 (1989): 58–59.

_____. Infectious complications of penile prosthesis surgery. *J. Urol.* 139 (1988): 953–955.

Kaufman, J. J. Penile prosthetic surgery under local anesthesia. *J. Urol.* 128 (1982): 1190–1191.

Kramarsky-Binkhorst, S. Female partner perception of Small-Carrion implant. *Urology* 12 (1978): 545–548.

Krauss, D. J., D. Bogin, and A. Culebras. The failed penile prosthetic implantation despite technical success. *J. Urol.* 129 (1983): 969–971.

Lewis, R. Penile prosthesis as a treatment for impotence. *Andrology Report* 2 (1993): 5–8.

Lewis, R. W. Long-term results of penile prosthesis surgery. *Urologic Clinics of North America* 22 (1985): 847–856.

Malloy, T. R., A. J. Wein, and V. L. Carpiniello. Comparison of the inflatable penile and the Small-Carrion prostheses in the surgical treatment of erectile impotence. *J. Urol.* 123 (1980): 678–679.

Montague, D. K. Experience with semirigid rod and inflatable penile prostheses. *J. Urol.* 129 (1983): 967–968.

Pedersen, B., L. Tiefer, M. Ruiz, and A. Melman. Evaluation of patients and partners 1 to 4 years after penile prosthesis surgery. *J. Urol.* 139 (1988): 956–958.

Rossier, A. B., and B. A. Fam. Indication and results of semirigid penile prostheses in spinal cord injury patients: Long-term followup. *J. Urol.* 131 (1984): 59–62.

Schlamowitz, K. E., L. E. Beutler, F. B. Scott, I. Karacan, and C. Ware. Reactions to the implantation of an inflatable penile prosthesis among psychogenically and organically impotent men. *J. Urol.* 129 (1983): 295–298.

Schover, L. R., and A. C. von Eschenbach. Sex therapy and the penile prosthesis: A synthesis. *J. Sex. Marital Ther.* 11 (1985): 57–66.

Scott, F. B., I. J. Fishman, and J. K. Light. A decade of experience with the inflatable penile prosthesis. *World J. Urol.* 1 (1983): 244–250.

References

Stanisic, T. H., J. C. Dean, J. M. Donovan, and L. E. Beutler. Clinical experience with a self-contained inflatable penile implant, the FlexiFlate. *J. Urol.* 139 (1988): 947–950.

Steege, J. F., A. L. Stout, and C. C. Carson. Patient satisfaction in Scott and Small-Carrion penile implant recipients: A study of 52 patients. *Archives of Sexual Behavior* 15 (1986): 393–399.

Stewart, T. D. Penile prosthesis: Potential value of medical psychiatric assessment and psychotherapy. *Psychother. Psychosom.* 44 (1985): 18–24.

Thomalla, J. V., S. T. Thompson, R. G. Rowland, and J. J. Mulcahy. Infectious complications of penile prosthetic implants. *J. Urol.* 138 (1987): 65–67.

Wilson, S. K., G. E. Wahman, and J. L. Lange. Eleven years of experience with the inflatable penile prosthesis. *J. Urol.* 139 (1988): 951–952.

CHAPTER 19. PENILE INJECTION

Althof, S. E., L. A. Turner, S. B. Levine et al. Intracavernosal injection in the treatment of impotence: A prospective study of sexual, psychological, and marital functioning. *J. Sex. Marital Ther.* 13 (1987): 155–167.

———. Why do so many people drop out from auto-injection therapy for impotence? *J. Sex. Marital Ther.* 15 (1989): 121–129.

Bahnson, R. R., and W. J. Catalona. Papaverine testing of impotent patients following nerve-sparing radical prostatectomy. *J. Urol.* 139 (1988): 773–774.

Brindley, G. S. Cavernosal alpha-blockade: A new technique for investigating and treating erectile impotence. *Brit. J. Psychiat.* 143 (1983): 332–337.

Buvat, J., M. Buvat-Herbaut, J. L. Dehaene, and A. Lemaire. Is intracavernous injection of papaverine a reliable screening test for vascular impotence? *J. Urol.* 135 (1986): 476–478.

Corriere, J. N., Jr., I. J. Fishman, G. S. Benson, and C. E. Carlton Jr. Development of fibrotic penile lesions secondary to the intracorporeal injection of vasoactive agents. *J. Urol.* 140 (1988): 615–617.

Girdley, F. M., R. C. Bruskewitz, J. Feyzi, P. H. Graversen, and T. C. Gasser. Intracavernous self-injection for impotence: A longterm therapeutic option? Experience in 78 patients. *J. Urol.* 140 (1988): 972–974.

Glina, S., A. C. Reichelt, P. P. Leao, and J. M. Dos Reis. Impact of cigarette smoking on papaverine-induced erection. *J. Urol.* 140 (1988): 523–524.

Hu, K. N., C. Burks, and W. C. Christy. Fibrosis of tunica albuginea: Complication of long-term intracavernous pharmacological self-injection. *J. Urol.* 138 (1987): 404–405.

Ishii, N., H. Watanabe, C. Irisawa et al. Intracavernous injection of prostaglandin El for the treatment of erectile impotence. *J. Urol.* 141 (1989): 323–325.

Juenemann, K. P., and P. Alken. Pharmacotherapy of erectile dysfunction: A review. *Int. J. Impotence Res.* 1 (1989): 71–93.

Levine, S. B., S. E. Althof, L. A. Turner et al. Side effects of self-administration of intracavernous papaverine and phentolamine for the treatment of impotence. *J. Urol.* 141 (1989): 54–57.

Linet, O. I., and F. G. Ogrinc. Efficacy and safety of intracavernosal alprostadil in men with erectile dysfunction. *N. Engl. J. Med.* 334 (1996): 873–877.

Padma-Nathan, H., A. Bennett, N. Gesundheidt et al. Treatment of erectile dysfunction by the medicated urethral system for erection (MUSE). *J. Urol.* 153 (1995): 472A, Abstract.

Sidi, A. A. Vasoactive intracavernous pharmacotherapy. *Urol. Clin. North Am.* 15 (1988): 95–101.

Sidi, A. A., J. S. Cameron, D. D. Dykstra, Y. Reinberg, and P. H. Lange. Vasoactive intracavernous pharmacotherapy for the treatment of erectile impotence in men with spinal cord injury. *J. Urol.* 138 (1987): 539–542.

Sidi, A. A., J. S. Cameron, L. M. Duffy, and P. H. Lange. Intracavernous drug-induced erections in the management of male erectile dysfunction: Experience with 100 patients. *J. Urol.* 135 (1986): 704–706.

Stackl, W., R. Hasun, and M. Marberger. Intracavernous injection of prostaglandin E, in impotent men. *J. Urol.* 140 (1988): 66–68.

Tullii, R. E., M. Degni, and A.F.C. Pinto. Fibrosis of the cavernous bodies following intracavernous auto-injection of vasoactive drugs. *Int. J. Impotence Res.* 1 (1989): 49–54.

Virag, R. About pharmacologically induced prolonged erection. *Lancet* 1 (1985): 519–520.

Wespes, E., C. Delcour, C. Rondeux, J. Struyven, and C. C. Schulman. The erectile angle: Objective criterion to evaluate the papaverine test in impotence. *J. Urol.* 138 (1987): 1171–1173.

Winter, C. C., and G. McDowell. Experience with 105 patients with priapism: Update review of all aspects. *J. Urol.* 140 (1988): 980–983.

Zorgniotti, A. W., and R. S. Lefleur. Auto-injection of the corpus cavernosum with a vasoactive drug combination for vasculogenic impotence. *J. Urol.* 133 (1985): 39–41.

CHAPTER 20. VACUUM DEVICES

Abbasi, A. A., A. S. Prasad, J. Ortega, E. Congco, and D. Oberleas. Gonadal function abnormalities in sickle cell anemia: Studies in adult male patients. *Ann. Int. Med.* 85 (1976): 601–605.

Almara Schiavo, R., and J. M. Pomerol Monseny. Penile erection using vacuum devices: Our experiences with 100 impotent patients with organic etiology. *Arch. Esp. Urol.* 46 (1993): 901–904.

Marmar, J. L., T. J. Debenedictis, and D. E. Praiss. The use of a vacuum constrictor device to augment a partial erection following an intracavernous injection. *J. Urol.* 140 (1988): 975–979.

Nadig, P. W. Six years' experience with the vacuum constriction device. *Int. J. Impotence Res.* 1 (1989): 55–58.

Nadig, P. W., J. C. Ware, and R. Blumoff. Noninvasive device to produce and maintain an erection-like state. *Urology* 27 (1986): 126–131.

van Thillo, E. L., and K. P. Delaere. The vacuum erection device: A noninvasive treatment for impotence. *Acta. Urol. Belg.* 60 (1992): 9–13.

Witherington, R. Vacuum constriction device for management of erectile impotence. *J. Urol.* 141 (1989): 320–322.

CHAPTER 21. THE LURE OF ALTERNATIVE MEDICINE

Abbasi, A. A., A. S. Prasad, P. Rabbani, and E. DuMouchelle. Experimental zinc deficiency in man: Effect on testicular function. *J. Lab. Clin. Med.* 96 (1980): 544–550.

Angell, M., and J. Kassirer. Alternative medicine: The risks of untested and unregulated remedies. *N. Engl. J. Med.* 339 (1998): 839–841.

Beigel, Y., I. Ostfeld, and N. Schoenfeld et al. Clinical problem solving: A leading question. *N. Engl. J. Med.* 339 (1998): 827–830.

Choi, H. K., D. H. Seong, and K. H. Rha. Clinical efficacy of Korean ginseng for erectile dysfunction. *Int. J. Impot. Res.* 7 (1995): 181–186.

Clark, L. C., G. S. Coombs, B. W. Turnbull et al. Effects of selenium supplementation for cancer prevention in patients with carcinoma of the skin. *JAMA* 276 (1996): 1957–1963.

Coppes, M. J., R. A. Anderson, and R. M. Egler et al. Alternative therapies for the treatment of childhood cancer. *N. Engl. J. Med.* 339 (1998): 846–847.

DiPaola, R. S., H. Zhang, G. H. Lambert et al. Clinical and biological activity of an estrogenic herbal combination (PC-SPES) in prostate cancer. *N. Engl. J. Med.* 339 (1998): 785–791.

Eisenberg, D. M., R. B. Davis, S. L. Ettner et al. Trends in alternative medicine use in the United States, 1990–1997: Results of a follow-up national survey. *JAMA* 280 (1998): 1569–1575.

Eisenberg, D. M., R. C. Kessler, C. Foster et al. Unconventional medicine in the United States: Prevalence, costs and patterns of use. *N. Engl. J. Med.* 328 (1993): 346–352.

Goldberg, Burton, ed. *Alternative medicine: The definitive guide.* Puyallup, WA: Future Medicine Publishing, 1993.

Grossman, E., T. Rosenthal, E. Peleg, C. Holmes, and D. S. Goldstein. Oral yohimbine increases blood pressure and sympathetic nervous outflow in hypertensive patients. *J. Cardiovasc. Pharmacol.* 22 (1993): 22–26.

Hartoma, T. R., K. Nahoul, and A. Netter. Zinc, plasma androgens and male sterility. *Lancet* 2 (1977): 1125–1126.

Hollander, E., and A. McCarley. Yohimbine treatment of sexual side effects induced by serotonin reuptake blockers. *J. Clin. Psychiatry* 53 (1992): 207–209.

Jacobsen, F. M. Fluoxetine induced sexual dysfunction and an open trial of yohimbine. *J. Clin. Psychiatry* 53 (1992): 119–122.

Joven, J., C. Villabona, J. Rubies-Prat et al. Hormonal profile and zinc levels in uremic men with gonadal dysfunction undergoing hemodialysis. *Clin. Chim. Acta.* 148 (1985): 239–245.

Kaptchuk, T. J., and D. M. Eisenberg. The persuasive appeal of alternative medicine. *Ann. Int. Med.* 129 (1998): 1061–1065.

Khedun, S. M., T. Vaicker, and B. Mahraraj. Zinc, hydrochlorothiazide and sexual dysfunction. *Centr. Afr. J. Med.* 41 (1995): 312–315.

King, D. S., R. L. Sharp, M. D. Vukovich, G. A. Brown et al. Efficacy of oral androstenedione on serum testosterone and to resistance training in young men. *JAMA* 281 (1999): 2020–2028.

Ko, R. J. Adulterants in Asian patent medicines. *N. Engl. J. Med.* 339 (1998): 847.

LoVecchio, F., S. C. Curry, and T. Bagnasco. Butyrolactone-induced central nervous system depression after ingestion of RenewTrient, a "dietary supplement." *N. Engl. J. Med.* 339 (1998): 847–848.

Mahajan, S. K., A. A. Abbasi, A. S. Prasad et al. Effect of oral zinc therapy on gonadal function in hemodialysis patients: A double-blind study. *Ann. Int. Med.* 97 (1982): 357–361.

Mahajan, S. K., A. S. Prasad, P. Rabbani, W. A. Briggs, and F. D. McDonald. Zinc deficiency: A reversible complication of uremia. *Am. J. Clin. Nutr.* 36 (1982): 1177–1183.

Margolis, R., P. Prieto, L. Stein, and S. Chinn. Statistical summary of 10,000 male cases using Afrodex in treatment of impotence. *Curr. Ther. Res.* 13 (1971): 616–622.

Montorsi, F., L. F. Strambi, G. Guazzoni et al. Effect of yohimbine-trazodone on psychogenic impotence: A randomized double-blind, placebo-controlled study. *Urology* 44 (1994): 732–736.

Morales, A., D.H.C. Surridge, P. G. Marshall, and J. Fenemore. Nonhormonal pharmacological treatment of organic impotence. *J. Urol.* 128 (1982): 45–47.

Slifman, N. R., et al. Brief report: Contamination of botanical dietary supplements by *Digitalis Lanata*. *N. Engl. J. Med.* 339 (1998): 806–811.

Yohimbine for male sexual dysfunction. *Medical Letter* 36 (1994): 115–116.

Yohimbine: Time for resurrection? Editorial. *Lancet* 2 (1986): 1194–1195.

Yoshizawa, K., W. C. Wiletti, S. J. Morris et al. Study of prediagnostic selenium level in toenails and the risk of advanced prostate cancer. *J. Natl. Cancer Inst.* 90 (1998): 1219–1224.

CHAPTER 22. THE SAGA OF DHEA

Arlt, W., F. Callies, J. C. van Vlijmen, I. Koehler et al. Dehydroepiandrosterone treatment in women with adrenal insufficiency. *N. Engl. J. Med.* 341 (1999): 1013–1020.

Barrett-Connor, E., K. T. Khaw, and S. S. Yen. A prospective study of dehydroepiandrosterone sulfate, mortality, and cardiovascular disease. *N. Engl. J. Med.* 315 (1986): 1519–1524.

Barrett-Connor, E., and S. Edelstein. A prospective study of dehydroepiandrosterone sulfate and cognitive function in an older population: The Rancho Bernardo Study. *J. Am. Geriatr. Soc.* 42 (1994): 420–423.

Bologa, L., J. Sharma, and E. Roberts. Dehydroepiandrosterone, and its sulfated derivative reduce neuronal death and enhance astrocytic differentiation in brain cell cultures. *J. Neurosci. Res.* 17 (1987): 225–234.

Kalmijn, S., L. J. Launer, R. P. Stolk et al. A prospective study on cortisol, dehydroepiandrosterone sulfate, and cognitive function in the elderly. *J. Clin. Endocrinol. Metab.* 83 (1998): 3487–3492.

Loria, R. M., T. H. Inge, S. S. Cook, A. K. Szakal, and W. Regelson. Protection against acute lethal viral infections with the native steroid dehydroepiandrosterone (DHEA). *J. Med. Virol.* 26 (1988): 301–314.

Nestler, J. E., J. N. Clore, and W. G. Blackard. Dehydroepiandrosterone: The "missing link" between hyperinsulinemia and atherosclerosis? *FASEB J.* 6 (1992): 3073–3075.

Schneider, L. S., M. Hinsey, and S. Lyness. Plasma dehydroepiandrosterone sulfate in Alzheimer's disease. *Biol. Psychiatry* 31 (1992): 205–208.

Shafagoj, Y., J. Opuku, D. Quereshi, W. Regelson, and M. Kalimi. Dehydroepiandrosterone prevents dexamethasone-induced hypertension in rats. *Am. J. Physiol.* 263 (1992): E210–213.

Straub, R. H., L. Konecna, S. Hrach et al. Serum dehydroepiandrosterone (DHEA) and DHEA sulfate are negatively correlated with serum interleukin-6 (IL-6), and DHEA inhibits IL-6 secretion from mononuclear cells in man *in vitro*: Possible link between endocrinosenescence and immunosenescence. *J. Clin. Endocrinol. Metab.* 83 (1998): 2012–2017.

Vermeulen, A. Dehydroepiandrosterone sulfate and aging. *Ann. N.Y. Acad. Sci.* 774 (1995): 121–125.

CHAPTER 23. THE PROSTATE AND ITS PROBLEMS

Bolt, J. W., C. Evans, and V. R. Marshall. Sexual dysfunction after prostatectomy. *Br. J. Urol.* 59 (1987): 319–322.

Finkle, A. L., and D. V. Prian. Sexual potency in elderly men before and after prostatectomy. *JAMA* 196 (1966): 139–143.

Gormley, G. J., E. Stoner, R. G. Bruskewitz et al. The effects of finasteride in men with benign prostatic hyperplasia. *N. Engl. J. Med.* 327 (1992): 1185–1191.

Lepor, H., W. D. Williford, M. J. Barry et al. The efficacy of terazosin, finasteride or both in benign prostatic hyperplasia. *N. Engl. J. Med.* 335 (1996): 533–539.

Lowe, F. C., R. L. McDaniel, J. J. Chmiel, and A. L. Hillman. Economic modeling to assess the costs of treatment with finasteride, terazosin and transurethral resection of the prostate for men with moderate to severe symptoms of benign prostatic hyperplasia. *Urology* 46 (1995): 477–483.

McConnell, J. D., R. Bruskewitz, P. Walsh et al. The effect of finasteride on the risk of acute urinary retention and the need for surgical treatment among men with benign prostatic hyperplasia. *N. Engl. J. Med.* 338 (1998): 557–563.

Moller-Nielsen, C., E. Lundhus, B. Moller-Madsen et al. Sexual life following "minimal" and "total" transurethral prostatic resection. *Urol. Int.* 40 (1985): 3–4.

Neal, D. E. Watchful waiting or drug therapy for benign prostatic hyperplasia. *Lancet* 350 (1997): 305–306.

Wasserman, M. D., C. P. Pollak, A. J. Spielman, and E. D. Weitzman. Impaired nocturnal erections and impotence following transurethral prostatectomy. *Urology* 15 (1980): 552–555.

Wilt, T. J., A. Ishani, G. Stark et al. Saw Palmetto extracts for treatment of benign prostatic hyperplasia: A systematic review. *JAMA* 280 (1998): 1604–1609.

CHAPTER 24. PROSTATE CANCER

Albertsen, P. C., J. A. Hanley, D. F. Gleason, and M. J. Barry. Competing risk analysis of men age 55–74 years at diagnosis for clinically localized prostate cancer. *JAMA* 280 (1998): 975–980.

Andriole, G. L., H. A. Guess, J. I. Epstein et al. Treatment with finasteride preserves usefulness of prostate-specific antigen in the detection of prostate cancer: Results of a randomized, double-blind, placebo-controlled clinical trial. *Urology* 52 (1998): 195–202.

Atala, A., M. Amin, and J. I. Harty. Diethylstilbesterol in treatment of postorchiectomy vaso-motor symptoms and its relationship with follicle-stimulating hormone, luteinizing hormone and testosterone. *Urology* 39 (1992): 108–110.

Beard, C. J., K. J. Propert, P. P. Rieker et al. Complications after treatment with external beam irradiation in early prostate cancer patients: A prospective multi-institutional outcomes study. *J. Clin. Oncol.* 15 (1997): 223–229.

Blasko, J. C., and P. H. Lange. Prostate cancer: The therapeutic challenge of locally advanced disease. *N. Engl. J. Med.* 337 (1997): 340–341.

Bolla, M., D. Gonzalez, P. Warde et al. Improved survival in patients with locally advanced prostate cancer treated with radiotherapy and goserelin. *N. Engl. J. Med.* 337 (1997): 295–300.

Catalona, W. J. Management of cancer of the prostate. *N. Engl. J. Med.* 331 (1994): 996–1004.

Messing, E. M., J. Manola, M. Sarodsky, G. Wilding et al. Immediate hormonal therapy compared with observation after radical prostatectomy and pelvic lymphadenopathy in men with node-positive prostate cancer. *N. Engl. J. Med.* 341 (1999): 1781–1788.

CHAPTER 25. THE FERTILE AND THE INFERTILE MAN

Charig, C. R., and J. S. Rundle. Flushing: Long-term side effect of orchiectomy in prostatic carcinoma. *Urology* 33 (1989): 175–178.

Coley, C. M., M. J. Barry, and A. G. Mulley. Screening for prostate cancer, part 3. *Ann. Intern. Med.* 126 (1997): 480–484.

Coley, C. M., M. J. Barry, C. Fleming, and A. G. Mulley. Early detection of prostate cancer. Part 1: Prior probability and effectiveness of tests. *Ann. Intern. Med.* 126 (1997): 394–406.

Coley, C. M., M. J. Barry, C. Fleming, M. C. Fahs, and A. G. Mulley. Early detection of prostate cancer. Part 2: Estimating the risks, benefits, and costs. *Ann. Intern. Med.* 126 (1997): 468–479.

Dearnaley, D. P., and J. Melia. Early prostate cancer: To treat or not to treat? *Lancet* 349 (1997): 892–893.

Eaton, A. C., and N. McGuire. Cyproterone acetate treatment of post-orchidectomy hot flushes: Double-blind crossover trial. *Lancet* 2 (1983): 1336–1337.

Feldman, J. M., R. W. Postelwaite, and J. F. Glenn. Hot flashes and sweats in men with testicular insufficiency. *Arch. Int. Med.* 136 (1976): 600–608.

Finkle, A. L., and S. P. Taylor. Sexual potency after radical prostatectomy. *J. Urol.* 125 (1981): 350–352.

Garnick, M. B., and W. F. Fair. Prostate cancer: Emerging concepts, parts 1 and 2. *Ann. Intern. Med.* 125 (1996): 117–125, 205–212.

Gerber, G. S., G. P. Zagaja, G. T. Bales et al. Saw Palmetto (Serenoa repens) in men with lower urinary tract symptoms: Effects on urodynamic parameters and voiding symptoms. *Urology* 51 (1998): 1003–1007.

Giovannucci, E. Selenium and risk of prostate cancer. *Lancet* 352 (1998): 755–756.

Johansson, J. E. Expectant management of early prostate cancer: Swedish experience. *J. Urol.* 152 (1994): 1753–1756.

Karling, P., M. Hammar, and E. Varenhorst. Prevalence and duration of hot flushes after surgical and medical castration in men with prostatic carcinoma. *J. Urol.* 152 (1994): 1170–1173.

Labrie, F., L. Cusan, J. L. Gomez, P. Diamond, and B. Candas. Combination of screening and preoperative endocrine therapy: The potential for an important decrease in prostate cancer mortality. *J. Clin. Endocrinol. Metab.* 80 (1995): 2002–2013.

Levison, V. The effect on fertility, libido and sexual function of postoperative radiotherapy and chemotherapy for cancer of the testicle. *Clin. Radiol.* 37 (1986): 161–164.

Loprinzi, C. L., J. C. Michalak, S. K. Quella et al. Megesterol acetate for the prevention of hot flashes. *N. Engl. J. Med.* 331(1994): 347–352.

Loprinzi, C. L., R. M. Goldberg, J. R. O'Fallon et al. Transdermal clonidine for ameliorating post-orchiectomy hot flashes. *J. Urol.* 151(1994): 634–636.

Lu-Yao, G. L., and R. E. Greenberg. Changes in prostate cancer incidence and treatment in USA. *Lancet* 343 (1994): 251–254.

Middleton, R. G. Prostate cancer: Are we screening and treating too much? *Ann. Intern. Med.* 126 (1997): 465–467.

Morgan, T. O., S. J. Jacobsen, W. F. McCarthy et al. Age specific ranges for prostate specific antigen in black men. *N. Engl. J. Med.* 335 (1996): 304–310.

Oesterling, J. E., S. J. Jacobsen, C. G. Chute et al. Serum prostatic specific antigen in a community based population of healthy men: Establishment of age specific ranges. *JAMA* 270 (1993): 800–804.

Palermo, G. D., J. Cohen, and Z. Rosenwaks. Intracytoplasmic sperm injection: A powerful tool to overcome fertilization failure. *Fertil. Steril.* 65 (1996): 899–908.

Palermo, G., H. Joris, P. Devroey, and A. C. Van Steirteghem. Pregnancies after intracytoplasmic injection of a single spermatozoon into an oocyte. *Lancet* 340 (1992): 17–18.

Prostate Cancer Trialists Collaborative Group. Maximum androgen blockade in advanced prostate cancer: An overview of 22 randomised trials with 3,283 deaths in 5,710 patients. *Lancet* 346 (1995): 265–269.

Silber, S. J. What forms of male infertility are there left to cure? *Human Reprod.* 10 (1995): 503–504.

Silber, S. J., J. Liu, Z. Nagy et al. The use of epididymal and testicular sperm for intracytopllasmic sperm injection: The genetic implications of male infertility. *Human Reprod.* 10 (1995): 2031–2043.

Smith, J. A. Editorial, Prostate cancer: If we only had more data. *J. Urol.* 152 (1994): 135.

Smith, J.A.J. A prospective comparison of treatments for symptomatic hot flushes following endocrine therapy for carcinoma of the prostate. *J. Urol.* 152 (1994): 132–134.

Spark, R. F. *The infertile male: The clinician's guide to diagnosis and treatment.* New York: Plenum, 1988.

Taplin, M. E., G. J. Bubley, T. D. Shuster et al. Mutation of the androgen-receptor gene in metastatic androgen-independent prostate cancer. *N. Engl. J. Med.* 332 (1995): 1393–1398.

Walsh, P. C. Radical prostatectomy, preservation of sexual function, cancer control: The controversy. *Urol. Clin. North Am.* 14 (1987): 663–673.

Walsh, P. C., J. I. Epstein, and F. C. Lowe. Potency following radical prostatectomy with wide unilateral excision of the neurovascular bundle. *J. Urol.* 138 (1987): 823–827.

Weldon, V. E., and F. R. Tavel. Potency-sparing radical perineal prostatectomy: Anatomy, surgical technique and initial results. *J. Urol.* 140 (1988): 559–562.

Woolf, S. H. Screening for prostate cancer with prostate specific antigen: An examination of the evidence. *N. Engl. J. Med.* 333 (1996): 1401–1405.

CHAPTER 26. IS THERE A MALE MENOPAUSE?

Bremner, W. J., M. V. Vitiello, and P. N. Prinz. Loss of circadian rhythmicity in blood testosterone levels with aging in normal men. *J. Clin. Endocrinol. Metab.* 56 (1983): 1278–1281.

Deslypere, J. P., and A. Vermeulen. Leydig cell function in normal men: Effect of age, lifestyle, residence, diet, and activity. *J. Clin. Endocrinol. Metab.* 59 (1984): 955–962.

Deslypere, J. P., J. M. Kaufman, T. Vermeulen, D. Vogelaers, J. L. Vandalem, and A. Vermeulen. Influence of age on pulsatile luteinizing hormone release and responsiveness of the gonadotrophs to sex hormone feedback in men. *J. Clin. Endocrinol. Metab.* 64 (1987): 68–73.

Hallberg, M. C., R. G. Wieland, E. M. Zorn, B. H. Furst, and J. M. Wieland. Impaired Leydig cell reserve and altered serum androgen binding in the aging male. *Fertil. Steril.* 27 (1976): 812–814.

Harman, S. M., and P. D. Tsitouras. Reproductive hormones in aging men. Part 1: Measurement of sex steroids, basal luteinizing hormone, and Leydig cell response to human chorionic gonadotropin. *J. Clin. Endocrinol. Metab.* 51 (1980): 35–40.

Harman, S. M., P. D. Tsitouras, P. T. Costa, and M. R. Blackman. Reproductive hormones in aging men. Part 2: Basal pituitary gonadotropins and gonadotropin responses to luteinizing hormone-releasing hormone. *J. Clin. Endocrinol. Metab.* 54 (1982): 547–551.

Heller, C. G., and G. B. Myers. The male climacteric, its symptomatology, diagnosis and treatment. *JAMA* 126 (1944): 472–477.

Kaplan, H. S. The concept of presbyrectia. *Int. J. Impotence Res.* 1 (1989): 59–65.

Karacan, I., R. L. Williams, J. I. Thornby, and P. J. Salis. Sleep-related penile tumescence as a function of age. *Am. J. Psychiatry* 132 (1975): 932–937.

Mulligan, T., S. M. Retchin, V. M. Chinchilli, and C. B. Bettinger. The role of aging and chronic disease in sexual dysfunction. *J. Am. Geriatr. Soc.* 36 (1988): 520–524.

Tsitouras, P. D., C. E. Martin, and S. M. Harman. Relationship of serum testosterone to sexual activity in healthy elderly men. *Gerontol.* 37 (1982): 288–293.

Urban, R. J., J. D. Veldhuis, R. M. Blizzard, and M. L. Dufau. Attenuated release of biologically active luteinizing hormone in healthy aging men. *J. Clin. Invest.* 81 (1988): 1020–1029.

Vermeulen, A., J. P. Deslypere, and J. M. Kaulman. Influence of antiopioids on luteinizing hormone pulsatility in aging men. *J. Clin. Endocrinol. Metab.* 68 (1989): 68–72.

Vermeulen, A., R. Rubens, and L. Verdonck. Testosterone secretion and metabolism in male senescence. *J. Clin. Endocrinol. Metab.* 34 (1972): 730–735.

Warner, B. A., M. L. Dufau, and R. J. Santen. Effects of aging and illness on the pituitary testicular axis in men: Qualitative as well as quantitative changes in luteinizing hormone. *J. Clin. Endocrinol. Metab.* 60 (1985): 263–268.

Werner, A. A. The male climacteric. *JAMA* 112 (1939): 1441–1443.

Winters, S. J., R. J. Sherins, and P. Troen. The gonadotropin-suppressive activity of androgen is increased in elderly men. *Metabolism* 33 (1984): 1052–1059.

Zumoff, B., G. W. Strain, J. Kream et al. Age variation of the 24-hour mean plasma concentrations of androgens, estrogens, and gonadotropins in normal adult men. *J. Clin. Endocrinol. Metab.* 54 (1982): 534–538.

CHAPTER 27. RESTORING YOUTHFUL HORMONE LEVELS IN MATURE MEN

Bhasin, S., C. J. Bagatell, W. B. Bremmer et al. Issues in testosterone replacement in older men. *J. Clin. Endocrinol. Metab.* 83 (1998): 3435–3448.

Davidson, J. M., J. J. Chen, L. Crapo, G. D. Gray, W. J. Greenleaf, and J. A. Catania. Hormonal changes and sexual function in aging men. *J. Clin. Endocrinol. Metab.* 57 (1983): 71–77.

Dollins, A. B., I. V. Zhdanova, R. J. Wurtman et al. Effect of inducing nocturnal serum melatonin levels in daytime on sleep, mood, body temperature and performance. *Proc. Natl. Acad. Sci.* 91 (1994): 1824–1828.

Garfinkel, D., M. Laudon, D. Not, and N. Zisapel. Improvement of sleep quality in elderly people by controlled release melatonin. *Lancet* 346 (1995): 541–544.

Neaves, W. B., L. Johnson, J. C. Porter, C. R. Parker Jr., and C. S. Petty. Leydig cell numbers, daily sperm production, and serum gonadotropin levels in aging men. *J. Clin. Endocrinol. Metab.* 59 (1984): 756–763.

Nieschlag, E., U. Lammers, C. W. Freischem, K. Langer, and E. J. Wickings. Reproductive functions in young fathers and grandfathers. *J. Clin. Endocrinol. Metab.* 55 (1982): 676–681.

Papadakis, M. A., D. Grady, D. Black et al. Growth hormone replacement in healthy older men improves body composition but not functional ability. *Ann. Int. Med.* 124 (1996): 708–716.

Piperaoli, W., and W. Regelson. *The melatonin miracle.* New York: Simon and Schuster, 1995.

Reppert, S. M., and D. R. Weaver. Melatonin madness. *Cell* 83 (1995): 1059–1062.

Rudman, D., A. G. Feller, H. S. Nagraj et al. Effects of growth hormone in men over 60 years old. *N. Engl. J. Med.* 323 (1990): 1–6.

Snyder, P. J., H. Preachey, P. Hannoush, J. A. Berlin et al. Effect of testosterone treatment on body composition and muscle strength in men over 65 years of age. *J. Clin. Endocrinol. Metab.* 84 (1999): 2647–2653.

Tenover, J. S. Effects of testosterone supplementation in the aging male. *J. Clin. Endocrinol. Metab.* 75 (1992): 1092–1098.

Tenover, J. S., A. M. Matsumoto, S. R. Plymate, and W. J. Bremner. The effects of aging in normal men on bioavailable testosterone and luteinizing hormone secretion: Response to clomiphene citrate. *J. Clin. Endocrinol. Metab.* 65 (1987): 1118–1126.

Vermeulen, A. Clinical review 24: Androgens in the aging male. *J. Clin. Endocrinol. Metab.* 73 (1991): 221–224.

Waldhauser, F., G. Weiszenbacher, E. Tatzer et al. Alterations in nocturnal serum melatonin levels in humans with growth and aging. *J. Clin. Endocrinol. Metab.* 66 (1988): 648–652.

CHAPTER 28. WHAT'S NEXT FOR MEN IN THE MILLENNIUM?

Constitution of the World Health Organization. *Handbook of basic documents.* 5th ed. Geneva: Palais des Nations (1952): 3–20.

Diokno, A. C., M. B. Brown, and A. R. Herzog. Sexual function in the elderly. *Arch. Int. Med.* 150 (1990): 197–200.

Heathcote, P. S., P. N. Mactaggart, R. J. Boston et al. Health-related quality of life in Australian men remaining disease free after radical prostatectomy. *Med. J. Aust.* 168 (1998): 483–486.

Klein, C. A., A. Prochazka, A. L. Spitzer, B. Gordon, and L. M. Glode. Spousal report of quality of life in treatment for localized prostate cancer. *Proc. Ann. Meet. Am. Soc. Oncol.* 15 (1996): 1630.

Lim, A. J., A. H. Brandon, and J. Fiedler et al. Quality of life: Radical prostatectomy versus radiation therapy for prostate cancer. *J. Urol.* 154 (1995): 1420–1425.

Litwin, M. S., R. J. Nied, and N. Dhanni. Health-related quality of life in men with erectile dysfunction. *J. Gen. Intern. Med.* 13 (1998): 158–166.

Lough, M. E., A. M. Lindsey, J. A. Shinn, and N. A. Stotts. Impact of symptom frequency and symptom distress on self-reported quality of life in heart transplant patients. *Heart & Lung* 16 (1987): 193–200.

Meyhoff, H. H., T. Hald, and J. Nording et al. A new patient weighted symptom score system (DAN-PSS-1). Clinical assessment of indications and outcomes of transurethral prostatectomy for uncomplicated benign prostatic hyperplasia. *Scand. J. Urol. Nephrol.* 27 (1993): 493–499.

Perez, E. D., T. Mulligan, and T. Wan. Why men are interested in an evaluation of a sexual problem. *J. Am. Geriatr. Soc.* 41 (1993): 233–237.

Tenover, J. L. Aging and male sexual function. In *The Handbook of Sexual Dysfunction,* chap. 8, pp. 39–42. San Francisco: American Society of Andrology, 1999.

Testa, M. A., and D. C. Simonson. Assessment of quality of life outcomes. *N. Engl. J. Med.* 334 (1996): 835–840.

Walsh, P. C., A. W. Partin, and J. I. Epstein. Case control and quality of life following anatomical radical retropubic prostatectomy: Results at 10 years. *J. Urol.* 152 (1994): 1831–1836.

Weinberger, M. H. Lowering blood pressure in patients without affecting quality of life. *Am. J. Med.* 89 (1989): 94–97.

Index

Psychogenic impotence
  compared with physiological, 16–17, 22
  penile prostheses and, 249
  performance anxiety and, 226–227
  psychologic problems and, 222
  Regi-Scan recordings and, 82
  using Viagra for, 229–230
  using yohimbine for, 10
  Viagra and, 107
  Viagra effectiveness and, 115
  yohimbine and, 10, 281–282
Psychologic factors, 221–237
  climacteric symptoms and, 364
  depression, 232–233
  ejaculation control exercises, 230
  evaluation and treatment of, 223–224
  Florida Sexual Health questionnaire and,
    233–237
  impotence and, 222
  in inhibited ejaculation, 44
  injuries to, 44
  insight therapy and, 230–232
  libido and, 36
  male impotence and, 16–17, 20
  medical history and, 47
  medications for, 229, 333
  nocturnal penile tumescence and, 78, 82,
    222
  penile injections and, 97, 225, 256
  penile prostheses and, 225, 248–249,
    250
  performance anxiety, 226–227
  primary impotence, 224–225
  secondary impotence, 226
  sensate focus exercises and, 227–229
  symptoms and diagnosis of, 222
  Viagra and, 229–230
Psychosis, 200, 203–204, 207–208
Psychotherapy
  depression and, 233
  impotence and, 225
Puberty. See also Adolescence
  delays in, 162
  reducing testosterone in precocious
    puberty, 183–184
  using steroids for delayed puberty,
    179–181
Pudendal nerve, 94–95
Pulsatile GnRH secretion. See
    Gonadotropin releasing hormone
    (GnRH)

Pulses
  doppler ultrasound recording of, 96–97
  evaluating blood flow with, 54
Pyospermia, 350
Pythagoras, 363

Quality of Life (QOL) issues
  costs, 392
  health related quality of life (HRQOL),
    390
  lifestyle pharacology and, 391
  male sexual satisfaction and, 394–395
  prostate surgery and, 395–396
  sexuality and, 390–394

Rabkin, Drs. Judith and Richard, 178
Radiation therapy
  impotence and incontinence following,
    344
  prostate cancer and, 343
  side effects of, 53, 337–338
Radical prostatectomy, 339, 343, 395
Radical retropubic prostatectomy (RRP),
    114
Rako, Dr. Susan, 176
Ranitidine (Zantac), 210
Rapid eye movement (REM) sleep, 24, 43,
    75–76
Reading, Dr. Anthony, 30
Reflex erections
  aging and, 369–370
  stimulation and inhibition of, 74–75
  stimulus-response reflex and, 74
  types of erections and, 36–38, 72
  Viagra and, 114
Refractory period, 40
Reglan, 147, 208
Renal disease. See Kidney disease
Repression
  of anger, 45
Resperine (Serpasil), 147, 200–201
Retinitis pigmentosa, 122
Retrograde ejaculation
  alcohol consumption and, 213
  BPH surgery and, 319, 324–325
  medications causing, 200
  occurrences of, 39–40
  orgasm phase problems and, 44–45
Rigi-Scan, 78–82
  abnormal readings of, 79
  alcohol consumption and, 79

Silicone implants. *See also* Penile prosthesis
    breast implants, 245–246
    penile prostheses, 24–25, 239, 245–246
Single photon emission computerized
        tomography (SPECT), 159
Sinusoids, 93
Situational erectile dysfunction, 30
Skin cancer
    selenium and, 289
Slag, Dr. Michael
    study on sexual dysfunction by, 31
Sleep-deprived electroencephalogram, 159
Sleep problems, 51
Small-Carrior prosthesis, 241
Small, Dr. Michael, 239
Smoking. *See* Cigarette smoking
Snap gauge, 78
Snyder, Dr. Peter, 378
Sodium overload, 196–197
Spectatoring
    performance anxiety and, 227
    Viagra and, 230
SPECT scan, 159
Sperm
    cervical mucus incompatibility and,
        354–355
    fertilization and, 347–348
    maturation of, 142–143
    motility of, 62, 348, 350
    production of, 39, 54, 142–143,
        348–349
    production problems, 349–350, 351–353
    semen analysis and, 349–350
    testosterone and, 173
    treatments for, 351–354
Spinal cord damage
    injuries to, 44
    neurogenic impotence and, 84–85
    sexuality after injuries to, 89
    syphilis and, 87
    Viagra and, 114–115
Spirochetes, 87
Spironolactone, 198–199
Squeeze technique, 44, 230
Start and stop technique, 44, 230
Stelazine, 147
Sterility, 349–350
Steroids. *See also* Anabolic androgenic
        steroids (AAS)
    androstenedione and, 285
    DHEA and, 299

Stimulus-response reflex, 74
Stimulus-response studies, 36–37
Stress
    hypertension and
    sexual dysfunction and, 49
Superfact, 208
Supplements
    availability of, 275
    costs of, 274
    FDA regulation and, 273–274
    list of, 294
Suramin, 208
Surgery. *See also* Penile prostheses
    for benign prostatic hyperplasia, 319,
        324–325
    for pituitary tumors, 146
    for prostate cancer, 339
    sexual side effects of, 52–53
    for varicoceles, 351–353
    for vasculogenic impotence, 92, 98–99, 225
    for venous incompetence, 43–44
Sympathetic nervous system, 253
Synarel, 208
Syphilis, 87
Systolic blood pressure, 39, 96

Tagamet, 209
Tamoxifen, 171
Tegretol, 159
Temporal lobe
    hormones and, 158–159
    sexual function of, 84
Temporal lobe epilepsy (TLE)
    neurogenic impotence and, 83
    symptoms and treatment of, 159
Tenover, Dr. J. Lisa, 377
Terazosin (Hytrin)
    combining with finasteride in prostate
        treatment, 321
    controlling BPH symptoms with,
        318–319
    cost of, 325
Testicles. *See also* Castration;
        Hypothalamic-pituitary-gonadal axis
    aging and, 367–368
    disorders of, 51, 143–145
    experimental evidence for role in sexual
        function, 21
    fetal development of, 140
    hormonal interaction with pituitary and
        hypothalmus, 141–142

Women's sexuality. *See* Female sexuality

Xanax, 209
X rays. *See also* Radiation therapy
  diagnostic, 97
  therapy with, 51, 53, 57, 329, 356

Yen, Dr. Samuel, 306, 309, 382
Yocon. *See* Yohimbine
Yohimbine
  as aphrodisiac, 103
  combining with trazodone, 282
  compared with Viagra, 102, 106

medication induced impotence and, 206,
  282–283
psychogenic impotence and, 10,
  281–282
side effects of, 282
studies on, 281
Yohimex. *See* Yohimbine

Zantac, 210
Zestril, 201
Zinc, 102, 279–280
Zoladex, 339
Zoloft, 204, 205, 206